Writtle

RECENT ADVANCES IN
ANIMAL NUTRITION — 2006

Recent Advances in Animal Nutrition

2006

P.C. Garnsworthy, PhD
J. Wiseman, PhD
University of Nottingham

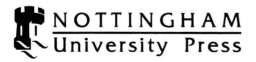

NOTTINGHAM
University Press

Nottingham University Press
Manor Farm, Main Street, Thrumpton
Nottingham, NG11 0AX, United Kingdom

NOTTINGHAM

First published 2007
© The several contributors names in the list of contents 2007

British Library Cataloguing in Publication Data
Recent Advances in Animal Nutrition — 2006:
University of Nottingham Feed Manufacturers
Conference (40th, 2006, Nottingham)
I. Garnsworthy, Philip C. II. Wiseman, J.

ISBN   978-1-904761-02-0

Disclaimer

Every reasonable effort has been made to ensure that the material in this book is true, correct, complete
and appropriate at the time of writing. Nevertheless the publishers, the editors and the authors do not
accept responsibility for any omission or error, or for any injury, damage, loss or financial
consequences arising from the use of the book.

Typeset by Nottingham University Press, Nottingham
Printed and bound by Cromwell Press, Trowbridge, Wiltshire

PREFACE

The 40th University of Nottingham Feed Conference was held at the Sutton Bonington Campus 13th – 15th September 2006. As befitted the 40th anniversary, delegates were accommodated in brand new accommodation – they were in fact the very first occupants – built to cater for rapidly expanding numbers of students in the School of Biosciences and our new School of Veterinary Medicine and Science. There is much happening at Sutton Bonington these days.

At the Anniversary Conference Dinner, Dr Brian Cooke presented a retrospective of 40 years of the Nottingham Conference. Brian was a 'member' at the first conference in 1967, so he was uniquely qualified to address delegates 40 years on!

A continuing practice of the conference has been to invite very well qualified speakers from anywhere in the World to address topics of importance to the feed industry. These topics are decided by members of the organising committee, who are from the commercial sector as well as the University.

The timing of specific sessions was influenced by the decision to hold our annual Cattle Fertility Conference the day before the Feed Conference. Many delegates had expressed a desire to attend the Fertility Conference and then the ruminant session of the Feed Conference. This worked particularly well, and will be repeated in 2007.

The first paper in the Ruminant Session was a collaboration between the University of Nottingham (Salter and Garnsworthy) and Cornel University USA (Bauman and Lock), and considered the topical theme of milk fatty acids with emphasis on trans fatty acids and conjugated linoleic acid, both of which have potential human health benefits. However it was pointed out that reducing concentrations of medium chain length saturated fatty acids could also have positive effects on human health.

The next paper combined experts from Canada (Lapierre, Ouellet, Berthiaume, Raggio and Doepel), France (Lemosquet) and New Zealand (Pacheco) in a discussion of enhancing efficiency of milk protein synthesis through providing balanced dietary amino acids.

Subsequently a paper (authors all from the same country – although 3000 miles apart - Thatcher, Silvestre, Bilby and Staples from Florida, and Santos from California) considered nutrient regulation of hormonal, humoral and cellular responses in postpartum lactating dairy cows. Declining dairy cow fertility is a major problem in many parts of the world.

The major impact of body condition score at calving on dairy cow performance and fertility was then discussed (Garnsworthy, Nottingham). It was concluded that lower targets are appropriate for high-merit cows.

The traditional objective in dairy farming is to produce one calf per annum and departures from this are thought to have a negative impact on herd performance. However, extended lactations are receiving considerable attention and were the subject of the next paper (MacMillan, Grainger and Auldist; Australia).

Papers in the General Session were concerned with micronutrients, legislation and feed by-products. Antioxidants are a key element of the body's defences and their value together with concentrations in food were described (Paganga, Southampton). Meat is regularly considered by many as being unhealthy due to its alleged high fat / cholesterol content and cancer-promoting potential. The next paper refuted these assertions and discussed the nutritional benefits arising from meat consumption (Biesalski, Germany). Two papers addressed EU matters: a paper on recent EU rulings was presented (Nelson, Raine and Oliver), followed by a paper reviewing the implications of EU enlargement on animal agriculture (Knowles).

The increasing importance of non-food/feed uses of plant raw materials is receiving increased attention, particularly in the context of utilisation of the co-products emerging from the biofuels industry. Two papers on this theme were organized. The first (Wilson) reviewed the implications of these developments on the animal feed industry and the second (Gibson and Karges, USA) considered the technicalities of co-product production in the context of optimization of their nutritional value.

The Non-ruminant Session commenced with a detailed review of the role of muscle glycogen on meat quality in pigs (Oksbjerg, Denmark) and continued with a paper on L-carnitine and its effect on prenatal muscle development and subsequent offspring performance in pigs (Woodworth, USA). With increasing concern over possible human infection associated with the H5N1 avian influenza virus, it was thought very opportune to include a paper (Connerton and Connerton, Nottingham) on zoonoses which identified the principal agents and the likely danger arising from them.

Nutrition x genotype interactions and recent developments in genetics were discussed (Hoste, Malton), followed by a comprehensive review of sow and boar nutrition in the light of the emergence of new genotypes (Close). Processing of raw materials for piglet diets is invariably defined simply in terms of the name of the process which is inadequate, as described in a paper (Doucet, White, Wiseman and Hill; Nottingham) on physicochemical changes to starch structure during processing of raw materials and their implications for starch digestibility in newly-weaned piglets. Finally, the conference returned to the theme of 'homegrown' legumes as raw materials for non-ruminants (Crépon, France).

We would like to thank all speakers and session chairmen (David Parker, Brian Cooke, Julian Wiseman, Tim Parr and Steve Jagger), together with members of the Programme Committee, for contributing to a very successful and innovative programme. We would also like to acknowledge the efficient administration (managed by Sue Golds), catering and support staff who ensure the smooth running of the conference.

The 2007 event will be held at the University of Nottingham Sutton Bonington Campus 4ᵗʰ – 7ᵗʰ September, immediately following the Cattle Fertility Conference on the 4ᵗʰ September. We look forward to renewing old acquaintances and making new friends.

P.C. Garnsworthy
J. Wiseman

DEDICATION

This book is dedicated to the memory of Bob Pickford and Des Cole who died this year. Both were closely associated with the Nottingham Feed Conference and made major contributions to the conference for many years.

Bob Pickford was a driving force behind the first Nutrition Conference for Feed Manufacturers held in 1967. His vision was for an annual forum that would facilitate translation of scientific ideas into commercial practice. There can be no doubt that this objective was achieved. Bob's dedicated support and enthusiasm helped to make the Feed Conference into an institution with a worldwide reputation for scientific excellence. He continued to serve on the Programme Committee right up until the conference this year.

Des Cole joined the Programme Committee in 1970 and acted as Chairman from 1984 to 1995. His extensive travels and attendance at conferences abroad provided Des with a wealth of ideas that helped to shape the format of the Nottingham Conference. He was particularly keen to maintain the reputation of a social gathering as well as a scientific meeting. Following his retirement from the University in 1995, Des continued his contact with the Conference through his publishing activities with Nottingham University Press.

CONTENTS

Preface

1   MILK FATTY ACIDS: IMPLICATIONS FOR HUMAN HEALTH   1
A.M. Salter[1], A.L. Lock[2], P.C. Garnsworthy[1] and D.E. Bauman[3]
[1]School of Biosciences, University of Nottingham, UK. [2]Department of Animal Science, University of Vermont, USA. [3]Department of Animal Science, Cornell University, USA

2   MILK PROTEIN: BIOLOGY SUPPORTS BALANCING RATIONS FOR AMINO ACIDS   19
H. Lapierre[1], G. Raggio[2], D.R. Ouellet[1], R. Berthiaume[1], S. Lemosquet[3], L. Doepel[4] and D. Pacheco[5]
[1]Dairy and Swine Research and Development Centre, Agriculture and Agri-Food Canada, Sherbrooke, QC, Canada, J1M 1Z3; [2]Dept. of Animal Science, Université Laval, Québec, QC, Canada, G1K 6P4; [3]I.N.R.A., UMR Production du Lait, 35590 Saint-Gilles, France; [4]Dept. of Agricultural, Food and Nutritional Science, University of Alberta, Edmonton, AL, Canada, T6G 2P5; [5]AgResearch, Palmerston North, New Zealand

3   NUTRIENT REGULATION OF HORMONAL, HUMORAL AND CELLULAR RESPONSES IN POSTPARTUM LACTATING DAIRY COWS: BUILDING BLOCKS FOR RESTORATION OF FERTILITY?   37
William W. Thatcher[1], Flavio T. Silvestre[1], Todd R. Bilby[1], Charles R. Staples[1], Jose E. P. Santos[2], Carlos A. Risco[3] and Leslie A. Maclaren[4]
[1]Department of Animal Sciences, University of Florida, Gainesville, FL, USA; [2]Veterinary Medicine Teaching and Research Center, University of California -Davis, Tulare, CA, USA; [3]Department of Large Animal Clinical Sciences, College of Veterinary Medicine, University of Florida, Gainesville, FL, USA, and [4]Department of Plant and Animal Sciences, Nova Scotia Agricultural College, Truro, Nova Scotia, Canada

4   BODY CONDITION SCORE IN DAIRY COWS: TARGETS FOR PRODUCTION AND FERTILITY   61
P.C. Garnsworthy
Division of Agricultural and Environmental Sciences, University of Nottingham School of Biosciences, Sutton Bonington Campus, Loughborough LE12 5RD, UK

**5   EXTENDED LACTATIONS IN INTENSIVE AND PASTURE-BASED
        DAIRYING**   87
K.L. Macmillan[1], C. Grainger[2], M.J. Auldist[2]
*[1]Department of Veterinary Science, University of Melbourne, Werribee,
3030, Australia; [2]Department of Primary Industries, Ellinbank, VIC 3821,
Australia*

6   ANTIOXIDANTS IN ANIMAL PRODUCTS   103
George Paganga
*AASC Ltd, Unit 5, Stanton Industrial Estate, Stanton Road,
Southampton SO15 4HU*

**7   MEAT AS A COMPONENT OF A HEALTHY DIET – ARE THERE ANY
        RISKS OR BENEFITS IF MEAT IS AVOIDED IN THE DIET?**   117
H.-K. Biesalski
*Universität Hohenheim, Institut für Biologische Chemie und
Ernährungswissenschaft, Garbenstrasse 30, 70593 Stuttgart, Germany*

8   INTERPRETATION AND APPLICATION OF EC RULINGS   153
Judith Nelson – Head of Feed Sector, AIC
Helen D Raine – Technology and Regulatory Affairs Director, ABNA Ltd
Tim Oliver – Legislation & Raw Materials Assessment Manager, ABN
P O Box 250, Oundle Road, Peterborough PE2 9PW, UK

**9   EUROPEAN UNION ENLARGEMENT: EFFECTS ON UK ANIMAL
        AGRICULTURE**   189
Andrew Knowles
*BPEX, PO Box 44, Winterhill House, Snowdon Drive, Milton Keynes,
MK6 1AX, UK*

**10   BY-PRODUCTS FROM NON-FOOD AGRICULTURE:
        IMPLICATIONS FOR THE FEED SUPPLY INDUSTRY**   199
Tim Wilson
ABNA, P O Box 250, Oundle Road, Peterborough PE2 9PW, UK

**11   BY-PRODUCTS FROM NON-FOOD AGRICULTURE:
        TECHNICALITIES OF NUTRITION AND QUALITY**   209
Matthew L. Gibson and and Kip Karges
*Dakota Gold Marketing, Dakota Gold Research Association,
Sioux Falls, South Dakota, USA*

**12   EFFECTS OF MANIPULATING MUSCLE GLYCOGEN ON MEAT
        QUALITY IN PIGS**   229
Niels Oksbjerg
*Danish Institute of Agricultural Sciences, Dept. of Food Science, Research
Centre Foulum, DK-8830 Tjele, Denmark*

13 **EFFECTS OF L-CARNITINE AND OTHER STRATEGIES TO INFLUENCE PRENATAL MUSCLE DEVELOPMENT AND SUBSEQUENT OFFSPRING PERFORMANCE** 243
Jason C. Woodworth
Lonza Inc, 1376 1500 Ave, Enterprise, Kansas 67441, USA

14 **POULTRY ZOONOSES** 255
Phillippa L. Connerton and Ian F. Connerton
Division of Food Sciences, University of Nottingham School of Biosciences, Sutton Bonington Campus, Loughborough, Leics LE12 5RD

15 **GENETICS AND NUTRITION: WHAT'S AROUND THE CORNER?** 275
Sam Hoste
Quantech Solutions, Orari Cottage, Howe Farm, Malton, North Yorks, YO17 6RG UK

16 **SOW AND BOAR NUTRITION: MODERN NUTRITION FOR MODERN GENOTYPES** 289
W H Close
Close Consultancy, Wokingham (Berkshire) will@closeconsultancy.com

17 **PHYSICOCHEMICAL CHANGES TO STARCH STRUCTURE DURING PROCESSING OF RAW MATERIALS AND THEIR IMPLICATIONS FOR STARCH DIGESTIBILITY IN NEWLY-WEANED PIGLETS** 313
Frederic J. Doucet, Gavin White, Julian Wiseman, Sandra E. Hill
School of Biosciences, University of Nottingham, Loughborough, LE12 5RD, UK

18 **NUTRITIONAL VALUE OF LEGUMES (PEA AND FABA BEAN) AND ECONOMICS OF THEIR USE** 331
Katell Crépon
Union Nationale Interprofessionnelle des Plantes riches en Protéines 12, avenue George V - PARIS

List of Participants 367

Index 373

1

MILK FATTY ACIDS: IMPLICATIONS FOR HUMAN HEALTH

A.M. SALTER[1], A.L. LOCK[2], P.C. GARNSWORTHY[1] AND D.E. BAUMAN[3]
[1]School of Biosciences, University of Nottingham, UK. [2]Department of Animal Science, University of Vermont, USA. [3]Department of Animal Science, Cornell University, USA

Introduction

Milk represents a complete source of nutrition for suckling animals. It has evolved to meet the energy and essential nutrient requirements of offspring up to the point of weaning. However, with the development of agriculture, man has exploited the potential of milk and dairy products as foods that can be consumed throughout the lifespan. Through breeding programmes and development of management techniques, milk from ruminant species has become a major staple of the human diet. In the British National Diet and Nutrition Survey (Hoare *et al.*, 2004), 94% of adults reported consuming milk during the previous seven days. Milk and milk products were estimated to contribute an average of approximately 10% of total energy, 14% of total fat and 24% of saturated fat to the British diet. It is the contribution to saturated fat intake that has caused concern to many human nutritionists. For many years it has been recognised that certain dietary saturated fatty acids have the potential to raise plasma cholesterol and thereby increase the risk of developing atherosclerotic cardiovascular disease (CVD). As a result, a reduction in intake of full-fat dairy products has been central to public health dietary recommendations around the world. However, the discovery of potential health benefits of a number of bioactive fatty acids, including conjugated linoleic acid (CLA), which is uniquely associated with ruminant meat and milk fat, has led to some reconsideration of the impact of dairy fat on human health.

The impact of dietary fatty acids on risk of developing cardiovascular disease

CVD mortality has declined dramatically in many industrialized countries since the 1970s. Figure 1 shows that death rates from coronary heart disease (CHD) in both the United Kingdom and the United States have declined over the last 40 years, particularly in men.

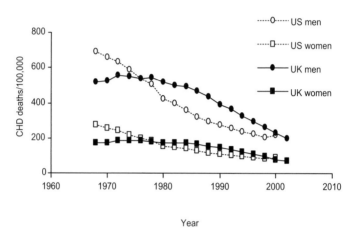

Figure 1. Age standardised death rates from CHD in the US and UK (Source: British Heart Foundation 2006a,b)

The reasons for these declines are not fully understood. However, they appear to be due to a combination of improved treatment of individuals and changes in risk factor levels within the whole population. In England and Wales, for example, it has been estimated that 42% of the decrease seen between 1981 and 2000 was due to improved treatment, and 58% was due to risk factor reductions within the population (Unal *et al.,* 2004). Of the risk factors, by far the biggest impact (48% of overall deaths) was from reduction in smoking, with lesser effects of reduced blood pressure (9.5%) and reduced cholesterol (9.6%). We may expect further significant reductions in CVD morbidity and mortality as the impact of increased use of highly effective cholesterol-lowering drugs (Statins) is fully realised (Salter 2005). However, at the present time specific dietary recommendations still continue to reinforce the avoidance of dairy fat (Litchtenstein *et al.,* 2006)

It is perhaps disappointing that reductions in plasma cholesterol have not been more manifest. Dietary recommendations aimed at reducing cholesterol have been central to the public health policies of most industrialized countries. As noted above, a reduction in intake of saturated fat has remained central to such policies. The basis of these recommendations lies in the widely accepted link between SFA intake, plasma cholesterol concentrations and risk of CVD. This was first demonstrated in the 1950s, when international comparisons showed that countries with lowest intakes of saturated fat also had the lowest population plasma cholesterol concentrations and lowest prevalence of CVD (Keys *et al.,* 1966). The influence of dietary fat composition on cholesterol concentrations was further established in a series of carefully controlled human feeding studies. From these experiments, equations were derived to predict the impact of changes in the amount and type of fat on plasma cholesterol (Keys *et al.,* 1965, Hegsted *et al.,*1965). Such findings on the effect of dietary fat on total plasma cholesterol led to generalized advice that population intakes of SFA with between 12-16 carbon atoms (lauric, myristic and palmitic acids) should be reduced. This inevitably affected dairy fat intake, which represents one of the main dietary sources of SFA. Figure 2 shows the dramatic changes in household consumption of liquid milk, indicating that since its introduction in the mid 1970s the consumption of reduced-fat (skimmed) milk has overtaken consumption of full fat milk.

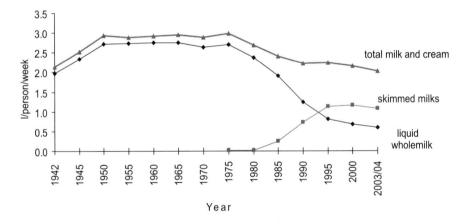

Figure 2. Household purchase of milk and milk products, 1942-2003/4, Great Britain (Source: British Heart Foundation 2006c)

Despite this dramatic change in pattern of milk consumption, however, total saturated fat (as a proportion of total energy intake) in the UK has remained remarkably constant (Figure 3). The reasons for this are not completely clear but they probably include a change in dietary sources of SFAs (with more being associated with processed food and pre-prepared meals) and the continuing decline in total energy expenditure leading to reduced energy intake. It could thus be argued that the continued policy of advocating a reduction in saturated fat intake has negatively influenced dairy fat consumption without having any real impact on the health of the nation.

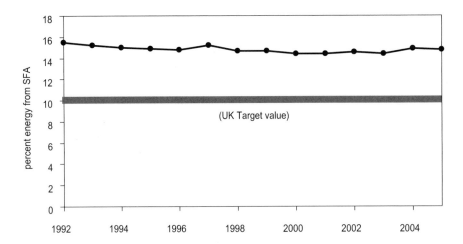

Figure 3. Saturated fat intake in the United Kingdom (Redrawn from British Heart Foundation 2006d)

It is important to recognise that milk does not contain only "cholesterol-raising" SFA. A typical fatty acid composition of bovine milk is shown in Figure 4. About 64% of the fatty acids found in milk fat are SFA. Of these, about 12% are short-chain SFA (C4:0-C10:0) and another 12% is stearic acid (C18:0). It is generally accepted that these particular SFAs have no effect on plasma cholesterol. The remaining SFA represent a mixture of lauric acid (C12:0), myristic acid (C14:0) and palmitic acid (C16:0).

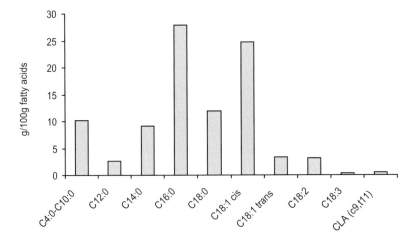

Figure 4. Fatty acid composition of cows milk (Data redrawn from Lock *et al.* (2005c))

Recent meta-analysis of human dietary studies (Mensink *et al.*, 2003) suggests that although lauric, myristic and palmitic acids each increase plasma concentration of the "pro-atherogenic" LDL cholesterol fraction, such adverse effects tend to be offset partially by an increase the "anti-atherogenic" HDL cholesterol fraction. In fact, compared to effects of dietary carbohydrates, their overall effect was small and, in the case of lauric acid, may actually be beneficial. This analysis therefore raises questions about the value of removing SFA from the diet if they are replaced simply by energy from carbohydrate. However, the same analysis confirms the benefits of *cis* monounsaturated (MUFA) and n-6 polyunsaturated fatty acids (PUFA). Thus, rather than reducing total milk fat consumption it may be potentially more beneficial to alter milk fatty acid composition.

Approximately 30% of fatty acids in milk are MUFA and 4% PUFA. The majority of these contain only *cis*-double bonds. A smaller proportion, approximately 4%, consists of fatty acids with one or more *trans*-double bonds. *Trans* fatty acids have been the subject of considerable interested in recent years and the meta-analysis of Mensink *et al.* (2003) suggests that they include the most potent cholesterol-raising dietary fatty acids. However, there are several isomers of *trans* C18:1 fatty acid and, as discussed below, those found in dairy products may not have the same impact on CVD risk as those found in hydrogenated vegetable oils. Furthermore, CLA isomers containing a mixture of *cis* and *trans* double bonds are found naturally only in ruminant meat and milk, and may have specific benefits to human health (Bauman *et al.*, 2006).

Regulation of milk fatty acid composition

The fatty acids in milk are a combination of those made *de novo* in the mammary gland, those mobilized from other body tissue, primarily adipose tissue, and those derived from the diet. It has been estimated that, in general, approximately 50% of bovine milk fat is derived from fatty acids taken up from plasma and of these, about 88% are derived from the diet (Grummer, 1991). However, specific sources of milk fatty acids vary depending on a number of factors, particularly stage of lactation.

As can be seen in Figure 5, the major product of *de novo* fatty acid synthesis is palmitic acid, with lesser amounts of the shorter chain saturated fatty acids being released from the fatty acid synthase (FAS) reaction. Relatively small amounts of myristic and palmitic acid are converted to their *cis* MUFA derivatives through the action of the enzyme, Stearoyl Coenzyme A Desaturase (SCD, also known as Δ9-desaturase). The absence of significant

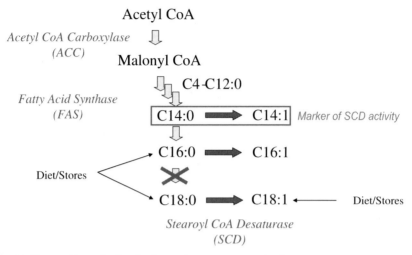

Figure 5. Fatty acid metabolism in the ruminant mammary gland

elongase activity in the ruminant mammary gland means that there is essentially no conversion of palmitic acid to stearic acid. The stearic acid in milk thus originates from either adipose tissue or indirectly from the diet. Biohydrogenation of dietary PUFA (largely n-6 linoleic acid and n-3 linolenic acid) within the rumen leads to a relatively high concentration of stearic acid being absorbed from the small intestine (Lock *et al.*, 2005b). In addition, a variety of intermediates in the biohydrogenation process, often containing *trans* double bonds, exit the rumen to be absorbed from the intestine, and can be found in relatively low concentrations in milk (Lock and Bauman 2004; Bauman and Lock 2006). Stearic acid is a major substrate for the action of SCD and approximately 60% of milk oleic acid (*cis*-9 C18:1) is formed in the mammary gland through the action of the SCD enzyme. The remainder of the oleic acid in milk represents that from the diet which has escaped biohydrogenation, and a further contribution from adipose tissue stores. Thus, manipulating the nature or proportion of milk fatty acids derived from the diet or adipose tissue could have an impact on the overall fatty acid composition of milk fat.

Manipulating the fatty acid content of milk fat through diet

Nutrition is the predominant environmental factor affecting milk fat and represents a practical tool to alter its yield and composition (Lock and Shingfield, 2004). It is well recognised that changing the type or amount of dietary fat fed to the ruminant can affect milk composition. For example, a recent study involving 26 dietary treatments showed that dietary oil concentration influenced milk fatty acids more than any other factor; increasing oil decreased SFA, and increased MUFA, CLA and trans fatty acids (TFA) (Garnsworthy, 2006). Manipulating the diet has been extensively explored as a potential way of increasing the PUFA content of milk. As discussed previously, the extent of such changes is limited by biohydrogenation of a large proportion of unsaturated fatty acids in the rumen (Lock *et al.*, 2005b). As has been previously reported at the Nottingham Feed Conference, various methods are available to protect unsaturated fatty acids from biohydrogenation (Garnsworthy, 1997; Ashes *et al.*, 2000). However, the extent of protection provided by current technologies is limited, allowing for only small increases in PUFA accumulation in milk. In recent years there has been particular interest in trying to increase the concentration of n-3 PUFA in milk. This is a result of the widely held view that in many industrialized countries the relative concentration of dietary n-3 PUFA, compared to n-6 PUFA, is low and may have detrimental effects on human health (Gebauer *et al.*, 2006). Many countries have made specific recommendations that n-3 PUFA intake should be increased. Although most of the known health benefits of n-3 PUFA relate to the very long chain highly unsaturated fatty acids, eicosapentaenoic acid (EPA) and docosahexaenoic acid (DHA), there has also been interest in increasing the concentration α-linolenic acid (ALA, C18:3) in milk as a possible precursor of these.

Feeding fish oil to dairy cattle leads to modest increases of EPA and DHA in milk. For example, Jones *et al.* (2000) showed that feeding up to 2% fish oil (dry matter basis) led to a dose dependent increase in EPA and DHA in milk. However, the transfer efficiency was estimated to be less than 7%. Speciality milk and dairy products are currently available that have been enriched with EPA and DHA through adding fish oil to the cow's diet. Adding large amounts of fish oil to the diet of ruminants, however, has a major impact on rumen function, interfering with biohydrogenation of unsaturated fatty acids and leading to accumulation of large quantities of *trans* fatty acids, which are subsequently absorbed by the animal and incorporated into milk (Loor *et al.*, 2005). This is often associated with a significant reduction in total milk fat concentration. A potentially more attractive alternative is to feed cows ALA, which can be converted to EPA and DHA through elongation and desaturation either in the tissues of the cow, or in the tissues of the consumer following consumption of ALA-enriched milk. In a recent study, ALA was increased by 50% in cows given extruded linseed (Garnsworthy, 2006). Unfortunately neither the dairy cow (Petit *et al.*, 2002) nor the consumer

(Arterburn *et al.,* 2006) is particularly efficient at converting ALA to EPA (which also limits production of DHA). From a human nutrition standpoint, using milk as a vehicle for delivering PUFA can be criticized due to the relatively high concentration of SFA associated with milk. At a time when most dietary advice is still aimed at reducing SFA intake by avoiding full fat dairy products, promoting milk as a source of PUFA, when sources low in SFA are available, may be difficult. Ideally any strategy for manipulating milk fatty acid composition should include reducing SFA content.

Stearoyl Coenzyme A Desaturase as a target for manipulating milk fatty acid composition

One of the primary influences on the fatty acid composition of milk is the relative contribution of *de novo* lipogenesis in the mammary gland compared to uptake of fatty acids from plasma (either of dietary origin or released from adipose tissue). As described above, newly synthesised fatty acids are saturated and mainly represent those believed to increase human plasma cholesterol (lauric, myristic and palmitic acid). Although a small proportion of these can be converted to their monounsaturated derivatives through the action of SCD, they represent relatively poor substrates for this enzyme. A large proportion of the fatty acids entering the mammary gland from the circulation is stearic acid. This is the preferred substrate of SCD and approximately two-thirds is converted into oleic acid (Shorten *et al.*, 2004). We have been specifically interested in the regulation of SCD in both adipose tissue and the mammary gland and the potential for manipulating SCD activity to alter fatty acid composition. The ratio of milk C14:1 to C14:0 is often used as an index of SCD activity because both fatty acids are exclusively synthesized de novo in the mammary gland. Previous work has shown considerable variability in this ratio among individual animals leading us to suggest that there may be significant genetic variability among animals (Lock and Garnsworthy, 2003; Lock *et al.*, 2005a; Garnsworthy, 2006). In a structured genetic study involving 2400 cows, the heritability of this ratio was approximately 0.3 (Garnsworthy & Royal, 2005). Furthermore, we have recently demonstrated that the C14:1/C14:0 ratio correlates well with concentration of SCD mRNA in somatic cells extracted from milk, and that between-cow variability seems to account for more variation in SCD mRNA than does stage of lactation or diet (Feng *et al.,* 2006). Thus, cows could potentially be selected for high mammary expression of SCD. However, whether this would have a significant impact on milk fatty acid composition remains to be established. Since two-thirds of stearic acid taken up into the mammary gland is already converted to oleic acid, even increasing SCD activity by as much 50% would have only a relatively modest impact on fatty acid composition of milk fat (Shorten *et al.*, 2004). However, as will be discussed below, increasing SCD activity may also have a significant impact on production of CLA in the mammary gland.

Trans fatty acids in milk

As discussed above, it has been suggested that *trans* fatty acids represent the most potent cholesterol raising component of the human diet. This had led to specific public health policies to reduce *trans* fatty acid intake and a number of countries, such as the USA, have recently introduced legislation requiring labelling of *trans* fatty acid content on all food products (Lock *et al.*, 2005d). Denmark has gone further by introducing legislation that limits the use of industrially-produced oils to no more than 2% of fat in human food products (Stender *et al.*, 2006).

The two primary sources of dietary TFA are partially hydrogenated vegetable oil and milk and meat products from ruminant animals. The former are produced by partial catalytic hydrogenation of vegetable and marine oils to render them solid/semi-solid at room temperature allowing their widespread use in the food industry, particularly in prepared foods (e.g. baked goods, frying fats and margarines). As already discussed, *trans* fatty acids in milk are products of incomplete biohydrogenation of PUFA by rumen microbes. Estimates for intakes of *trans* fatty acids, and their source, vary considerably from country to country. In the USA, prior to the introduction of labelling legislation, about 80% was derived from PHVO (US Food and Drug Administration 2003). In many countries in Europe, a higher proportion (abut 50%) comes from dairy fat (Hulshof *et al.*, 1999). The recent requirements for labelling of *trans* fatty acid content of food has led to an increased interest in the relative effects of *trans* fatty acids of ruminant origin compared to those in PHVO. In fact, the chemical nature of the *trans* fats in these two sources varies substantially (Lock *et al* 2005d).

Partial-hydrogenation of vegetable oils can result in oils containing variable amounts of *trans* fatty acids, representing up to 60% of total fatty acids. These are predominantly *trans* C18:1 with an even distribution of *trans*-9, *trans*-10, *trans*-11 and *trans*-12 18:1 isomers (Figure 6; Craig-Schmidt, 1992; Emken, 1995). Ruminant derived lipids typically contain 1 to 8% of their total fatty acids as *trans* fatty acids (Craig-Schmidt 1998), and these are also predominantly *trans* C18:1 (Emken 1995). In ruminant fat, vaccenic acid (*trans*-11 18:1; VA) is the most common *trans* C18:1, typically accounting

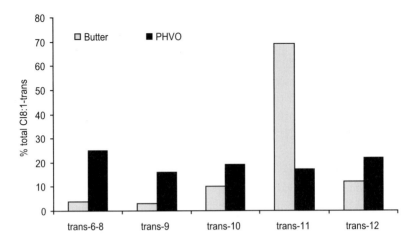

Figure 6. Distribution of *trans* 18:1 fatty acids in ruminant fat and partially hydrogenated vegetable oils (PHVO) (Redrawn from data in Lock *et al.* (2005c))

for 60 to 80% of total *trans* fatty acids (Emken, 1995; Craig-Schmidt, 1998). The double bond position can significantly influence the metabolism and physiological effects of *trans* fatty acids, suggesting that differences in distribution between ruminant and industrial sources may be of significance in relation to human health effects. Lock *at al.* (2005d) recently reviewed the evidence that *trans* fatty acids of ruminant origin may have different effects on human health than those from PHVO. Much of the evidence that *trans* fatty acids are associated with adverse changes in plasma lipoproteins and increased risk of CVD arises from large epidemiological studies that have not distinguished between ruminant and PHVO sources. Where such analysis is possible, it is usually *trans* fatty acids from PHVO that are associated with adverse effects, whereas those from ruminants have shown no association with CVD risk (Lock *et al.*, 2005d).

A possible explanation for differential effects of TFA from ruminants and PHVO is that VA can be converted to *cis*-9, *trans*-11 CLA (rumenic acid; RA), through the action of SCD. Several studies have established that humans are capable of this conversion (Salminen *et al.*, 1998; Adlof *et al.*, 2000; Turpeinen *et al.*, 2002); Turpeinen *et al.* (2002) estimated that a minimum of 20% of VA was converted to RA in humans, thereby doubling RA supply. As described below, RA has been associated with a range of potential health benefits including anti-atherogenic and anti-carcinogenic actions. RA content of milk can be increased by manipulating the diet of the cow, and such increases are usually associated with even greater increases in VA content. Since VA can be converted to RA in the tissues of the consumer, this particular *trans* fatty acid may actually benefit human health.

Conjugated linoleic acid in milk

The last decade has seen enormous interest in the potential effects of CLA on human health. Much of this has focussed on the *trans*-10, *cis* 12 C18:2 isomer and its ability to reduce body fat deposition. This isomer normally occurs in only small amounts in the human food chain and studies have focused on chemically produced supplements. The dramatic effects of this isomer that were initially reported in mice have failed to be reproduced in human studies. Of greater interest to the dairy industry is RA, which occurs naturally in ruminant milk. As reported previously at the Nottingham Feed Conference, RA production can be increased by manipulating the diet of the cow (Bauman *et al.*, 2001). Feeding dairy cows a typical commercial diet supplemented with PUFA–rich plant oil can result in production of milk in which the RA content may approach 5% of total fatty acids, with RA representing 90% of the CLA (Bauman *et al.*, 2000; Bauman and Lock, 2006). As indicated in Figure 7, the basis for such manipulation is altered activity of the rumen microbial population so that biohydrogenation of PUFA is incomplete and there is an accumulation of intermediates including VA and RA. The majority of RA in milk fat is synthesized endogenously from VA in the mammary gland, and the normal ratio of VA to RA in milk fat is approximately 3:1 (Bauman & Lock 2006).

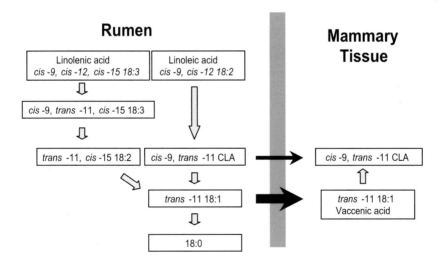

Figure 7. CLA production in the ruminant (Adapted from Bauman *et al.*, 2001)

A number of studies utilizing animal models of human disease have suggested potential health benefits of RA/VA-enriched milk fat (reviewed by Lock *et al.*, 2005d). Ip *et al.* (1999) demonstrated that dietary consumption of a RA/

VA-enriched butter was effective in reducing the number and incidence of mammary tumors in a rat model. In that study it was noted that tissue concentrations of RA were greater in rats fed RA/VA-enriched butter than in rats fed a comparable amount of synthetic RA, possibly due to endogenous synthesis of RA from VA in the butter (Ip *et al.*, 1999). This was supported by a subsequent study in which feeding rats increasing amounts of pure VA resulted in a progressive increase in tissue concentrations of RA with a corresponding reduction in the number of premalignant mammary lesions, an early marker for mammary cancer (Banni *et al.*, 2001). Lock *et al.* (2004) investigated this further using sterculic oil to inhibit SCD, thereby blocking endogenous synthesis of RA. Addition of sterculic oil to a diet containing RA/VA-enriched butter markedly attenuated the biological effects of VA on tissue content of RA and the number and growth of premalignant lesions, indicating that the bioactive effects of VA were mostly, perhaps exclusively, through its conversion to RA.

Although animal experiments appear promising, assessing the role of RA/VA in prevention of cancer in humans is difficult because there is a lack of consensus on biomarkers for most types of cancer. Therefore, epidemiological data remain inconclusive (Bauman *et al.*, 2005, Lock *et al.*, 2005d).

Numerous investigations with animal models have also examined the effects of CLA isomers on atherosclerosis and related variables. The majority of these studies have utilized synthetic sources of CLA to examine cholesterol metabolism, and results indicate that dietary CLA can suppress dietary-cholesterol-induced atherosclerosis and, in some incidences, alter plasma cholesterol concentrations (see review by Bauman *et al.*, 2005). As with cancer studies, promising results from animal experiments are not always supported by human epidemiological studies. Recent evidence suggests that *cis*-9, *trans*-11 and *trans*-10, *cis*-12 CLA have opposing effects on plasma triacylglycerol and on the ratios of LDL:HDL cholesterol and total cholesterol:HDL, with *cis*-9,*trans*-11 CLA demonstrating a relative hypolipidaemic effect and *trans*-10, *cis*-12 CLA a hyperlipidaemic effect (Tricon *et al.*, 2004).

A recent study examined the effects of RA/VA-enriched butter in Golden Syrian hamsters fed high fat (20%), high cholesterol (0.2%) diets (Lock *et al.*, 2005c). The VA/RA-enriched butter had a number of beneficial effects on CVD-related variables, including reduced total and pro-atherogenic plasma cholesterol levels (VLDL and LDL), suggesting that RA may modify production of atherogenic lipoproteins by the liver. Of particular interest was that hamsters fed RA/VA-enriched butter had lower plasma VLDL and LDL cholesterol concentrations than hamsters fed an equivalent diet containing *trans* fatty acids from PHVO. This further suggests that VA found in dairy products may have beneficial effects, compared to other *trans* C18:1 isomers, due to conversion to RA through the action of SCD.

The effects of RA/VA-enriched dairy products on blood lipids in healthy human subjects have recently been reported (Tricon *et al.,* 2006). Consumption of RA/VA-enriched milk increased total intake of RA 9.4-fold and VA 15–fold. This change in dietary intake had no significant effect on plasma LDL or HDL cholesterol concentration. Thus, although the study failed to indicate a beneficial effect of RA/VA–enriched milk on plasma lipids, it also failed to demonstrate any significant adverse effects of a diet enriched in VA. This is indirect evidence that the effects of *trans* fatty acids on LDL and HDL cholesterol might be restricted to those isomers more abundant in PHVO than in dairy fat. This is another example where promising animal responses are not always translated into equivalent human responses.

Conclusions

It is clear that in many countries, including the UK, several decades of nutritional advice aimed at reducing dietary saturated fat intake have dramatically reduced intake of full-fat dairy products. However, these changes appear to have had little impact on total SFA consumption when expressed as a proportion of total energy intake. Despite this, CVD death rates have continued to decline.

It is possible to achieve limited increases the PUFA content of milk by feeding PUFA rich diets to dairy cows, particularly if PUFA are protected from biohydrogenation in the rumen. Although this has led to a limited availability of n-3 PUFA enriched milk to the consumer, the value of such milk can be challenged because of its relatively high SFA content.

The most recent threat to the dairy industry could be a global move toward labelling of the *trans* fatty acid content of foods. With a reduction in the use of PHVO, dairy fat will become the largest source of dietary *trans* fatty acids. However, growing evidence suggests VA, that the predominant isomer found in milk fat, may actually be beneficial rather than detrimental to human health. A major challenge is, however, to persuade legislators and the public to recognise this distinction.

The last decade has seen a proliferation in potential health claims attributed to CLA. Growing evidence suggests that RA, the major CLA isomer associated with dairy fat, continues to hold some promise as an anti-carcinogenic and possibly anti-atherogenic component of milk fat. Further human feeding trials are required to confirm these benefits. At a time when death rates from CVD are in decline, and highly effective cholesterol lowering drugs are available, the potential benefits of consuming RA, and possibly VA, may ultimately challenge the continued recommendation to avoid dairy fat consumption.

References

Adlof, R.O., Duval, S. and Emken, E.A. (2000) Biosynthesis of conjugated linoleic acid in humans. *Lipids* **35**: 131-135.

Arterburn, L.M., Bailey Hall, E. and Oken, H (2006) Distribution, interconversion, and dose response of n-3 fatty acids in humans. *American Journal of Clinical Nutrition* **83**(suppl) 1467S-76S.

Ashes, J.R., Gulati, S.K., Kitessa, S.M., Fleck, E., and Scott, T.W. (2000) Utilization of rumen protected n-3 fatty acids by ruminants. In *Recent Advances in Animal Nutrition -2000* (Edited by P.C. Garnsworthy & J. Wiseman), pp 33-44. Nottingham University Press, Nottingham

Banni, S., Angioni, E., Murru, E., Carta, G., Melis, M.P., Bauman, D.E., Dong, Y. and Ip, C. (2001), Vaccenic acid feeding increases tissue levels of conjugated linoleic acid and suppresses development of premalignant lesions in rat mammary gland. *Nutrition and Cancer* **41**, 91-97.

Bauman, D.E., Barbano, D.M., Dwyer, D.A. and Griinari, J.M. (2000), Technical note, Production of butter with enhanced conjugated linoleic acid for use in biomedical studies with animal models. *Journal of Dairy Science* **83**, 2422-2425.

Bauman, D.E., Corl, B.A., Baumgard, L.H. and Griinari, J.M. (2001) Conjugated linoleic acid (CLA) and the dairy cow. In *Recent Advances in Animal Nutrition -2001* (Edited by P.C. Garnsworthy & J. Wiseman), pp 33-44. Nottingham University Press, Nottingham

Bauman, D.E. and Lock A.L. (2006) Conjugated linoleic acid: biosynthesis and nutritional significance. In: P.F. Fox and P.L.H. McSweeney (Eds.) *Advanced Dairy Chemistry, Volume 2: Lipids*, 3rd Edition. pp. 93-136. Springer, New York, NY, USA.

Bauman, D.E., Lock, A.L. Corl, B.A. Ip, C. Salter, A.M. and Parodi, P.W. (2006) Milk fatty acids and human health: potential role of conjugated linoleic acid and *trans* fatty acids. In: K. Sejrsen, T. Hvelplund, and M. O. Nielsen (Eds.) *Ruminant Physiology: Digestion, Metabolism and Impact of Nutrition on Gene Expression, Immunology and Stress*. pp. 529-561. Wageningen Academic Publishers, Wageningen, The Netherlands.

British Heath Foundation (2006a) Age-standardised death rates per 100,000 population from CHD, men, 1968-2002, selected countries, the World

(Table). http://www.heartstats.org/temp/Tabsp1.5spmenspweb06.xls.

British Heath Foundation (2006b) Age-standardised death rates per 100,000 population from CHD, women, 1968-2002, selected countries, the World (Table). http://www.heartstats.org/temp/Tabsp1.5spwomensp web06.xls .

British Heath Foundation (2006c) Household purchase of milk and milk products, 1942-2003/04, United Kingdom (Figure) http:// www.heartstats.org/temp/PspFigsp5.6bspweb06.ppt

British Heath Foundation (2006d) Consumption of total and saturated fat, adults aged 16 and above, 1975-2003/04, Great Britain, with Choosing a Better Diet targets (Figure) http://www.heartstats.org/temp/ FIGsp5.2aspweb06.xls

Craig-Schmidt, M.C. (1992) Fatty acid isomers in foods. In *Fatty Acids in Foods and their Health Implications* (Ed. C.K. Chow). Marcel Dekker Inc., New York, NY, pp 363-396.

Craig-Schmidt, M.C. (1998) World wide consumption of *trans* fatty acids. In *Trans Fatty Acids in Human Nutrition* (Eds. J.-L. Sebedio and W.W. Christie). The Oily Press, Dundee, Scotland, pp. 59-114.

Emken, E.A. (1995) *Trans* fatty acids and coronary heart disease risk, physicochemical properties, intake, and metabolism. *American Journal of Clinical Nutrition* **62**, 659S-669S.

Feng, S., Salter, A.M. and Garnsworthy, P.C. (2006) Use of milk somatic cells to study Stearoyl–CoA Desaturase activity in the bovine mammary gland. 4th Euro Fed Lipid Congress. Oils, Fats and Lipids for a Healthier Future: The Need for Interdisciplinary Approaches. pp252.

Garnsworthy, P.C. (1997) Fats in dairy cow diets. In *Recent Advances in Animal Nutrition -1997* pp 33-44 Edited by P.C. Garnsworthy & J. Wiseman. Nottingham University Press, Nottingham.

Garnsworthy, P.C. (2006) Nutritional and genetic influences on milk fatty acid composition in dairy cows. *Proceedings XIIth Animal Science Congress, Asian-Australasian Association of Animal Production Societies*, BEXCO Busan, Korea.

Garnsworthy, P.C. and Royal, M.D. (2005) Heritability of Ä9-desaturase enzyme activity in Holstein-Friesian dairy cows. In: *Proceedings of the 26th World Congress and Exhibition of the International Society for Fat Research, Prague.*

Gebauer, S.K., Psota, T.L., Harris, W.S. and Kris-Etherton, P.M. (2006) n-3 Fatty acid dietary recommendations and food sources to achieve essentiality and cardiovascular benefits. *American Journal of Clinical Nutrition* 83(Suppl): 1526S-1535S.

Grummer, R.R. (1991) Effect of feed on the composition of milk fat. *Journal of Dairy Science* **74**:3244–3257.

Hegsted. D.M., McGandy, R.B., Myers, M.L. and Stare, F.J. (1965) Quantitative effects of dietary fat on serum cholesterol in man. *Am. J. Clin. Nutr.* **17**: 281-295.

Hoare, J., Henderson, L., Bates, C.J., Prentice, A., Birch, M., Swan, G. and Farron, M. (2004) The *National Diet & Nutrition Survey: adults aged 19 to 64 years.* Volume 5. HMSO London.

Hulshof, K.F.A.M., Erp-Baart, M.A., Anttolainen, M., Becker, W., Church, S.M., Couet, C., Hermann-Kunz, E., Kesteloot, H., Leth, T., Martins, I., Moreiras, O., Moschandreas, J., Pizzoferrato, L., Rimestad, A.H., Thorgeirsdottir, H., van Amelsvoort, J.M.M., Aro, A., Kafatos, A.G., Lanzmann-Petithory, D. and van Poppel, G. (1999) Intake of fatty acids in Western Europe with emphasis on *trans* fatty acids: The TRANSFAIR study. *European Journal of Clinical Nutrition* **53**, 143-157.

Ip, C., Banni, S., Angioni, E., Carta, G., McGinley, J., Thompson, H.J., Barbano, D. and Bauman, D.E. (1999) Conjugated linoleic acid-enriched butter fat alters mammary gland morphogenesis and reduces cancer risk in rats. *Journal of Nutrition* **129**:2135-2142.

Jones, D.F., Weiss, W.P. and Palmquist, D.L. (2000) Influence of dietary tallow and fish oil on milk composition. *Journal of Dairy Science* **83**: 2024-2026.

Keys, A., Anderson, J.T. and Grande, F. (1965) Serum cholesterol response to changes in diet. IV. Particular saturated fatty acids in the diet. *Metabolism* **14**: 776-787.

Keys, A., Aravanis, C., Blackburn, H.W. *et al.* (1966) Epidemiological studies related to coronary heart disease: characteristics of men aged 40-59 in seven countries. *Acta Med Scand Suppl.* **460**:1-392.

Lichtenstein, A.H., Appel, L.J., Brands, M. *et al* (2006) Diet and lifestyle recommendations revision 2006. A scientific statement from the American Heart Association Scientific Nutrition Committee. *Circulation* **114**: 82-96.

Lock, A.L. and Bauman, D.E. (2004) Modifying milk fat composition of dairy cows to enhance fatty acids beneficial to human health. *Lipids* **39**: 1197-1206.

Lock, A.L., Bauman, D.E. and Garnsworthy, P.C. (2005a) Effect of production variables on the *cis*-9, *trans*-11 conjugated linoleic acid content of cows' milk. *Journal of Dairy Science* **88**: 2714-2717.

Lock, A.L., Corl, B.A., Barbano, D.M., Bauman, D.E. and Ip, C. (2004) The anticarcinogenic effect of *trans*-11 18:1 is dependent on its conversion to *cis*-9, *trans*-11 CLA by Delta 9-desaturase in rats. *Journal of Nutrition* **134**: 2698-2704.

Lock, A.L. and Garnsworthy, P.C. (2003) Seasonal variation in milk conjugated linoleic acid and Δ⁹-desaturase activity in dairy cows. *Livestock Production Science* **79**: 47-59.

Lock, A.L., Harvatine, K.J., Ipharraguerre, I.R., Van Amburgh, M.E., Drackley, J.K. and Bauman, D.E. (2005b) The dynamics of fat digestion in lactating dairy cows: what does the literature tell us? *Proceedings of Cornell Nutrition Conference* pp. 83-94.

Lock, A.L., Horne, C.A.M., Bauman, D.E. and A.M. Salter (2005c) Effect of butter enriched in conjugated linoleic acid (CLA) and vaccenic acid on plasma lipoproteins and tissue fatty acid composition in the cholesterol-fed hamster. *Journal of Nutrition* **135**: 1934-1939.

Lock, A.L., Parodi, P.W. and Bauman, D.E. (2005d) The biology of *trans* fatty acids: implications for human health and the dairy industry. *Australian Journal of Dairy Technology* **60**: 134-142.

Lock, A.L. and Shingfield, K.J. (2004) Optimising milk composition. In: E. Kebreab, J. Mills, and D. Beever (Eds.) *UK Dairying: Using Science to Meet Consumers' Needs*. pp. 107-188. Nottingham University Press, Nottingham, UK.

Loor J.J., Ueda K., Ferlay A., Chilliard Y. and Doreau M. (2005) Intestinal flow and digestibility of trans fatty acids and conjugated linoleic acids (CLA) in dairy cows fed a high-concentrate diet supplemented with fish oil, linseed oil, or sunflower oil. *Animal Feed Science and Technology* **119**: 203-225.

Mensink, R.P., Zock, P.L., Kester, A.D.M. and Katan, M.B. (2003) Effects of dietary fatty acids and carbohydrates on the ration of serum total to HDL cholesterol and on serum lipids and apolipoproteins: a meta-analysis of 60 controlled trials. *American Journal of Clinical Nutrition* **77**:1146-55.

Petit, H.V., Dewhurst, R.J., Scollan, N.D., Proulx, J.G., Khalid, M., Hareign, W., Twagiramungu, H. and Mann, G.E. (2002) Milk production and composition, ovarian function, and prostaglandin secretion of dairy cows fed omega-3 fats. *Journal of Dairy Science* **85**: 889-899.

Unal, B., Critichley, J.A and Capewell, S. (2004) Explaining the decline in coronary heart disease mortality in England and Wales between 1981 and 2000. *Circulation* **109**: 1101-1107.

Salminen, I., Mutanen, M., Jauhiainen, M. and Aro, A. (1998) Dietary *trans* fatty acids increase conjugated linoleic acid levels in human serum. *Journal of Nutritional Biochemistry* **9**: 93-98.

Salter, A.M. (2005) The role of diet in preventing cardiovascular disease in the "post statin" era. *Proceedings of the Cornell Nutrition Conference 2005.*

Salter, A.M., Daniel, Z.C.T.R., Wynn, R.J., Locki, A.L., Garnworthy, P.C. and Buttery, P.J. (2002) Manipulating the fatty acid compositon of animal products. What has and what might be achieved? In *Recent Advances in Animal Nutrition -2002*, pp 33-44 Edited by P.C. Garnsworthy & J. Wiseman. Nottingham University Press, Nottingham.

Shorten, P.R., Pleasants, T.B. and Upreti, G.C. (2004) A mathematical model for mammary fatty acid synthesis and trglyceride assembly: the role of stearoyl CoA desaturase (SCD). *Journal of Dairy Research* **71**: 385-397.

Stender, S., Dyerberg, J., Bysted, A., Leth, T. and Astrup, A. (2006) A trans world journey. *Atherosclerosis supplements* **7**: 47-52

Tricon, S., Burdge, G.C., Jones, E.L., Russell, J.J., El-Khazen, S., Moretti, E., Hall, W.L., Gerry, A.B., Leake, D.S., Grimble, R.F., Williams, C.M., Calder, P.C. and Yaqoob, P. (2006) Effects of dairy products naturally enriched with *cis*-9,*trans*-11 conjugated linoleic acid on the blood lipid profile in healthy middle-aged men. *American Journal of Clinical Nutrition* **83**: 744-753.

Tricon, S., Burdge, G.C., Kew, S., Banerjee, T., Russell, J.J., Jones, E.L., Grimble, R.F., Williams, C.M., Yaqoob, P. and Calder, P.C. (2004) Opposing effects of *cis*-9, *trans*-11 and *trans*-10, *cis*-12 conjugated linoleic acid on blood lipids in healthy humans. *American Journal of Clinical Nutrition* **80**: 614-62.

Turpeinen, A.M., Mutanen, M., Aro, A., Salminen, I., Basu, S., Palmquist, D.L. and Griinari, J. M. (2002) Bioconversion of vaccenic acid to conjugated linoleic acid in humans. *American Journal of Clinical Investigation* **76**:504-510.

US Food and Drug Administration (2003) Questions and answers about *trans* fat nutrition labeling. www.cfsan.fda.gov/~dms/qatrans2.html.2003

2

MILK PROTEIN: BIOLOGY SUPPORTS BALANCING RATIONS FOR AMINO ACIDS

H. LAPIERRE[1], G. RAGGIO[2], D.R. OUELLET[1], R. BERTHIAUME[1], S. LEMOSQUET[3], L. DOEPEL[4] AND D. PACHECO[5]

[1]*Dairy and Swine Research and Development Centre, Agriculture and Agri-Food Canada, Sherbrooke, QC, Canada, J1M 1Z3;* [2]*Dept. of Animal Science, Université Laval, Québec, QC, Canada, G1K 6P4;* [3]*I.N.R.A., UMR Production du Lait, 35590 Saint-Gilles, France;* [4]*Dept. of Agricultural, Food and Nutritional Science, University of Alberta, Edmonton, AL, Canada, T6G 2P5;* [5]*AgResearch, Palmerston North, New Zealand.*

Introduction

Over the last decade, there has been a renewed interest to increase the efficiency of transfer of the crude protein fed to the dairy cow into milk true protein. Such increased efficiency would help to reach two high-currency objectives: increase the competitiveness of dairy producers and dairy products in a global market, and limit the impact of livestock production on the environment. Part of the excretion of nitrogen (N), which is the protein not used by the animal, is recognized to contribute to N_2O formation, a greenhouse gas, and to ammonia emission leading to the formation of fine particulate matters, largely responsible for the deterioration of the quality of air.

To increase efficiency, we need to improve the match between supply and requirements, and we need to refine our estimations of both. Big improvements have been achieved in recent decades to refine our assessment of protein supply to dairy cows: we moved from crude protein to degradable and undegradable protein. These represent a combination of partial requirements for rumen microflora and for the cow itself. A last step was then achieved to determine the amount of protein ultimately available and used by the animal itself, the metabolizable protein (MP). This is the sum of undegradable protein and microbial protein (INRA, 1989 (PDI system); AFRC, 1993; Fox *et al.*, 2004 (CNCPS system)), sometimes with endogenous protein included (NRC, 2001). To estimate MP available to dairy cows, complex rumen sub-models have been developed to combine rumen degradability of protein and energy, rate of passage, etc. These predictions yield not only the flow of MP, but also the flow of individual amino acids (AA). Two questions then arise: 1) Should we consider individual AA? and 2) How is AA supply used for milk production?

In this chapter, we will limit our considerations to essential AA. They are called "essential" because the dairy cow cannot synthesize them and therefore, they need to be supplied from the combination of rumen undegradable protein (RUP) and microbial protein. Essential AA include histidine, isoleucine, leucine, lysine, methionine, phenylalanine, threonine, tryptophan and valine. This does not deny the importance of the non-essential AA. The polypeptide chains constituting proteins contain both essential and non-essential AA, but the non-essential AA can be synthesized by the dairy cow. However, there is a sub-group within the non-essential AA for which synthesis is not sufficient to support high levels of production; these are called semi-essential. Arginine is the most typical AA of this group as de novo synthesis of arginine could represent up to 0.40 of total supply to the animal (Doepel *et al.*, 2004). Histidine could theoretically also be synthesized by the mammal, but its synthetic pathway has limited capacity and therefore endogenous synthesis is usually ignored. It has also been suggested that glutamine may be classified as semi-essential under certain circumstances, especially around calving (Doepel *et al.*, 2004; Meijer *et al.*, 1995). Data are scarce on non-essential AA metabolism (especially to quantify *de novo* synthesis and therefore having an accurate estimate of their true total supply to the dairy cow), so the discussion will be limited to the fate of essential AA.

Why should we consider individual AA?

At the tissue level, it is clear that the raw material used by cells to build proteins is free AA. Therefore, an estimation of requirements in terms of AA theoretically would cover exactly what is being used by the animal. If the supply of protein always contain the same proportions of AA, and all AA had similar metabolic fate, then we would not need to partition supply and requirement of MP into individual AA. This is clearly not the case, as discussed below.

SUPPLY OF AA

Comparison of profiles for individual AA from microbial protein and different feed ingredients (supplying RUP) reveals the disparity in their AA composition and strongly suggests potential variations in the profile of AA supplied to a dairy cow (Figure 1, NRC 2001). Indeed, large variations in the proportion of individual AA in duodenal protein have been reported (Figure 2, NRC 2001). This clearly indicates that MP cannot be considered as a homogenous entity and needs to be better defined in terms of its AA to really assess what is provided to the dairy cow.

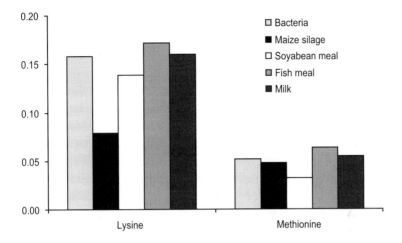

Figure 1. Lysine and methionine content (proportion of essential AA) of feed ingredients, bacteria and milk.

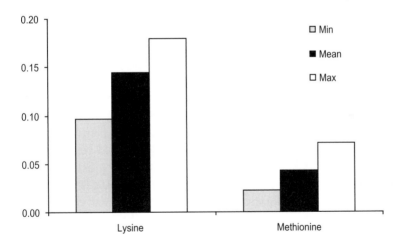

Figure 2. Concentration of lysine and methionine (proportion of essential AA) in duodenal protein from studies used by NRC (2001) to develop equations predicting duodenal AA flow.

Once it is recognized that the proportion of AA in duodenal digesta can vary widely, the first challenge becomes to predict adequately the supply of individual AA. A number of rumen sub-models have been developed to predict fractions of feed that by-pass the rumen, utilisation of degradable N and energy for microbial growth, and subsequent passage into the duodenum, in order to estimate total flow of crude protein to the duodenum. Models use different approaches to estimate flow of individual AA available to the dairy cow, either assigning an AA composition to each duodenal fraction, RUP, microbial protein (e.g. CNCPS) and endogenous protein when considered, or using regression equations to link the percentage of an essential AA in duodenal protein to the percentage of this AA in RUP and the percentage of RUP in duodenal protein (NRC, 2001). Estimated duodenal flow combined with a digestibility factor estimates the amount of AA available to the animal. As discussed later, not all of the duodenal flow represents a net input of AA to the dairy cow. In dairy cows, up to 0.20 of duodenal N flow originates from endogenous proteins (Ouellet *et al.*, 2002; 2005). At the entrance to the duodenum, endogenous proteins comprise mainly mucoproteins, saliva, sloughed epithelial cells and enzyme secretions into the abomasum (Tamminga *et al.*, 1995). This endogenous fraction constitutes a recycling of AA previously absorbed from the small intestine, returned to the gut tissue via arterial circulation and used to build proteins that are returned into the lumen of the gut prior to the duodenum. As such, they do not represent a net input of AA for the animal, but are just a form of recycling.

In summary, the proportion of essential AA in duodenal protein will vary greatly, depending mainly on source of RUP and its degradability in the rumen.

UTILISATION OF AA ACROSS TISSUES

In dairy cows, metabolism of AA has been studied mainly across the mammary gland (an obvious target) and also across the splanchnic tissues, despite the complex surgical preparations needed to conduct these studies. The splanchnic tissues comprising the portal-drained viscera (gut, spleen, pancreas and associated mesenteric fat) plus the liver have been extensively studied because of their high metabolic activity. In dairy cows, despite the fact that these tissues contribute less than 0.10 of body mass (Gibb *et al.*, 1992), they account for close to 0.50 of whole body oxygen consumption (Huntington, 1990) and contribute close to 0.50 to whole body protein synthesis (Lapierre *et al.*, 2002).

Net utilisation of essential AA across the gut

Measurement of net utilisation of essential AA across the gut is not an easy task. In other tissues, AA are only supplied from the blood source and can be more easily quantified. However, net supply of AA to the gut also requires quantification of AA digested from the lumen of the small intestine. First attempts to determine net utilisation of AA across the portal-drained viscera were in sheep, where disappearance across the small intestine was compared with the amount of AA absorbed in the portal vein: recovery in the portal vein of the amount that had disappeared from the small intestine ranged from 0.19 for histidine to 0.69 for lysine, suggesting a huge net utilisation of AA by the gut (Tagari and Bergman, 1978). More recent data in sheep (MacRae *et al.*, 1997) and in dairy cows (Berthiaume *et al.*, 2001) reported higher recoveries than in the first study, ranging from 0.43 (threonine) to 0.95 (histidine). However, this ratio does not really represent what is being lost through passage across the gut. As discussed above, part of the small intestinal disappearance is not a net supply. Endogenous proteins secreted prior to the duodenum have been made from AA provided by arterial supply and their digestion and absorption do not contribute to net supply. Therefore, without any net utilisation of AA by the gut tissue, portal absorption will always be less than apparent disappearance from the small intestine.

True losses of AA across the gut will be through oxidation and those endogenous secretions that are not reabsorbed and therefore secreted in the faeces. There are limited data in ruminants on endogenous protein secretions and gut oxidation; both processes being challenging to measure directly. However, recent studies reported oxidation across the portal-drained viscera of leucine in dairy cows (Lapierre at al., 2002) and of leucine and methionine but not of lysine and phenylalanine in sheep (Lobley *et al.*, 2003). Phenylalanine was also observed not to be oxidized across the gut in dairy cows (Reynolds *et al.*, 2000). In dairy cows, indirect measurements (comparing estimated flow of digested AA and measured portal absorption) have suggested substantial losses of branched-chained AA (isoleucine, leucine and valine), probably via oxidation, and of threonine, most likely due to its high concentration in endogenous secretions (Lapierre *et al.*, 2006). A more complete review of AA utilisation by the portal-drained viscera across farm species is in Lobley and Lapierre (2003). An additional loss of AA through gut metabolism is endogenous secretions that are not reabsorbed and are excreted in the faeces. Quantification of these losses is also challenging and there is no general agreement between predictive systems as to what they are and on which basis they should be calculated (dry matter intake, body weight, or protein intake). Recent work has shown that they can represent up to 0.30 of N in faeces and that they may be related to fibre content of the diet (Ouellet *et al.*, 2002; 2005). More work is needed to elucidate the true loss of AA through this metabolic fate in high yielding dairy cows.

Overall, despite the fact that exact amounts and regulatory mechanisms are still unknown, there is enough evidence to suggest significant net utilisation of some essential AA by gut tissues, mainly through oxidation and losses of endogenous proteins in the faeces, at a rate that differs among AA.

Net utilisation of essential AA across the liver

Due to its anatomical location and vascular structure, AA metabolism across the liver may be "simpler" to determine and analyse than across the gut. From a database of studies where N transfers across the splanchnic tissues had been studied (22 treatments), the liver removed 0.45 of total AA absorbed (AA being measured individually or as alpha-amino-N; Lapierre *et al.*, 2005a). We have to be very cautious in the interpretation of this number before we apply it to all AA; a ratio of 0.45 might not apply to all AA under all circumstances. This removal encompasses all AA, essential and non-essential. The liver removes AA for a number of purposes. Among other functions, the liver plays the important role of avoiding hyperaminoacidaemia and therefore extracts excess AA through urea synthesis, uses AA for synthesis of proteins (some of which are then exported to the plasma) and also uses some AA, mainly non-essential, for synthesis of glucose. These different roles of the liver already suggest variable and different hepatic removal of different AA.

To better estimate the fate of individual AA across the liver, another database was used, in which net splanchnic flux of individual AA had been measured (14 treatments; Lapierre *et al.*, 2005a). Two groups of essential AA were quite distinctive in their behaviour across the splanchnic tissues and related well with the groups described by Mepham (1982) according to their metabolism across the mammary gland. Amino acids from Group 1, for which mammary uptake is approximately equal to secretion in milk protein, are substantially removed by the liver, and post-liver supply is approximately equal to mammary uptake. Histidine, methionine, phenylalanine, and tryptophan are included in this group. On average, hepatic removal relative to net portal absorption varied from 0.36 for methionine to 0.48 for phenylalanine (Lapierre *et al.*, 2005a). In contrast, AA from Group 2, already identified as those for which mammary uptake exceeds milk output, are, on a net basis, barely removed by the liver, and post-liver supply is higher than mammary uptake. Group 2 consists of the branched-chain AA (isoleucine, leucine and valine) and lysine. Therefore, despite the fact that the liver is the major site of ureagenesis, not all of the excess essential AA is, on a net basis, extracted by the liver. They can be deaminated elsewhere in the body and the N returned to the liver through shuttles like alanine or glutamine prior to excretion of the N as urea. The distribution of enzymes responsible for AA catabolism is directly linked with the two groups described above. For Group 1 AA, degradative enzymes are predominantly restricted to the liver; for Group 2 AA, the enzymes responsible for catabolism are widely distributed across tissues, including liver, muscle, fat, gut and mammary gland (Lobley and Lapierre, 2003).

Net utilisation of essential AA across the mammary gland

As described by Mepham (1982) and discussed in the previous section, AA of Group 1 (histidine, methionine, phenylalanine and tryptophan), are all taken up as free AA from blood circulation and incorporated into milk protein. For AA of Group 2 (isoleucine, leucine, valine and lysine), uptake usually exceeds output. These observations have been made in connection with splanchnic measurements (Berthiaume *et al.*, 2006; Raggio *et al.*, 2004) and also in studies of mammary metabolism in dairy cows (Cant *et al.*, 1993; Guinard and Rulquin, 1994; Pacheco, 2000; Raggio *et al.*, 2006). It should be stated here that mammary uptake of non-essential AA (except arginine) is usually not sufficient to support the amount of non-essential AA used to make milk protein, i.e. there must be synthesis of non-essential AA within the mammary gland. Effectively, it has been shown that N from lysine taken up by the mammary gland in excess of milk protein was used for synthesis of non-essential AA within the mammary gland (Lapierre *et al.*, 2003).

Figure 3 summarizes the fate of two AA representative of Group 1 (methionine) and Group 2 (lysine) across the splanchnic tissues and the mammary gland (Lapierre *et al.*, 2005a). Overall, it is clear that metabolism of AA varies among AA and between tissues. Therefore we need to refine our definition of supply and requirement to the AA level and not just their aggregate, the proteins. Such an approach has been proven to be beneficial in monogastrics, in terms of animal performance, production cost and reducing the impact of livestock on the environment.

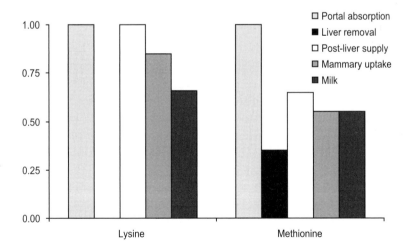

Figure 3. Net flux of two essential AA representative of Group 1 (methionine) and Group 2 (lysine) in dairy cows, relative to portal absorption.

How: fixed or variable efficiency of transfer?

As both the proportional contribution to duodenal flow and the metabolic fate across the gut, the liver and the mammary gland vary markedly among essential AA, it appears necessary to consider individual AA in dairy nutrition. However, it is not enough to determine adequately the supply of MP or individual AA. The next question becomes: "How will these AA be used for milk production?" Actually, after a tremendous amount of work has been done to estimate supply of MP and AA, their estimated metabolic utilisation is quite simple: a fixed efficiency! It is assumed in most of the predictive models (AFRC, 1993; NRC, 2001; CNCPS (Fox *et al.* 2004)) that the theoretical portion of the supply for maintenance is used with a fixed efficiency, and that the supply left for productive purposes is also used with a fixed efficiency. The NRC (2001) applies a fixed conversion factor of 0.67 from MP to protein used for maintenance or milk; CNCPS uses a different factor among AA, but a fixed factor within either maintenance or lactation. For CNCPS, efficiency of utilisation of AA for lactation is based on an average uptake:output ratio of AA across the mammary gland. Therefore, these models estimate a fixed return of increased protein supply into milk protein until requirements are reached, after which the response is zero. These efficiency factors are unlikely to be fixed across protein intakes (if energy is sufficient); few biological systems work in a linear fashion with a zero response once a threshold is reached.

EXPERIMENTAL EVIDENCE OF VARIABLE EFFICIENCY

With the increased interest in N efficiency, recent studies have shown that reducing N supply increases efficiency of N utilisation (Wright *et al.*, 1998; Castillo *et al.*, 2001; Raggio *et al.*, 2004). The AFRC (1998) Technical Committee on Responses to Nutrients reported that "It may be argued that the net efficiency with which absorbed AA are used for milk production (k_{nl}) should be regarded not as a constant but as a variable to be predicted within the feeding system for attributes both of the diets (balance of AA supplied) and the cow (efficiency of use of ideal AA mixture)."

However, caution is needed when interpreting studies where apparent efficiency of N utilization has been increased. Increased apparent efficiency of N utilisation could be real (a lower supply of protein decreases AA catabolism across the tissues) or artificial (reduced N intake results in a negative N balance which would artificially increase N efficiency through temporary utilisation of body protein, but this would obviously not be sustainable in practical farming). To help solve this issue, a study was performed to measure net tissue AA metabolism at different protein intakes in dairy cows (Raggio *et al.*, 2004). First, milk protein yield achieved by these cows was higher than predicted (802 vs 714 g/d) at low protein intake (127 g/kg CP, 1922 g/d MP) and lower than predicted (902 vs 1100 g/d) at high intake (166 g/kg CP, 2517 g MP/d; NRC, 2001). Second, post-liver supply of essential AA was sufficient for milk protein yield, which suggests that utilisation of body protein (i.e. negative N balance) was not the reason for the increased efficiency, except for histidine whose supply could have come from muscular dipeptides. As shown in Figure 4, removal of AA (methionine as an example of Group 1 and lysine as an example of Group 2) increased at a proportional rate higher than increased portal absorption. This increased removal occurred across the liver for Group 1 and across the mammary gland and peripheral tissues for Group 2, resulting in a decreased efficiency at higher protein intake. This increased removal of AA was linked directly with a more than doubled urinary-N excretion at the high protein intake (urinary-N 165 g N/d) compared with the low protein intake (urinary-N 79 g N/d). For lysine, the ratio of milk protein output to portal absorption averaged 0.68 for low protein supply and 0.56 for high protein supply; for methionine, the ratio was 0.66 for low protein supply and 0.52 for high protein supply. If estimated requirements for maintenance are removed to obtain efficiency for lactation, efficiencies of lactation are 0.96 for lysine at low protein supply, 0.71 for lysine at high protein supply, 0.95 for methionine at low protein supply, and 0.66 for methionine at high protein supply.

Clearly, at lower protein supply, the animal has the capacity to reduce AA catabolism. Indeed, in dairy cows, increased MP supply increased oxidation of leucine across the gut, the liver (Lapierre *et al.*, 2002) and the mammary gland (Bequette *et al.*, 1996; Raggio *et al.*, 2006). It has also been observed that mammary uptake of AA from Group 2 in excess of the needs for AA output into milk protein increased as protein supply increased (e.g. Guinard and Rulquin, 1994, Raggio *et al.*, 2004 and 2006). This indirectly suggests increased catabolism of these AA in the mammary gland, although this excess of uptake of AA from Group 2 relative to milk output is not essential to maintain milk protein output (Bequette *et al.*, 1996; Lapierre *et al.*, 2005b).

Studies measuring directly the fate of AA across tissues have shown that the dairy cow has the possibility to decrease catabolism of AA as supply is reduced. This decrease is observed whether the site of catabolism of essential AA is the liver or other tissues, including the gut and the mammary gland.

(a)

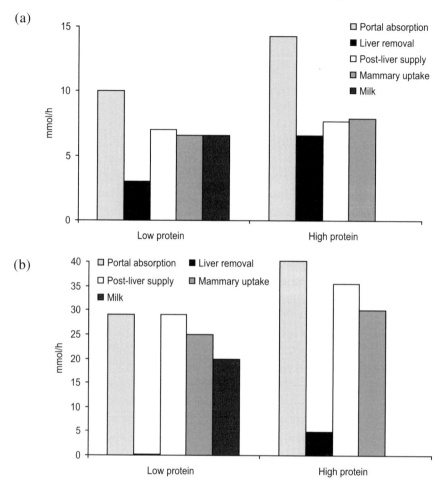

(b)

Figure 4. Net flux of two essential AA representative of Group 1 (a- methionine) and Group 2 (b-lysine) in dairy cows at two protein feeding levels.

ESTIMATION OF THIS VARIABLE EFFICIENCY

It is clear that efficiency of utilisation of absorbed AA should not be a fixed factor, but efficiency factors presented above were estimated from only one study. In an effort to predict efficiency in relation to supply, a database (59 trials) was built by compiling all published reports where AA had been infused post-ruminally (Doepel *et al.*, 2004). Linear and non-linear models were tested to relate milk AA-protein output to AA supply (with just the control treatment relying on a predictive model to estimate digestible AA). A segmented-linear model (fixed efficiency followed by zero response when requirements are met - Figure 5a) and a logistic model (Figure 5b) were similar in their reliability (Doepel *et al.*, 2004). The logistic model, however, offers the possibility to estimate variable efficiency of transfer, which decreased as protein supply increased (Table 1). These estimates were close to the efficiencies estimated in the study of Raggio *et al.* (2004), discussed in the previous section. From estimation of the optimum supply for individual AA (Doepel *et al.*, 2004), an ideal profile of EAA was determined. Despite the fact that this theoretical calculation has many limitations, especially as AA were usually infused in groups rather than individually in most of the studies, the requirements estimated with this approach were identical to those obtained previously by Schwab *et al.* (1992 a and b) or by Rulquin *et al.* (1993) for lysine (0.072 of MP) and methionine (0.025 of MP).

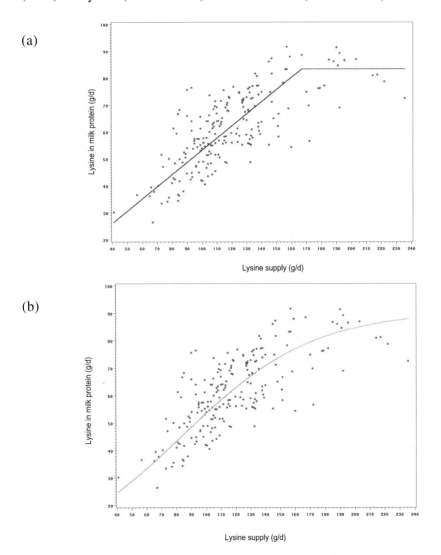

Figure 5. Segment-linear (a) and logistic (b) models of lysine in milk protein as a function of lysine supply.

Table 1. Efficiency of utilisation of AA for lactation after discounting maintenance requirements from total AA supply.

AA	Linear model (fixed)	Logistic model Proportion of optimum supply			
		0.50	*0.75*	*1.00*	*1.25*
Lysine	0.77	0.90	0.76	0.68	0.60
Methionine	0.80	0.89	0.75	0.66	0.59

Adapted from Doepel *et al.*, 2004

Although not perfect, a first step has been made to propose variable efficiencies of AA use for lactation, which decrease as supply increases. This should help to improve prediction of milk protein output with alterations in protein supply. However, this approach maintains a fixed efficiency for utilization of absorbed AA towards maintenance functions. Such a situation, with variable efficiency of utilization of AA for production and fixed efficiency for maintenance, is somewhat artificial, as removal of each AA across the different tissues will be a single function. Therefore, the animal will not change efficiency of utilisation for one metabolic function and not for the other. In a near future, we may need to rethink our estimation of maintenance requirements in line with a new approach for the efficiency of lactation.

VARIATION OF EFFICIENCY: REGULATION OF UTILISATION OF AA ACROSS TISSUES

There is no clear evidence on the mechanisms regulating AA extraction across the gut, the liver and the mammary gland, and if this removal is regulating milk protein output or is regulated by mammary gland anabolism (Hanigan *et al.*, 2005; Lapierre *et al.*, 2005a). Because post-liver supply of Group 1 AA equals milk protein output, it becomes tempting to suggest that the liver has the role of regulator and only what passes through the liver can be used by the mammary gland. However, we have to remember that these are static net measurements. If the liver removes a high proportion of what is absorbed, total inflow to the liver is much higher than absorption alone. The proportion of total inflow (i.e., arterial plus portal inflow) actually removed by the liver in dairy cows is 0.03 for histidine, 0.09 for methionine and 0.08 for phenylalanine (Lapierre *et al.*, 2005a). Conceptually, this allows absorbed AA to circulate around the body a few times, being "seen" by the mammary gland and giving it the opportunity to capture them before they are removed by the liver. Thus, mammary gland anabolism and capture of AA would also affect gut and liver removal.

What are the signals bridging mammary, gut and hepatic metabolism? In the fed situation, milk protein output of Group 1 AA is directly related to post-liver supply; in this case, hepatic removal is highly correlated with concentrations (portal or arterial), portal-arterial difference or liver influx (Hanigan *et al.*, 2005; Lapierre *et al.*, 2005a). However, when AA are infused into a jugular vein, the relation between hepatic removal and portal-arterial difference is totally lost and removal is then linked only with concentration or inflow (Berthiaume *et al.*, 2002). In addition, the mechanism regulating extraction of Group 2 AA across the mammary gland in excess of requirements for milk protein synthesis is unknown. It is not clear if this is just an obligate mechanism due to the location of degradative enzymes for these AA to remove them when they are in excess, or if this excess uptake has some underlying purpose. A recent study where milk protein production was enhanced with protein (casein) showed that mammary uptake of Group 2 AA is enhanced to support increased milk protein production more than uptake of non-essential AA, whereas propionate supply increased uptake of non-essential AA. These results suggest that the "choice" of the mammary gland to increase its excess of Group 2 AA rather than taking up non-essential AA may serve two purposes: to supply N and carbon skeletons for synthesis of non-essential AA plus an extra supply of carbon skeletons to be used as an energy source within the mammary gland (Raggio *et al.*, 2006). At whole body level, the "choice" could be driven by coordination of utilization of N and carbon skeletons between organs (VanMilgen, 2002) with complementarities for metabolism of groups of AA between the liver and peripheral tissues (including the mammary gland). Hormonal cross-talking probably drives this coordination (Berthiaume *et al.*, 2003), but no clues have yet been identified clearly.

Conclusion

In conclusion, the biology beyond the rumen clearly indicates why we need to consider individual AA. The proportion of AA in duodenal protein flow and their metabolic fate across the gut, the liver and the mammary gland vary greatly among individual AA. In addition, decreased efficiency of transfer of absorbed AA into milk protein with increased protein supply, supported by empirical observations, is directly related to increased extraction of AA for non-productive purposes across different tissues. Catabolism and therefore efficiency of each AA across different tissues is altered depending on its supply. We still need to determine the key factors regulating how efficiency of transfer of absorbed AA into milk protein increases with decreased supply (and vice-versa) to improve prediction of milk output. The real challenge for nutritionists will be to determine to which level of total MP, and with which balance of individual AA supply, this optimal efficiency can be achieved, i.e. efficiency reducing feed cost and excretion of N into the environment with no detrimental effect on milk protein yield.

References

AFRC Technical Committee on Responses to Nutrients. (1993). *Energy and Protein Requirements of Ruminants*, p 159.   CAB International, Wallingford, Oxon, UK.

AFRC Technical Committee on Responses to Nutrients. (1998). *Response in the Yield of Milk Constituents to the Intake of Nutrients by Dairy Cows*, report No. 11, p 112. Edited by G. Alderman.   CAB International, Wallingford, Oxon, UK.

Bequette, B.J., Metcalf, J.A., Wray-Cahen, D., Backwell, F.R., Sutton, J.D., Lomax, M.A., MacRae, J.C. and Lobley, G.E. (1996) Leucine and protein metabolism in the lactating dairy cow mammary gland: responses to supplemental dietary crude protein intake. *Journal of Dairy Research*, **63**, 209-222.

Berthiaume, R., Dubreuil, P., Stevenson, M., McBride, B.W. and Lapierre, H. (2001) Intestinal disappearance, mesenteric and portal appearance of amino acids in dairy cows fed ruminally protected methionine. *Journal of Dairy Science,* **84**, 194-203.

Bethiaume, R., Thivierge, M.C., Lobley, G.E., Dubreuil, P., Babkine, M. and Lapierre, H. (2002) Effect of a jugular infusion of essential amino acids on splanchnic metabolism in dairy cows fed a protein deficient diet. *Journal of Animal Science,* 80 / *Journal of Dairy Science,* **85**, Supplement 1, 72 -73.

Bethiaume, R., Thivierge, M.C., Lobley, G.E., Dubreuil, P., Babkine, M. and Lapierre, H. (2003) Effect of a jugular infusion of essential AA on splanchnic metabolism of glucose and hormones in dairy cows fed a protein deficient diet. In *Progress in research on energy and protein metabolism*, pp.125-128.   Edited by. W.B. Souffrant and C.C. Metges. EAAP plublication No.109

Berthiaume, R., Thivierge, M.C., Patton, R.A., Dubreuil, P., Stevenson, M., McBride, B.W. and Lapierre, H. (2006) Effect of ruminally protected methionine on splanchnic metabolism of amino acids in lactating dairy cows. *Journal of Dairy Science,* **89**, 1621-1634.

Cant, J.P., DePeters, E.J. and Baldwin, R.L. (1993) Mammary amino acid utilization in dairy cows fed fat and its relationship to milk protein depression. *Journal of Dairy Science,* **76**, 762-774.

Castillo, A.R., Kebreab, E., Beever, D.E., Barbi, J.H., Sutton, J.D., Kirby, H.C. and France, J. (2001) The effect of protein supplementation on nitrogen utilization in lactating dairy cows fed grass silage diets. *Journal of Animal Science,* **79**, 247-253.

Cornell Net Carbohydrate and Protein System, version 5.0.34. Cornell University, Ithaca NY.

Doepel, L., Pacheco, D., Kennelly, J.J., Hanigan, M.D., López, I.F. and Lapierre, H. (2004) Milk protein synthesis as a function of amino acid supply. *Journal of Dairy Science,* **87**, 1279-1297.

Fox, D.G., Tedeschi, L.O., Tylutki, T.P., Russell, J.B., Van Amburgh, M.E., Chase, L.E., Pell, A.N. and Overton, T.R. (2004) The Cornell net carbohydrate and protein system model for evaluating herd nutrition and nutrient excretion. *Animal and Feed Science Technology*, **112**, 29-78.

Gibb, M.J., Ivings, W.E,. Dhanoa, M.S. and Sutton, J.D. (1992) Changes in body components of autumn-calving Holstein-Friesian cows over the first 29 weeks of lactation. *Animal Production*, **55**, 339-360.

Guinard, J. and Rulquin H. (1994) Effect of graded levels of duodenal infusions of casein on mammary uptake in lactating cows. 2. Individual amino acids. *Journal of Dairy Science,* **77**, 3304-3315.

Hanigan, M.D. (2005) Quantitative aspects of splanchnic metabolism in the ruminant. *Animal Production,* **80**, 23-32.

Huntington, G.B. (1990) Energy metabolism in the digestive tract and liver of cattle: influence of physiological state and nutrition. *Reproduction Nutrition Development*, **30**, 35-47.

Institut National de la Recherche Agronomique INRA. (1989) Ruminant Nutrition: recommended allowances and feed tables. Edited by R. Jarrige and J. Libbey. Eurotext, Paris, France.

Lapierre, H., Blouin, J.P., Bernier J.F., Reynolds, C.K., Dubreuil P. and Lobley, G.E. (2002) Effect of diet quality on whole body and splanchnic protein metabolism in lactating dairy cows. *Journal of Dairy Science,* **85**, 2631-2641.

Lapierre, H., Milne E., Renaud, J. and Lobley G.E. (2003) Lysine utilization by the mammary gland. In *Progress in research on energy and protein metabolism,* pp.777-780. Edited by W.B. Souffrant and C.C. Metges. EAAP plublication No.109.

Lapierre, H., Berthiaume, R., Raggio, G., Thivierge, M.C., Doepel, L.,

Pacheco, D., Dubreuil, P. and Lobley, G.E. (2005a) The route of absorbed nitrogen into milk protein. *Animal Science*, **80**, 11-22.

Lapierre, H., Doepel, L., Milne, E. and Lobley, G.E. (2005b) Effect of lysine (Lys) supply on its utilization by the mammary gland. *Journal of Animal Science, ***83** / *Journal of Dairy Science, ***88** Supplement 1, 89.

Lapierre, H., Pacheco, D., Berthiaume, R., Ouellet, D.R., Schwab, C., Dubreuil, P., Holtrop, G. and Lobley, G.E. (2006) What is the true supply of amino acids? *Journal of Dairy Science, ***89**, E Supplement, E1-E14.

Lobley, G.E. and Lapierre, H. (2003) Post-absorptive metabolism of amino acids. In *Progress in research on energy and protein metabolism*, pp.737-756. Edited by W.B. Souffrant and C.C. Metges. EAAP plublication No.109.

Lobley, G.E., Shen X., Le, G., Bremner, D.M., Milne, E., Graham, C.A., Anderson, S.E. and. Dennison, N. (2003) Oxidation of essential amino acids by the ovine gastrointestinal tract. *British Journal of Nutrition,* **89**, 617-629.

Macrae, J.C., Bruce, L.A., Brown, D.S., Farningham, D.A. and Franklin, M. (1997) Absorption of amino acids from the intestine and their net flux across the mesenteric- and portal-drained viscera of lambs. *Journal of Animal Science,* **75**, 3307-3314.

Meijer, G.A.L., de Visser, H., van der Meulen, J., van der Koelen, C.J. and Klop, A. (1995) Effect of glutamine or propionate infused into the abomasum on milk yield, milk composition, nitrogen retention and net flux of amino acids across the udder of high yielding dairy cows. In *Proceedings of the Seventh Symposium on protein metabolism and nutrition*, pp. 157-160. Edited by A.F. Nunes, A.V. Portugal, J.P. Costa and J.R. Ribeiro. Estacoa Zootechnica National, Santerm, Portugal.

Mepham, T.B. (1982) Amino acid utilization by lactating mammary gland. *Journal of Dairy Science,* **65**, 287-298.

National Research Council. (2001) Nutrient requirements of dairy cattle. 7th revised edition. Edited by National Academy of Sciences, Washington, DC.

Ouellet, D.R., Demers, M., Zuur, G., Lobley, G.E., Seoane, J.R., Nolan, J.V. and Lapierre, H. (2002) Effect of dietary fiber on endogenous nitrogen flows in lactating dairy cows. *Journal of Dairy Science,* **85**, 3013-3025.

Ouellet, D.R., Berthiaume, R., Holtrop, G., Lobley, G.E., Martineau, R. and Lapierre, H. (2005) Endogenous nitrogen (EN) flows: Effect of methods of conservation of timothy in lactating dairy cows. *Journal of Animal Science, ***83** / *Journal of Dairy Science, ***88**, Supplement 1, 317.

Pacheco, D. (2000) Amino acid utilisation by the mammary gland of dairy cows fed fresh forage. Ph.D. Thesis, Departement of Animal Science. Massey University, New Zealand.

Raggio, G., Pacheco, D., Berthiaume, R., Lobley, G.E., Pellerin, D., Allard, G., Dubreuil, P. and Lapierre, H. (2004) Effect of metabolizable protein on splanchnic flux of amino acids in lactating dairy cows. *Journal of Dairy Science,* **87**, 3461-3472.

Raggio, G., Lemosquet, S., Lobley, G.E., Rulquin, H. and Lapierre, H. (2006) Effect of casein and propionate supply on mammary gland protein metabolism. *Journal of Dairy Science,* **89**, 4340-4351.

Reynolds, C.K., Crompton, L.A., Bequette, B.J., France, J., Beever, D.E. and MacRae, J.C. (2000) Effects of diet protein level and abomasal amino acid infusion on phenylalanine and tyrosine metabolism in lactating dairy cows. *Journal of Animal Science, 78 / Journal of Dairy Science,* **83**, Supplement 1, 298-299. (Abstract)

Rulquin, H., Pisulewski, P.M., Vérité, R. and Guinard, J. (1993) Milk production and composition as a function of postruminal lysine and methionine supply: a nutrient-response approach. *Livestock Production Science*, **37**, 69-90.

Schwab, C.G., Bozak, C.K., Whitehouse, N.L. and Mesbah, M.M.A. (1992a) Amino acid limitation and flow to duodenum at four stages of lactation. 1. Sequence of lysine and methionine limitation. *Journal of Dairy Science,* **75**, 3486-3502.

Schwab, C.G., Bozak C.K., Whitehouse, N.L. and Olson, V.M. (1992b) Amino acid limitation and flow to the duodenum at four stages of lactation: 2. Extent of lysine limitation. *Journal of Dairy Science,* **75**, 3503-3518.

Tagari, H. and Bergman, E.N. (1978) Intestinal disappearance and portal blood appearance of amino acids in sheep. *Journal of Nutrition*, **108**, 790-803.

Tamminga, S., Schulze, H., VanBruchem, J. and Huisman, J. (1995) Nutritional significance of endogenous n-losses along the gastrointestinal-tract of farm-animals. *Arch Tierernahr,* **48**, 9-22.

Van Milgen, J. (2002) Modeling biochemical aspects of energy metabolism in mammals. *Journal of Nutrition,* **132**, 3195-3202.

Wright, T.C., Moscardini S., Luimes P.H., Susmel P. and McBride B.W. (1998) Effects of rumen-degradable protein and feed intake on nitrogen balance and milk protein production in dairy cows. *Journal of Dairy Science,* **81**, 784-793.

3

NUTRIENT REGULATION OF HORMONAL, HUMORAL AND CELLULAR RESPONSES IN POSTPARTUM LACTATING DAIRY COWS: BUILDING BLOCKS FOR RESTORATION OF FERTILITY?

WILLIAM W. THATCHER[1], FLAVIO T. SILVESTRE[1], TODD R. BILBY[1], CHARLES R. STAPLES[1], JOSE E. P. SANTOS[2], MAURICO E. BENZAQUEN[3], CARLOS A. RISCO[3] AND LESLIE A. MACLAREN[4]

[1]Department of Animal Sciences, University of Florida, Gainesville, FL, USA; [2]Veterinary Medicine Teaching and Research Center, University of California -Davis, Tulare, CA, USA; [3]Department of Large Animal Clinical Sciences, College of Veterinary Medicine, University of Florida, Gainesville, FL, USA, and [4]Department of Plant and Animal Sciences, Nova Scotia Agricultural College, Truro, Nova Scotia, Canada

Introduction

Reproductive performance of lactating dairy cows worldwide has decreased markedly in association with selection for milk yield over the last 25 years. This condition is referred to as an "infertility syndrome" that hopefully is reversible with the application of current technology across the disciplines of dairy management, nutrition, herd health, genetics and physiology. Reproductive management systems have been developed that allow for a first service insemination rate following a synchronized ovulation of 35 to 40% under commercial conditions (Moore and Thatcher, 2006). However, it is evident that many of the cows presented for service are anovulatory and are not in a state to achieve optimal fertility. In a summary of nine studies from five dairy farms in California (Rutigliano and Santos, 2005), interrelationships among parity, body condition score (BCS; 1 to 5 scale), milk yield, AI protocol (inseminated at oestrus or Timed AI (TAI)), and cyclicity (cyclic or anovular) were evaluated for their impacts on pregnancy rate (PR) and embryonic survival to the first postpartum AI (n = 5,767). Cows were inseminated following a pre-synchronized (two PGF2α injections given 14 d apart) TAI protocol or oestrous synchronization protocol initiated 12 to 14 days after pre-synchronization. Occurrence of cyclicity was greater (P < 0.001) for multiparous than primiparous cows (81.8 vs 69.5%) at 65 d postpartum. Cyclicity was also influenced (P < 0.01) by milking frequency (twice = 82.7% vs thrice = 68.7%), BCS both at calving and AI, BCS change, and milk yield. However, milk yield, BCS at calving, and AI protocol had no effect on PR at 30 and 58 days after AI or on pregnancy loss. As expected, more (P < 0.001) cyclic than anovular cows were pregnant at 30 (40.0 vs 28.3%) and 58 (34.2 vs 23.0%) days after AI, and cows that were anovulatory prior to oestrus synchronization tended (P = 0.09) to experience greater pregnancy loss (14.5 vs 18.6%) between 30 and 58 days of gestation. Pregnancy loss was highest (22.5 vs 16.8 vs 12.2%; P < 0.01) and conception rate at day 58 lowest (21.7 vs 30.4 vs 35.6%; P < 0.01) in cows that lost > 1 unit of BCS than those that lost < 1 or experienced no change in BCS from calving to AI, respectively. Likewise, cows having a greater BCS at the actual time of AI (> 3.75 vs 3.0 to 3.5 vs < 2.75) had better (P < 0.01) conception rates at 30 (46.4 vs 40.1 vs 33.9%, respectively) and 58 (41.8 vs 34.6 vs 27.9%) days after AI. Consequently, minimizing losses of BCS after calving and improving cyclicity early postpartum are expected to increase PR and enhance embryonic survival. The challenge is to manage body condition in healthy cows, with an inherent high dry matter intake, so that they have sufficient energy stores at parturition to meet the demands of ensuing negative energy status without a predisposition to fatty livers and metabolic disturbances and have sufficient body condition at the beginning of the breeding period such that they are cycling and able to sustain a pregnancy. These associations emphasise the importance of nutritional management from the time of "dry-off" to the time of insemination, which is critical to herd reproductive performance.

The focus of this chapter is to identify those physiological windows during the periparturient and postpartum periods that appear to be amenable to nutritional management that may improve subsequent fertility during the insemination period.

Parturient health events

METRITIS AND ENDOMETRITIS

Puerperal metritis (PM) is a serious condition in dairy cows since it affects production, fertility, and can be life-threatening. A better understanding of calving-related factors that predispose cows to PM would aid in the prevention, diagnosis, and treatment of this condition. A prospective longitudinal study was conducted with a 1000-cow dairy farm in north Florida between August 1, 2002 and April 15, 2003 to evaluate the effect of calving status, parity, and season on the incidence of postpartum PM in lactating dairy cows, and the role of rectal temperature as a predictor of this condition (Benzaquen, Risco, Archbald, Melendez, Thatcher and Thatcher, 2006). The farm employed a postpartum health monitoring program. Cows with a normal calving status

(Nc) were those without any calving-related problems. Cows with an abnormal calving status (Ac) were those with dystocia, retained foetal membranes with or without dystocia, or twins at calving. Daily rectal temperature (RT) of all cows was taken between 0700 and 0900 h from days 3 to 13 post partum, and a health examination was performed by the on-farm veterinarian. Cows that appeared sick (depressed, eyes tented, etc.) or had a rectal temperature > 39.5°C were examined for septic metritis. The criterion for diagnosis of septic metritis was the presence of a watery, brown-coloured, fetid discharge from the vulva (noted after palpating the uterus rectally), with or without a rectal temperature > 39.5°C. Cows diagnosed with septic metritis were treated with systemic antibiotics, anti-inflammatory agents, calcium, and energy supplements. The environmental thermal heat index (THI) was calculated using the daily ambient temperature and percent relative humidity recorded at the closest weather station. Two seasons were defined, based on mean THI, as the following: a cool season from October to April (THI < 76.2) and a warm season from May to September (THI ≥ 76.2).

A total of 450 parturitions were evaluated. Cows with Nc had a lower incidence of PM compared to cows with an Ac status (13 vs. 41%; P < 0.001). A season by parity interaction was detected. During the cool season, primiparous cows had the highest incidence of PM (39.4%) compared with primiparous cows in the warm season (12.7%). In contrast, the incidence of PM in multiparous cows did not differ between the cool (11%) and warm (18%) seasons. The reasons for the parity difference are speculative; perhaps foetal stunting during the hot season in Florida reduced the incidence of dystocia, whereas larger calves born in the winter season increased occurrence of dystocia and subsequent PM in primiparous heifers. The RT of cows that were diagnosed with PM increased 24 h before diagnosis of PM and reached a maximum RT of 39.2°C ± 0.05 on day 0 (i.e., day of diagnosis). In cows with PM and fever at diagnosis, the RT started to increase between 72 to 48 h before the diagnosis of PM and continued to increase to a maximum RT of 39.7°C ± 0.09 on day 0. However, for cows with PM and no fever at diagnosis, no daily incremental increases of RT before the diagnosis of PM were detected; however, the RT on day 0 (38.9°C ± 0.08) was different from cows without PM (38.5°C ± 0.04; P < 0.001). Cows without PM had a stable RT during the first 13 days postpartum (mean of 38.6°C ± 0.01.)

All cows were examined for clinical endometritis between 20 and 30 days postpartum. The criterion used to diagnose clinical endometritis was one of the following conditions associated or not with each other: cervical diameter greater than 6.0 cm; asymmetry of the uterine horns with fluid content and/ or pus present at the vulva following rectal manipulation of the uterus. The overall incidence of clinical endometritis was 24%. Cows of Ac status were more frequently diagnosed (40.6%) with clinical endometritis than those of Nc status (17.7%; P < 0.001). A higher incidence of clinical endometritis was detected for those cows diagnosed with PM (38.2%) compared to cows without PM (20.2%; P < 0.005). There was no difference in accumulated PR by 150 days postpartum (mean = 50%) between normal cows and cows experiencing PM. However, a seasonal effect was detected (cool season of 60% > warm season of 22%; P < 0.02).

REPEAT BREEDERS

The status of the uterus in lactating dairy cows at the time of insemination probably contributes to the infertility syndrome of lactating dairy cows. A vivid example is the repeat breeder cow that appears to be clinically normal regarding the reproductive tract but has repeated normal cycles and fails to conceive. A proportion of repeat breeder cows have distinct alterations in spatial endometrial architecture characterized by walled-off and occluded uterine glands, degeneration of the glandular epithelium, thickening of the underlying stroma, and infiltration of either eosinophils or lymphocytes or both (Cupps, 1973). It was hypothesized that this localized condition was a carry over from prior inflammatory responses to metritis and endometritis in the early postpartum period. This uterine condition may be related to the report that 41% of normally lactating dairy cows (i.e., cows that did not experience either external discharges on the tail, perineum and vulva or internally diagnosed by vaginoscopy between 20 to 33 days postpartum) were diagnosed with subclinical endometritis at 34 to 47 days postpartum and experienced a lower PR to first insemination (Kasimanickam, Duffield, Foster, Gartley, Leslie, Walton and Johnson, 2004). Is there a parallel between the repeat breeder and the high producing population of today's cows regarding similar uterine statuses that compromise embryo survival? Recent findings indicate that repeat breeder cows have an abnormal pattern of epidermal growth factor (EGF) concentrations in endometrial tissue during the oestrous cycle and that treatment involving exposure to oestradiol may restore a normal secretory pattern and fertility (Katagiri and Takahashi, 2005). Perhaps the physiological status of lactation and high production has associated homeorhetic regulatory effects that alter the local inflammatory status within the uterus. Perhaps the anti-inflammatory effects of long chain n-3 polyunsaturated fatty acids, administered via the diet, may have a therapeutic role during the breeding period.

Nutritional alteration of periparturient reproductive events

POSTPARTUM IMMUNOSUPPRESSION AND RESPONSE TO
ORGANIC SELENIUM

During the immediate postpartum period, the cow's immune system is challenged severely (Goff, 2006), and the innate and humoral defence systems are reduced. The incidence of diseases and disorders can be high during this time period and have a negative impact on reproductive performance. For example the likelihood of pregnancy (odds ratio) was reduced if cows had retained foetal membranes (RFM) or lost one unit of BCS (Loeffler, de Vries and Schukken, 1999). Reduction in adaptive and innate immunity at parturition increases the risk of health disorders such as RFM, metritis, and mastitis. Selenium has long been associated with immunity. Cattle supplemented with Se-yeast had an 18% increase of Se in plasma in comparison to sodium selenite in some studies (Weiss, 2003). The state of Florida, USA is in a selenium deficient area, and lactating dairy cows are exposed to a seasonal period of heat stress that affects reproductive performance and health.

We have conducted an experiment to evaluate a supplemental source of organic selenium on reproductive and immune responses by dairy cows (Silvestre, Silvestre, Santos, Risco, Staples and Thatcher, 2006; Silvestre, Silvestre, Crawford, Santos, Staples, and Thatcher, 2006). Objectives were to evaluate effects of organic Se on PR at the first and second postpartum AI services, uterine health, and milk yield during the summer heat stress period. Cows were assigned (23 ± 8 days prepartum) to diets of organic Se (Se-yeast [SY; Sel-Plex®, Alltech; n = 289] or inorganic sodium Se [SS; n = 285]) fed at 0.3 ppm (DM basis) for > 81 days postpartum. Rectal temperature was recorded each morning for 10 days postpartum (dpp). Vaginoscopies were performed at 5 and 10 dpp. Cows within diet were assigned randomly to 2 reproductive management programs (Presynch-Ovsynch vs CIDR-Ovsynch [i.e., Ovsynch began 3 days after withdrawal of a 7 day-CIDR]). All cows were resynchronized for a second service with Ovsynch at 20 to 23 days after first service. An ultrasound pregnancy diagnosis was conducted at 27 to 30 days after first TAI. Cows in oestrus following Presynchs were AI up to the second TAI service. Strategic blood sampling determined anovulatory status at Ovsynch and ovulatory response after TAI to first service. The PR at second service was determined by rectal palpation at ~ 42 dpp. Blood was sampled for Se (n = 20 cows/diet) at -25, 0, 7, 14, 21, and 37 dpp. Plasma Se increased in SY-fed cows (0.087 vs 0.069 ± 0.004 μg/ml; $P < 0.01$). Milk yield (35.6 kg/d for 81 days), milk somatic cells (291,618 cells/ml), and frequencies of retained foetal membrane (9.7%), mastitis (14.4%), anovulation (17.7%), and synchronized ovulation after TAI (82.5%) were not affected by diet or reproductive program. Diet failed to alter first service PR at ~ 30 days post AI (SY, 24.9% [62/249] vs SS, 23.6% [62/262]) or pregnancy losses between ~ 30 and ~ 55 days post AI (SY, 39.3% vs SS, 37.1%.) These low pregnancy rates and high embryonic losses are typical of cows managed during the summer heat stress period of Florida. Diet altered second service PR [SY, 17% (34/199) vs SS, 11.3% (24/211); P < 0.05]. The benefit of SY on second service pregnancy rate is intriguing. We hypothesize that cows of the SY group were better able to re-establish an embryo-trophic environment at second service following either early or late embryonic losses. Diet altered frequency of multiparous cows detected with > 1 event of fever (rectal temperature > 39.5°C; SY, 13.3% [25/188] vs SS, 25.5% [46/181]; P < 0.05) but the SY effect was not observed in primiparous cows which had a much higher frequency of fever (40.5%). Vaginoscopy discharge scores at 5 and 10 dpp were better for the SY group; namely, 47.1 (217/460) vs 35.0% (153/437) clear, 43.4 [200/460] vs 47.8% [209/437]) mucopurulent, and 9.3 (43/460) vs 17.1% (75/437) purulent for SY and SS groups, respectively (P < 0.05). Feeding organic Se (Se-yeast, Sel-Plex®) improved uterine health and second service PR during summer.

Innate immunity (i.e., neutrophil function) was determined by phagocytic and oxidative burst capacity of neutrophils in whole blood using a dual colour flow cytometric method. Samples were collected from a subsample of 36 cows at -26 dpp and 40 cows at 0, 7, 14, 21 and 37 dpp and analyzed for neutrophil function. Adaptive immunity (ability to induce an antibody response) was monitored with anti-IgG to Ovalbumin (Ovalb) following vaccination with Ovalb antigen (1 mg [i.m.]) dissolved in an E. coli J5 endotoxemia preventive vaccine at -60 and -22 ± 6 dpp (day of initiating SY [n = 38] and SS [n = 47] diets) and again at parturition (day 0) with Ovalb dissolved in PBS with Quil-A adjuvant. Serum samples were collected on days of immunization and at 21 and 42 dpp.

Percentage of gated neutrophils that phagocytized E. coli and underwent oxidative burst did not differ between dietary groups at -26 dpp (44.6 ± 4.6%). For subsequent samples, a diet by parity by day interaction was detected (P < 0.05); namely, SY improved neutrophil function at parturition in multiparous cows (42 ± 6.14% vs 24.3 ± 7.2%; Figure 1) and at 7, 14 and 37 dpp in primiparous cows (53.9 vs 30.7%, 58.6 vs 41.9%, and 53.4 vs 34.8%, respectively; pooled SE = 6.8%; Figure 2). It is clear that neutrophil function is suppressed in multiparous cows at the time of parturition and it is not restored until between 7 to 14 days postpartum (Figure 1). In contrast, the primiparous cows did not have a restoration in neutrophil function until

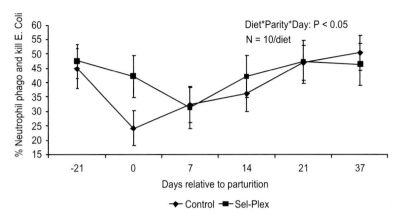

Figure 1. Phagocytosis and killing activity of neutrophils in whole blood from periparturient multiparous dairy cows fed an inorganic selenium (control) or organic selenium (Sel-Plex®) supplements.

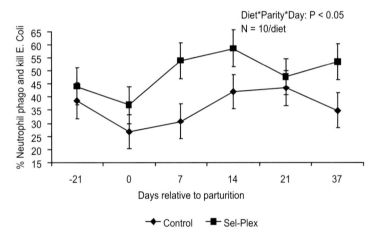

Figure 2. Phagocytosis and killing activity of neutrophils in whole blood from periparturient primiparous dairy cows fed an inorganic selenium (control) or organic selenium (Sel-Plex®) supplements.

between 14 to 21 days postpartum (Figure 2). Organic Se improved phagocytosis and killing activity of neutrophils in both multiparous and primiparous cows (Figures 1 and 2). However, the primiparous cows seemed to be more responsive in that SY stimulated neutrophil function throughout 0 to 21 dpp whereas, SY stimulation in multiparous cows was evident on only the day of parturition. In most of our postpartum experiments, we detect distinct differences between primiparous and multiparous cows for a multiplicity of physiological and biochemical responses.

Anti-IgG to Ovalb did not differ between dietary groups at -60 and -22 dpp (0.18 ± 0.01 and 0.97 ± 0.04 OD). Although Anti-IgG to Ovalb concentration did not differ between dietary groups for primiparous cows (1.40 ± 0.08 OD), concentrations were higher in SY cows at 21 and 42 dpp (1.91 ± 0.1 vs 1.24 ± 0.07; 1.44 ± 0.7 vs 0.99 ± 0.07 OD, respectively; P < 0.01). Thus our measurement of adaptive immunity was improved in multiparous dairy cows in response to SY but not in primiparous cows.

Our findings indicated that feeding Se as organic Se (Se-yeast, Sel-Plex®), beginning at 26 days prepartum, elevated plasma Se concentrations, increased neutrophil function at the time of parturition, improved immuno-responsiveness in multiparous cows, improved uterine health, and increased second service PR during summer in an environment that is Se deficient.

FEEDING FAT DURING THE PERIPARTURIENT PERIOD

Staples and Thatcher (2006) summarized extensively the effects of fatty acids and fatty acid supplements on reproductive performance of lactating dairy cows at the Nottingham Feed Conference. It is clear that dietary fat effects are not simply due to energy, but that specific nutraceutical effects probably are manifested whereby certain fatty acids interact as substrates for specific enzymes (e.g., PGHS-2) and also interact with peroxisome proliferator-activated receptors (PPARs) to regulate gene expression. The essential polyunsaturated fatty acids, linoleic (18:2n-6) and α-linolenic (18:3n-3), undergo steps of chain elongation and desaturation forming differential n-6 products, such as dihomo-gamma linolenic (20:3n-6) and arachadonic (20:4n-6) acids, and n-3 products such as eicosapentaenoic acid (EPA; 20:5n-3). These specific long-chain polyunsaturated fatty acids produce eicosonaoid products of the prostaglandin series PGF1, PGF2 and PGF3, respectively, as well as various thromboxanes, leukotrienes, lipoxins, hydroperoxy-eicosatetraenoic acids and hydroxyeicosatetraenoic acids (HETE) that regulate inflammation and immunity. Clearly, the early postpartum period represents a time when the immune system is suppressed severely and there are major inflammatory processes underway in association with regression of the uterus and reabsorption of uterine tissues. Several of the eicosonaoids exert pro-inflammatory actions (e.g., PGE_2), and $PGF_2\alpha$ appears to be involved as well with neutrophil function as related to phagocytosis of bacteria. Consequently, feeding fatty acids (e.g., linoleic acid) during the periparturient period that act as precursors for the biosynthesis of prostaglandins of the 2 series may benefit the health of the cow postpartum. Later on in the postpartum period, it may be reasonable to feed fatty acids (e.g., EPA) that lead to biosynthesis of fatty acids that are anti-inflammatory in nature. This would reduce possible residual inflammatory responses in the uterus associated with carryover effects of subclinical endometritis or, as reported in repeat breeder cows (Cupps, 1973), and also reduce potential luteolytic peaks at the time that the conceptus is suppressing $PGF_2\alpha$ secretion in order to maintain the corpus luteum for pregnancy maintenance.

A study examined whether feeding of calcium salts of fatty acids (~ 28% linoleic acid and 4% linolenic acid) would have modulatory effects on postpartum dynamics of $PGF_2\alpha$ secretion, metabolites, hormones, cow health, milk production, and reproductive performance (Cullens, Staples, Bilby, Silvestre, Bartolome, Sozzi, Badinga, Thatcher and Arthington 2004). Primiparous (n = 22) and multiparous (n = 25) Holstein cows were used in a completely randomized block design to determine the effects of timing of initiation of fat supplementation (Megalac-R, Church and Dwight Co. Inc., Princeton, N.J.) on cow performance over the first 14 weeks postpartum. The four dietary treatments were: 1) Control (no supplemental fat source; Treatment 1) and Treatments 2-4 with Megalac-R supplementation (2% of dietary dry matter) beginning at 28 days prior to expected calving date (Treatment 2), at day of parturition (Treatment 3), or at 28 days in milk (Treatment 4). Cows fed Megalac-R received ~204 g per day during the prepartum period and ~328 g per day in the postpartum period. The study was designed to be carried out in the summer heat stress period of Florida. Blood samples were collected thrice weekly from calving until 10 weeks after parturition. An Ovsynch program was begun between 5 and 10 days of the cycle on 62 dpp with AI occurring at 72 dpp. Orthogonal contrasts tested for treatments were 1 vs. (2 + 3 + 4), 2 vs. (3 + 4), and 3 vs. 4. Mean milk production was 38.1, 41.5, 36.5, and 37.1 kg/d, tending to be greater (P = 0.06) for cows fed fat starting in the prepartum period compared with the postpartum period (Treatment 2 versus Treatments 3 and 4). Pattern of plasma progesterone concentrations accumulated from calving to 79 dpp did not differ among treatments. Of cows that ovulated to the Ovsynch protocol, cows fed fat tended (Treatment 1 versus Treatments 2, 3 and 4; P = 0.09) to experience better first service conception rate than controls (27.8 [3/11], 40.0 [4/10], 70 [7/10], and 63.6% [7/11]).

Plasma profiles of PGFM (Figure 3) for the first 12 dpp differed among groups; namely, those fed Megalac-R beginning prepartum (Treatment 2) versus cows fed Megalac-R beginning at parturition (Treatment 3) plus those not fed Megalac-R during the first 12 days after parturition (Treatments 1 and 4). Our interpretation is that cows fed Megalac-R prepartum had their lipid pools enriched in linoleic acid and that the greater pool of linoleic acid increased substrate concentrations of arachidonic acid, the precursor for

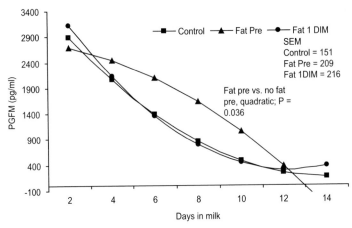

Figure 3. Effect of supplementation with a Ca salt of fatty acids enriched with linoleic acid, beginning pre-partum (28 days prior to expected calving date) or postpartum (one day in milk [DIM]), on plasma prostaglandin $F_{2\acute{a}}$ metabolite (PGFM) concentrations during the early postpartum period of dairy cows.

synthesis of $PGF_{2\alpha}$ and other PG2 series prostaglandins that would be pro-inflammatory. Associated with the parturition process is marked stimulation of uterine $PGF_{2\alpha}$ secretion primarily from the caruncular tissue. The increased potential for the uterus and cells of the immune system to secrete prostaglandins because of supplemental feeding of linoleic acid–calcium salts may enhance the postpartum uterine health and immuno-competence of the cow. This is somewhat supported by examining the frequency of health disorders in the cows that were fed Megalac-R prepartum compared with control cows and cows fed Megalac-R postpartum. Initiation of fat feeding (Megalac-R®) in the period immediately prior to calving resulted in fewer health problems (mastitis, retained foetal membranes, or metritis) in the first 10 days postpartum compared with cows not fed fat prepartum (1/12 vs. 15/35).

In an additional study, dairy cows (n = 154) supplemented with a calcium salt blend of linoleic acid and monoenoic trans C18:1 fatty acids (EnerG I Transition Formula®) or a calcium salt of palm oil (EnerG II®) (Virtus Nutrition) from 25 days before calving until 60 dpp were TAI and flushed 5 days after AI with recovered structures evaluated (Cerri, Bruno, Chebel, Galvao, Rutgliano, Juchem, Thatcher, Luchini, and Santos, 2004). Cows fed EnerG II Transition Formula® tended to have (P = 0.11) a greater fertilization rate (87 vs 73%), had more accessory sperm per structure collected (34 vs. 21), and tended to have (P = 0.06) a greater proportion of embryos classified as high quality (73 vs. 51%). In a larger set of cows (n = 397), conception rate at first AI was greater for cows fed the linoleic and trans acid salt (33.5 vs 25.6%) (Juchem, Cerri, Bruno, Galvao, Lemos, Villasenor, Coscioni, Rutgliano, Thatcher, Luchini and Santos, 2004). Development of bovine embryos appeared to be affected by feeding particular sources and amounts of fatty acids. Whether this was due to direct effects on the ova-follicular environment, the embryos, or the intra-oviductal/uterine environments needs further investigation.

EFFECT OF EXOGENOUS BST ON MATERNAL ENDOCRINE AND EMBRYONIC RESPONSES UNTIL DAY 17:

We have extended our investigations involving bST and feeding of Ca salts of fatty acids to the period approaching pregnancy recognition associated with CL maintenance at day 17 after oestrus in lactating dairy cows. Our objective was to examine the effects of bST injection (500 mg; Posilac, Monsanto) and Ca salts of fatty acids enriched with fish oil on endocrine responses, ovarian-uterine function, expression of various genes in the uterus, and conceptus development on day 17 after oestrus in cyclic and pregnant lactating dairy cows (Bilby, Sozzi, Lopez, Silvestre, Ealy, Staples and Thatcher, 2006). The study was conducted from September 2002 until February 2003. Two diets were fed in which the oil of whole cottonseed (15% of dietary DM; control diet) was compared with oil prepared as a Ca salt containing fish oil (CaSFO) as one of the primary oils (1.9% of dietary DM; Virtus Nutrition). Formulated concentrations of ether extract (5.7%), non-structural carbohydrate (36%), crude protein (18%), and net energy for lactation (1.7 Mcal/kg [7.1 MJ/kg]) were similar between diets (100% DM basis). Ingredients (maize silage, alfalfa hay, cottonseed hulls, ground maize, citrus pulp, soyabean meal, expeller soyabean meal, whole cottonseeds, calcium salt of fat, and mineral/vitamin premix) were fed as a totally mixed ration twice daily. All cows (n = 35) were fed the control diet for the first 10 dpp. Starting on day 11 of lactation, 8 cows were temporarily assigned to a transition diet containing 0.95% CaSFO to initially adjust cows to eating CaSFO. On day 18 postpartum, the CaSFO was increased to 1.9% of dietary DM on which cows remained for the duration of the experiment. Ad libitum feed intakes were measured daily on a group basis. Daily feed intake by cows fed CaSFO averaged 20.9 kg DM/cow over the entire period of feeding. Calculated intake of EPA and DHA was 7.4 g/d for each fatty acid (14.8 g/d total). Cows were milked thrice daily and individual milk weights recorded daily.

The following experimental protocol was implemented relative to sequential treatments to evaluate effects of CaSFO and Control diets in cyclic cows, effects of cyclic versus pregnancy status in cows fed the control diet, and effects of bST across cyclic-diets and cyclic-pregnant control groups (Bilby, Sozzi, Lopez, Silvestre, Ealy, Staples and Thatcher, 2006). All cows were presynchronized and started an Ovsynch protocol at approximately 7 days after a detected oestrus. Cows assigned to bST treatment received an injection of bST at the TAI and 11 days later. The second injection at day 11 was to ensure that GH concentration would be sustained until the time of slaughter on day 17. All cows that were designated for slaughter had to have ovulated and formed a CL when evaluated at day 7 following the second GnRH injection of the Ovsynch protocol.

Pregnancy rate for lactating cows was higher in bST-treated (83% [5/6]) than in control (40% [4/10]) cows (OR =7.499, 95% Confidence Limits 0.798 – 175.519; Chi-Square = 2.9, P < 0.09) (Bilby, Sozzi, Lopez, Silvestre, Ealy, Staples and Thatcher, 2006*).* This difference at day 17 is only a trend, but it agrees with the significant bST stimulation of pregnancy rate reported from numerous field experiments (Morales-Roura, Zarco, Hernandez-Ceron and Rodriguez, 2001; Moreira, Risco, Pires, Ambrose, Drost and Thatcher, 2000; Moreira, Risco, Mattos, Lopes and Thatcher, 2001; Santos, Juchem, Cerri, Galvão, Chebel, Thatcher, Dei and Bilby, 2004). When conceptuses were flushed from the uterus, bST treatment increased length of extra-embryonic membranes (45 vs 34 cm; P < 0.09) and the amount of Interferon-τ in the uterine flushings (9.4 vs 5.3 μg; P < 0.05). Interferon-τ is secreted by the trophoectoderm cells of the extra-embryonic membranes. Indeed, when the content of Interferon-τ in the uterine flushing was adjusted for length of extra-embryonic membranes as a covariate, difference due to bST was no longer significant. Thus a greater uterine pool size of Interferon-τ in bST-treated cows appeared to be due to a greater size of conceptuses at day 17.

Responses of plasma GH and IGF-1 among the groups treated with bST were interesting (Bilby, Sozzi, Lopez, Silvestre, Ealy, Staples and Thatcher, 2006). Injection of bST stimulated plasma GH concentrations as expected. Concentrations of GH were higher in cows that were pregnant compared to cyclic cows. Both groups of lactating dairy cows received the same injection doses of bST. However, those cows that conceived (5/6), and had a conceptus present at day 17, had higher concentrations of GH compared with cyclic cows. It is interesting that cyclic cows fed CaSFO also had higher plasma GH concentrations than control-cyclic cows P < 0.05). These differences were readily apparent by 8 days after first bST injection, and all groups had a temporal elevation associated with the second injection on day 11, but differences due to pregnancy and diets were maintained.

The overall mean concentrations of plasma IGF-1 for the six experimental groups clearly reflected stimulation due to bST (Bilby, Sozzi, Lopez, Silvestre, Ealy, Staples and Thatcher, 2006). Among the pregnant cows, bST stimulated a 79% increase in IGF-1 that may have contributed to the bST increase in conceptus development and Interferon-τ responses. The bST-induced increase in cyclic control cows was not as large. Pregnant control cows treated with bST had higher sustained concentrations of IGF-1 than cyclic control cows between 10 and 17 days after GnRH. This difference might have contributed to the greater degree of conceptus development in bST-treated cows. Although GH in plasma was markedly elevated in cyclic cows fed CaSFO that received bST, their concentrations of IGF-1 remained relatively low throughout the sampling period. This reflects potential dietary effects of fat feeding on endocrine and metabolic responses in lactating dairy cows. Perhaps the higher milk production and lower plasma concentrations of insulin in cows fed CaSFO (Bilby, Sozzi, Lopez, Silvestre, Ealy, Staples and Thatcher, 2006) altered liver responsiveness to exogenous bST to reduce peripheral secretion of IGF-1 compared with control-fed cyclic cows treated with bST.

We have examined endometrial steady state concentrations of mRNA for a variety of genes and endometrial proteins that may be involved in maintenance of pregnancy and as components of the IGF-family (Bilby, Guzeloglu, MacLaren, Staples and Thatcher, 2006). Although expression of PGHS-2 mRNA did not differ among treatments, the quantity of PGHS-2 protein was elevated in pregnancy. However, expression of the oxytocin receptor (OTR) and the amount of ER (oestradiol receptor) α protein were decreased in pregnant cows versus cyclic cows at day 17. The increased amount of PGHS-2 protein in endometrium of pregnant cows may reflect the need for the synthesis of prostaglandins for proliferative and immuno-modulatory effects, but the ability to secrete $PGF_{2\alpha}$ in a pulsatile luteolytic manner is attenuated (Thatcher, Moreira, Santos, Mattos, Lopes, Pancarci and Risco, 2001) and consistent with decreased expression of the OTR and ERa protein of the present study. Treatment with bST appeared to favour antiluteolytic responses in that PGES mRNA was elevated in both cyclic and pregnant cows treated with bST, and PGFS mRNA was decreased in endometrial tissue of pregnant cows that were treated with bST.

Localized expression of IGF-1 mRNA was decreased in endometrial tissue of pregnant compared to cyclic cows (Figure 4), and this decrease was apparent even though peripheral concentrations of IGF-1 were elevated in bST-treated cows and in particular bST-treated pregnant cows. Among the cyclic cows, feeding of CaSFO reduced expression of IGF-1 mRNA in a manner mimicking the decrease detected for pregnancy. Localized expression of IGF-2 mRNA within the endometrium is elevated in pregnancy, and bST stimulated this expression in both cyclic and pregnant cows (Figure 5). Feeding of CaSFO stimulated endometrial expression of IGF-2 in cyclic cows, and the increased expression was comparable to that achieved with bST in cyclic cows not fed CaSFO and to the increase in IGF-2 mRNA expression of pregnant cows (Figure 5).

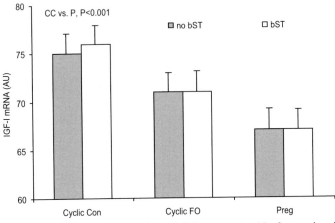

Figure 4. Abundance of IGF-1 mRNA in endometrial tissues at day 17 of a synchronized oestrous cycle. in cyclic cows fed a control (Cyclic Con) diet, or cyclic cows fed a FO (Cyclic FO) diet, or pregnant cows fed a control diet (Preg) with or without bST treatment at day 0 and 11 of the synchronized oestrous cycle.

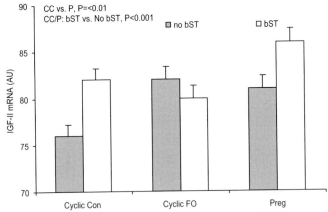

Figure 5. Abundance of IGF-II mRNA in endometrial tissues at day 17 of a synchronized oestrous cycle. in cyclic cows fed a control (Cyclic Con) diet, or cyclic cows fed a FO (Cyclic FO) diet, or pregnant cows fed a control diet (Preg) with or without bST treatment at day 0 and 11 of the synchronized oestrous cycle.

Early embryonic development that ultimately leads to maintenance of pregnancy is dependent upon conceptus-maternal communication.   Both suboptimal responsiveness of the endometrium to interferon-τ and inadequate secretion of interferon-τ probably contribute to embryonic mortality and reduced PR. Peripheral orchestraters of oviductal and endometrial environments are the steroid hormones, such as progesterone and perhaps protein hormones such as GH and IGF-1, which may in turn regulate local growth factors in a paracrine fashion within the endometrium and conceptus, as well as cross-talk between these tissues. Clearly, interferon-τ induces a number of genes (Wolf, Arnold, Bauersachs,Beier, Blum, Einspanier, Frohlich, Herrler, Hiendleder, Kolle, Prelle, Reichenbach, Stojkovic, Wenigerkind, Sinowatz, 2003) within the endometrium (i.e., signal tranducer and activator of transcription factors [e.g., STAT 1 and 2], Interferon regulatory factor -1, Interferon stimulated gene 17, MX protein, granulocyte-chemotactic protein-2, and 2',5'-oligoadenylate synthetase) which implies that interferon-τ supports maintenance of pregnancy via a multiplicity of potential mechanisms. In the present study (Bilby, Guzeloglu, MacLaren, Staples and Thatcher, 2006), bST alters endometrial gene expression of PGES mRNA, PGFS mRNA, ERα protein, IGF-2 mRNA and IGFBP2 mRNA in cyclic and pregnant cows, and, in some instances, differentially between pregnant and cyclic states (e.g., IGFBP-2 mRNA; PGFS mRNA and ERα protein). The present study also shows that fatty acids in fish oil appear to act as nutraceuticals to decrease expression of IGF-1 mRNA and enhance expression of IGF-2 mRNA in a manner comparable to bST. These are potentially complex systems indicating that pharmaceutical and nutraceutical treatments may influence embryo-maternal interactions in a manner to perhaps improve conception rate and embryo survival.

A multiplicity of additional dietary fish oil effects were detected on extra-uterine and, in particular, uterine responses that warrant further description. In a comparison of fatty acid concentrations among various tissues, the endometrium and liver had highest concentrations of C18:2n-6, C20:4n-6, C18:3n-3, EPA, and DHA compared to milk fat, mammary tissue, muscle, and both subcutaneous and internal fat tissues (Figure 6; Bilby, Jenkins, Staples, Thatcher, 2006). An important observation was that the CaSFO diet reduced concentrations of arachidonic acid (C20:4n-6) (Figure 7A) and preferentially increased concentrations of EPA and DHA in the endometrium (Figure 7B). Thus it is clear that EPA and DHA fatty acids of the CaSFO diet are absorbed from the gastrointestinal tract and are preferentially taken up in the endometrial tissue.

The peroxisome proliferator-activated receptors (PPARs) are a family of nuclear receptors activated by specific fatty acids, eicosanoids and peroxisome proliferators. Previous studies have shown that they are involved in regulation of genes affecting steroid and prostaglandin synthesis

(MacLaren, Guzeloglu, Michel, and Thatcher, 2006). Northern blot analysis indicated that PPARα and PPARδ mRNAs were expressed in endometrium from cyclic and pregnant Holstein cows at day 17 following oestrus on all treatments. Western blot experiments confirmed the presence of PPARα and

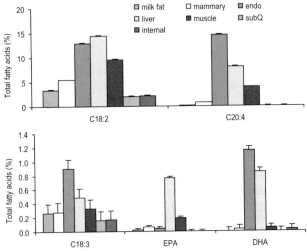

Figure 6. Concentrations of C18:2n-6, C20:4n-6, C18:3n-3, EPA and DHA as a percentage of total fatty acids in milk fat, mammary, endometrium (endo), liver, muscle, subcutaneous (subQ) and internal fat tissues collected at day 17 of a synchronized oestrous cycle.

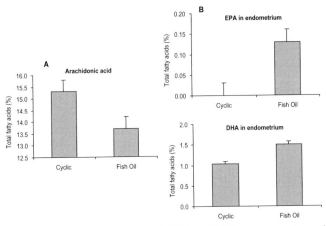

Figure 7. Concentrations of arachadonic (20:4n-6), EPA and DHA as a percentage of total fatty acids in endometrial tissue collected at day 17 of a synchronized oestrous cycle from cyclic cows fed control (Cyclic) or fish oil diets. .

PPARδ protein in bovine endometrium (MacLaren and Thatcher, in preparation). Treatment with bST was associated with increased PPARδ mRNA levels in pregnant but not cyclic cows, suggesting that the effect may be mediated by the embryo (Figure 8). Supplementation with n-3 PUFA-rich

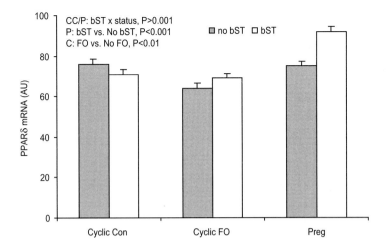

Figure 8. Abundance of PPARä mRNA in endometrial tissues at day 17 of a synchronized oestrous cycle in cyclic cows fed a control (Cyclic Con) diet, or cyclic cows fed a FO (Cyclic FO) diet, or pregnant cows fed a control diet (Preg), with or without bST treatment at day 0 and 11 of the synchronized oestrous cycle.

fish oil was associated with reduced steady state concentrations of PPARδ mRNA (Figure 8). In contrast, the CaSFO diet did not alter abundance of PPARα mRNA; however, bST did stimulate PPARα mRNA abundance in pregnant cows but not in cyclic cows fed the control diets (data not shown). Immunohistochemistry to localize PPARδ indicated that the protein is expressed in the luminal epithelium, glandular epithelium, subepithelial stroma and, to a lesser extent, in the adluminal stroma. The decrease in abundance of PPARδ mRNA associated with cows fed the CaSFO diet also was reflected with immunolocalization in that there was a reduction in moderate staining intensity of PPARδ protein in the luminal epithelium of cows fed FO with or without bST treatment (Figure 9).

In latter stages of the oestrous cycle, the decrease in progesterone receptors and the increase in ER-α receptors led to an induction of oxytocin receptors and PGHS-2. Consequently, PGF2α is secreted in a pulsatile pattern to cause luteolysis. This system undergoes an antilutelytic pathway in the presence of a conceptus as described above (i.e., decrease in ER-α and oxytocin receptors) that leads to maintenance of the corpus luteum in pregnancy. In the present study, feeding CaSFO appeared to induce subtle antiluteolytic effects when examining immunohistochemistry spatial responses for the progesterone and oestradiol-α receptors and PGHS-2 proteins. Staining for progesterone receptors in the superficial glandular epithelial cells of the cyclic cows at day 17 indicated that CaSFO increased moderate and heavy staining (Figure 10). Conversely, moderate to heavy staining intensity for the ER-α receptor was reduced in the luminal epithelial cells of CaSFO-fed cows (Figure 11). This antiluteolytic pattern

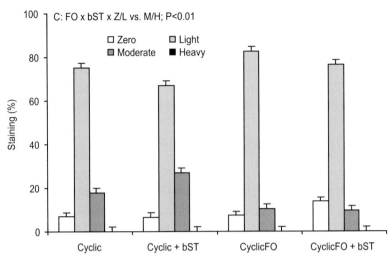

Figure 9. Percent staining (zero, light, moderate and heavy) of PPARα receptor protein in endometrial luminal epithelium collected on day 17 of a synchronized oestrous cycle in cyclic cows fed a control (Cyclic) or FO (Cyclic FO) diets and injected with or without bST.

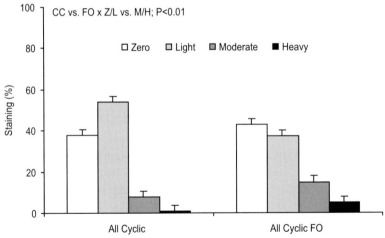

Figure 10. Percent staining (zero, light, moderate and heavy) of progesterone receptor protein in endometrial superficial glandular epithelium collected on day 17 of a synchronized oestrous cycle in all (+/- bST) cyclic cows fed a control (All Cyclic) or FO (All Cyclic FO) diets.

was associated with an attenuated effector response, reflected by a decrease in heavy staining for PGHS-2 protein in theluminal epithelium (Figure 12). Perhaps activation of the PPARδ receptor attenuates expression of the progesterone receptor and enhances expression of the ER-α receptor and PGHS-2 protein. It is clear that EPA antagonizes the stimulatory effects of arachidonic acid on $PGF_{2\alpha}$ secretion. If such an antagonism exists, then EPA via the diet would reduce the

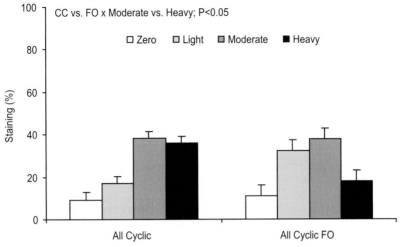

Figure 11. Percent staining (zero, light, moderate and heavy) of oestradiol-α receptor protein in endometrial luminal epithelium collected on day 17 of a synchronized oestrous cycle in all (+/- bST) cyclic cows fed a control (All Cyclic) or FO (All Cyclic FO) diets.

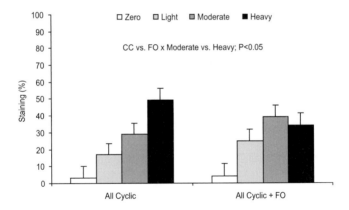

Figure 12. Percent staining (zero, light, moderate and heavy) of PGHS-2 protein in endometrial luminal epithelium collected on day 17 of a synchronized oestrous cycle in all (+/- bST) cyclic cows fed a control (All Cyclic) or FO (All Cyclic FO) diets.

presence of PPARδ receptor or compete with arachidonic acid for the receptor, resulting in counter arachidonic effects that would increase the progesterone receptor and decrease both the ER-α receptor and PGHS-2 protein within the luminal epithelial cells. As a consequence, a dietary manipulation of a nutraceutical has possibly augmented cellular and intracellular processes to sustain embryo development or pregnancy.

Summary

Major advancements have been made for programmed reproductive management. However, reproductive performance is not optimal. It is clear that major attention needs to focus on management of the lactating dairy cow during the peripartum and postpartum period to optimize the transition from the non-lactating to the lactating state in a manner that improves general health, immune function, and restoration of subsequent reproductive competence. Development of programs to optimize health, lactational, and reproductive performance will entail integration of herd health, nutrition and reproductive management programs. Growing evidence indicates that the design and delivery of supplemental organic selenium and unsaturated fatty acids (specifically linoleic acid, linolenic acid, EPA, and DHA) to the lower gut for absorption may target tissues to alter reproductive function and fertility. Changes in reproductive responses can be affected by fat supplementation involving potential alterations in ovarian, uterine, and conceptus sensitivity to metabolic hormones such as bST, insulin-like growth factor-I and gonadotrophins (LH and FSH). In addition, the specific alteration of eicosanoids at certain physiological windows (e.g., periparturient and breeding periods) as well as organic selenium may benefit health (e.g., innate and adaptive immuno-responses) and subsequent reproductive competence and performance of lactating dairy cows that are dealing with the homeorhetic processes of lactation that appear to antagonize reproduction.. The impacts of these nutraceutical agents on inter- and intracellular processes for efficient function of reproductive processes in the lactating dairy cow warrant a high priority for investigation. Indeed this area of investigation needs to be supported by nutritional, pharmaceutical, and governmental entities to deal with the infertility syndrome of lactating dairy cows. Furthermore, this unique animal model has major implications for application to human health.

Acknowledgements

We would like to acknowledge: Alltech Inc. for donation of Sel-Plex® and partial financial support, Virtus Nutrition for donation of EnerG II Reproduction formula for experimental purposes, Church and Dwight Inc. for donation of Megalac-R® and partial financial support, Florida-Georgia Milk Checkoff Program, and the partial financial support received by the NRI Competitive Grant Program-USDA, grants no. 98-35203-6367 and no.2004-35203-14137.

References

Benzaquen, M.E., Risco, C.A., Archbald, L.F., Melendez, P., Thatcher, M-J., Thatcher, W.W. (2006) Rectal Temperature, Calving-Related Factors and the Incidence of Puerperal Metritis in Postpartum Dairy Cows. *Journal of Dairy Science* In Press.

Bilby, T. R., Guzeloglu, A., MacLaren, L. A., Staples, C. R., Thatcher, W.W. (2006) Pregnancy, bST and omega-3 fatty acids in lactating dairy cows: II. Gene expression related to maintenance of pregnancy. *Journal of Dairy Science* **89**, 3375–3385.

Bilby, T.R., Jenkins, T., Staples, C.R., Thatcher, W.W. (2006) Pregnancy, bST and omega-3 fatty acids in lactating dairy cows: III. Fatty acid distribution. *Journal of Dairy Science* **89**, 3386–3399.

Bilby, T.R., Sozzi, A., Lopez, M.M., Silvestre, F., Ealy, A.D., Staples, C.R., Thatcher, W.W. (2006) Pregnancy, bST and omega-3 fatty acids in lactating dairy cows: I. ovarian, conceptus and growth hormone – IGF system response. *Journal of Dairy Science* **89**, 3360–3374.

Cerri R.L.A., Bruno, R.G.S., Chebel, R.C., Galvao, K.N., Rutgliano, H., Juchem, S.O., Thatcher, W.W., Luchini, D., Santos, J.E.P. (2004) Effect of fat sources differing in fatty acid profile on fertilization rate and embryo quality in lactating dairy cows. *Journal of Dairy Science* **87**, Suppl. 1, 297.

Cullens, F.M., Staples, C.R., Bilby, T.R., Silvestre, F., Bartolome, J., Sozzi, A., Badinga, L., Thatcher, W.W., Arthington, J.D. (2004) Effect of timing of initiation of fat supplementation on milk production, plasma hormones and metabolites, and conception rates of Holstein cows in summer. *Journal of Dairy Science* **86**, Suppl. 1, 308.

Cupps, P.T. (1973) Uterine changes associated with impaired fertility in the dairy cow. *Journal of Dairy Science* **56**, 878-884.

Goff, J. P. (2006) Major Advances in Our Understanding of Nutritional Influences on Bovine Health. *Journal of Dairy Science* **89**, 1292–1301

Juchem, S.O., Cerri, R.L.A., Bruno, R., Galvao, K.N., Lemos, E.W., Villasenor, M., Coscioni, A.C., Rutgliano, H.M., Thatcher, W.W., Luchini, D., Santos, J.E.P., (2004) Effect of feeding Ca salts of palm oil (PO) or a blend of linoleic and monoenoic trans fatty acids (LTFA) on uterine involution and reproductive performance in Holstein cows. *Journal of Dairy Science* **87**, Suppl. 1, 310.

Kasimanickam, R., Duffield, T.F., Foster, R.A., Gartley, C.J., Leslie, K.E., Walton, J.S., Johnson, W.H. (2004) Endometrial cytology and ultrasonography for the detection of subclinical endometritis in postpartum dairy cows. *Theriogenology* **62**, 9-23.

Katagiri, S. and Takahasi, Y. (2005) Potential relationship between normalization of endometrial epidermal growth factor profile and restoration of fertility in repeat breeder cows. *Animal Reprod. Sci.* **95**:54-66.

Loeffler, S.H., de Vries, M.J. and Schukken, Y.H. (1999) The effects of time of disease occurrence, milk yield, and body condition on fertility of dairy cows. *Journal of Dairy Science* **82**, 2589-2604.

MacLaren, L.A., Guzeloglu, A., Michel, A.F. and Thatcher W.W. (2006) Peroxisome proliferatior-activated receptor (PPAR) expression in cultured bovine endometrial cells and response to omega-3 fatty acid, growth hormone and agonist stimulation in relation to series 2 prostaglandin production. *Domestic Animal Endocrinology* 30:155-169.

Moore, K., Thatcher, W.W. (2006) Major Advances Associated with Reproduction in Dairy Cattle. *Journal of Dairy Science* **89**, 1254–1266.

Morales-Roura, J.S., Zarco, L., Hernandez-Ceron, J. Rodriguez, G. (2001) Effect of short-term treatment with bovine Somatotropin at estrus on conception rate and luteal function of repeat-breeding dairy cows. *Theriogenology* **55**, 1831-1841.

Moreira, F., Risco, C.A., Pires, M.F.A., Ambrose, J.D., Drost, M., Thatcher, W.W. (2000) Use of bovine somatotropin in lactating dairy cows receiving timed artificial insemination. *Journal of Dairy Science* **83**, 1237-1247.

Moreira, F.C.O., Risco, C.A., Mattos, R., Lopes, F., Thatcher, W.W. (2001) Effects of presynchronization and bovine somatotropin on pregnancy rates to a timed artificial insemination protocol in lactating dairy cows. *Journal of Dairy Science* **84**, 1646-1659.

Rutigliano, H.M., Santos, J.E.P. (2005) Interrelationships among parity, body condition score (BCS), milk yield, AI protocol, and cyclicity with embryonic survival in lactating dairy cows. *Journal of Dairy Science* **88**, Suppl 1:39.

Santos, J.E.P., Juchem, S.O., Cerri, R.L.A., Galvão, K.N., Chebel, R.C., Thatcher, W.W., Dei, C.S., Bilby, C.R. (2004) Effect of bST and reproductive management on reproductive performance of Holstein dairy cows. *Journal of Dairy Science* **87**, 868-88.

Silvestre, F.T., Silvestre, D.T., Crawford, C., Santos, J.E.P., Staples, C.R., Thatcher. W.W. (2006) Effect of selenium (Se) source on innate and adaptive immunity of periparturient dairy cows. *Biol. Repro.* 39th Annual Meeting. Special Issue. page 132.

Silvestre, F.T., Silvestre, D.T., Santos, J.E.P., Risco, C., Staples, C.R., Thatcher, W.W. (2006) Effects of selenium (Se) sources on dairy cows. *Journal of Animal Science* **89** (Suppl 1.):52.

Staples, C.R., Thatcher, W.W. (2006) Effects of fatty acids on reproduction of dairy cows. Pages 229-256 in *Recent Advances in Animal Nutrition 2005*. P.C. Garnsworthy and J. Wiseman, eds. Nottingham University Press, Nottingham, UK.

Thatcher, W.W., Moreira, F., Santos, J.E.P., Mattos, R.C., Lopes, F.L., Pancarci, S.M.,. Risco, C.A. (2001) Effects of hormonal treatments on reproductive performance and embryo production. *Theriogenology* **55**, 75-89.

Weiss, W. P. (2003) Selenium nutrition of dairy cows: comparing responses to organic and inorganic selenium forms. *Proceedings of Alltech's 19th Annual Symposium*. Nottingham University Press, Nottingham. p. 333-343.

Wolf, E., Arnold, G.J., Bauersachs, S., Beier, H.M., Blum, H., Einspanier, R., Frohlich, T., Herrler, A., Hiendleder, S., Kolle, S., Prelle, K., Reichenbach, H.D., Stojkovic, M., Wenigerkind, H., Sinowatz, F. (2003) Embryo-maternal communication in bovine - strategies for deciphering a complex cross-talk. *Reproduction Domestic Animals* **38**:276-89.

4

BODY CONDITION SCORE IN DAIRY COWS: TARGETS FOR PRODUCTION AND FERTILITY

P.C. GARNSWORTHY

Division of Agricultural and Environmental Sciences, University of Nottingham School of Biosciences, Sutton Bonington Campus, Loughborough LE12 5RD, UK

Introduction

Body condition score (BCS) is probably the most useful management tool available to dairy producers for assessing the nutritional status of cows. It provides a rapid indication of levels of body fat reserves at almost zero cost. Body fat reserves play an important biological role in early lactation by buffering the cow against feed shortages whilst she partitions energy mainly towards milk output. However, rapid mobilisation of body fat reserves causes fertility and health problems. It is important, therefore, that appropriate targets for BCS are established, based on the underlying biology of the cow.

The current chapter discusses the use of BCS for assessing body fatness; relationships among BCS, feed intake and negative energy balance; implications of BCS changes for cow health and fertility; and BCS targets at different stages of lactation. Importantly, it will address the question of whether BCS targets should be updated for modern dairy cows.

Body condition scoring systems

Several body condition scoring systems were introduced in the 1970s and 1980s. Lowman, Scott and Somerville (1973) adapted a system used previously for scoring beef cattle, which involves palpation of the lumbar vertebrae and around the tail head. A scale of 1 to 4 was proposed; 1 corresponds to a cow that looks emaciated, has sharp bones and has no palpable fat cover around the tail head; 4 corresponds to a cow that is excessively fat and the spinous processes of the lumbar vertebrae cannot be felt. A similar system with a scale of 0 to 5 was proposed by Mulvany (1977) in the UK. In Australia, a scale of 1 to 8 was introduced by Earle (1976). In the United States, a scale of 1 to 5 was proposed by Wildman *et al.* (1982). In New Zealand, a scale of 1 to 10 was introduced in 1993 by the Livestock Improvement Corporation (Stockdale, 2001). Different systems place different emphasis on fat cover felt in different anatomical regions; the US system uses visual appraisal with no requirement to palpate cows. Variations among scoring systems can lead to confusion when comparing targets and responses.

The majority of publications in the past decade have used a 1 to 5 scale. A 1 to 5 scale is used also by the UK Department for Environment Food and Rural Affairs in its advisory leaflet on body condition scoring (Defra, 2001), which is cited by the official welfare code for cattle (Defra, 2003). For these reasons, a 1 to 5 scale will be used in the current review, unless specified otherwise. Photographs and descriptions of this scale are available online (see Defra, 2001 and Ferguson, 2006). The following equations were used to convert other scales to a 1 to 5 scale:

1-4 scale: $BCS \times 4/3 - 1/3$
0-5 scale: $BCS \times 4/5 + 1$
1-8 scale: $BCS \times 4/7 + 3/7$
1-9 scale: $BCS/2 + 1/2$
1-10 scale: $BCS \times 4/9 + 5/9$

The use of simple mathematical conversions between scales might not be accurate if scales are not linear across the whole range of scores. Roche *et al.* (2004) compared a body condition scoring system used in New Zealand (1 to 10 scale) with systems used in USA (1 to 5 scale), Ireland (1 to 5 scale) and Australia (1 to 8 scale). Although there were significant correlations among systems, scores tended to converge at the bottom of the scales. Unfortunately, the study included no cows outside the range 2 to 4.25 (1-5 scale), and different scoring systems were confounded with different operators. Nevertheless, the study highlights the need for some caution in comparisons of studies that have used different scales. At present, however, there is insufficient information available to justify anything other than simple mathematical conversion to a 1-5 scale.

Ferguson *et al.* (2006) compared scores of four observers for 57 cows ranging in BCS from 2.0 to 4.5 and found significant, but small, differences between observers; the greatest difference in mean BCS between observers was 0.29 units. In an earlier study, Ferguson *et al.* (1994) compared scores given to 225 cows by four observers and found that 58 % of the time all observers gave the same score to the same cow. An additional 33% of the time observers gave plus or minus 0.25 to the same cow. Scores among observers were highly correlated ($r = 0.76$ to 0.88). In another recent study, Kristensen *et al.* (2006) compared scores of six highly-trained instructors and 51 practicing veterinarians. Each individual scored approximately 20 cows twice, giving a total of 2,230 scores. Between scoring sessions, the instructors gave training to the veterinarians. Instructors agreed with each other 83% of the time, and repeated scores agreed 72 to 95% of the time. Scores given by veterinarians were more variable and generally lower than instructors' scores at the first session. Following training, however, veterinarians' scores became more homogenous and similar to the instructors' scores. It was concluded that a limited amount of training brought about substantial improvement in the validity and precision of BCS determined by practicing veterinarians, compared with BCS recorded on the same cows by highly trained classifiers.

Although BCS is positively related to live weight, cows in early lactation can often maintain or gain live weight whilst BCS is declining, due to the effect of gut fill on live weight (Garnsworthy, 1988). For this reason, BCS is better than live weight as an indicator of body fat reserves. Several studies have reported strong relationships between BCS and body fat content. For example, Wright and Russel (1984) reported a strong positive relationship between BCS and total fat content in non-pregnant, non-lactating, Friesian cows, as did Garnsworthy *et al.* (1986). Similarly, Otto *et al.* (1991) found that one unit of BCS increase for cull cows corresponded to an increase of 12.65% ether extract (a chemical measure of fat content).

Some reports suggest that the relationship between BCS and fat content might not be linear at the lower end of the scale. Gregory *et al.* (1998) found that over the range of 1.4 to 8.0 (1-8 scale), BCS was positively related to weight of internal fat depots, proportion of fat in a sample joint, and muscle to bone ratio in the sample joint of cull cows; however below BCS 3 (1-8 scale), cows had limited body fat reserves and there was little change in body fat with change in BCS. In a recent study of 146 lactating Holstein-Friesian cows, Yan *et al.* (2005) found that BCS was not related to empty body concentration of crude protein, but BCS was significantly ($P < 0.001$) related to empty body concentrations of lipid (Lipid ($g/kg^{0.75}$) = 271.7 BCS − 233.7; $R^2 = 0.57$) and energy (Energy ($MJ/kg^{0.75}$) = 10.06 BCS + 9.9; $R^2 = 0.58$). Although only linear relationships were reported, their figures indicate little change in body fat with change in BCS when BCS was below 2, supporting the observations of Gregory *et al.* (1998).

Body condition score, dry matter intake and energy balance

Early recommendations (e.g. Lowman *et al.*, 1973) were for minimum BCS (1-4 scale) of 3.5 at calving, 2.5 at mating and 3.0 at drying off. These recommendations were based on observations that dry matter intake normally increases at a slower rate than milk yield in early lactation. Under these circumstances, energy output in milk exceeds energy intake from feed, and the cow is in 'negative energy balance'. Cows in negative energy balance mobilise body fat reserves to support milk production. Increasing body fat reserves at calving, by increasing prepartum feed supply, allowed greater fat mobilisation and higher milk yields postpartum (Broster, 1971). This explains the relatively high BCS recommendation of 3.5 at calving; the philosophy was to 'steam up' cows before calving so that they could 'milk off their backs' after calving.

Studies in the 1980s, however, showed that body fat has a negative feedback effect on feed intake. In two experiments, Garnsworthy and Topps (1982) controlled the energy intake of cows before calving so that cows calved with BCS (1-4 scale) of 1.7 (Thin), 2.7 (Medium) or 3.7 (Fat). After calving, all cows were offered a high-energy total-mixed ration (TMR) *ad libitum*. There was no effect of BCS at calving on milk yield. Over the first 12 weeks of lactation, cows that were fat at calving lost 0.9-1.0 BCS units; cows with medium BCS at calving lost 0.5-0.6 BCS units; cows that were thin at calving gained 0.4-0.5 BCS units. BCS tended to converge at 2.5 in week 12-15 of lactation (Figure 1a), suggesting that cows have a target BCS that they try to attain in early lactation. Although milk yield peaked in week 6 of lactation for all groups of cows (Figure 1b), maximum dry matter intake was reached in week 15 for fat cows, week 11 for medium cows and week 9 for thin cows (Figure 1c). This suggested that feed intake was controlled by physiological feedback mechanisms and that level of body fat had a direct effect on feed intake.

Numerous studies in the 1980s and early 1990s (reviewed by Garnsworthy, 1988; Broster and Broster, 1998) confirmed the strong negative relationship between BCS at calving and change in BCS during early lactation (Figure 2). Each individual dairy cow has a genetically-programmed target BCS that she attempts to reach approximately 10 to 12 weeks after calving. If her BCS is above this target, feed intake is reduced and she loses condition; if her BCS is below this target, feed intake is increased and she gains condition. The biological drive for a cow to attain a target BCS appears to be as strong as the drive to attain a genetically-programmed peak milk yield. The philosophy of getting cows in 'good condition' at calving is, therefore, counter productive. Instead of a high BCS at calving compensating for low feed intake in early lactation, it actually reduces feed intake further and exacerbates negative energy balance.

To quantify effects of BCS on feed intake in early lactation, Garnsworthy (1994) examined data from 143 cows in 8 experiments where weekly values were available for milk yield, BCS and dry matter intake over the first 17

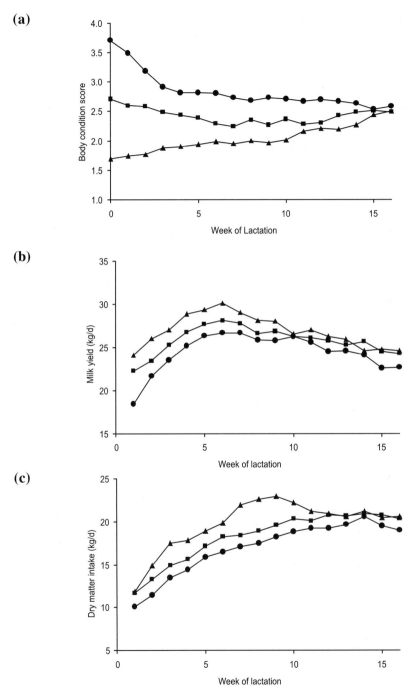

Figure 1. Changes in BCS (a), milk yield (b) and dry matter intake (c) for cows calving at BCS (1-4 scale) >3.5 (●), 2.5 – 3.0 (■), or <2.0 (▲). Data are combined means of Experiments 1 and 2 from Garnsworthy and Topps (1982).

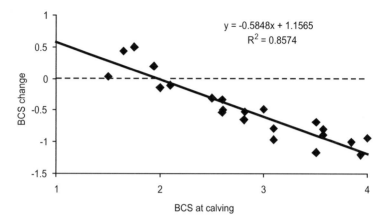

Figure 2. Relationship between BCS at calving and change in BCS over the first 10 – 12 weeks of lactation. Data (1 – 4 scale) are group means from review by Garnsworthy (1988), and were originally published in Land and Leaver (1980; 1981), Garnsworthy and Topps (1982), Treacher *et al.* (1986), Garnsworthy and Jones (1987) and Bourchier *et al.* (1987)

weeks of lactation. The model assumed that intake would be related primarily to milk energy output, but would be modified by a feedback factor related to the difference between current BCS and target BCS. For high-energy diets (>11.5 MJ ME/kg DM), the best equation for predicting dry matter intake (kg/d) was 0.458n + 0.538Y - 0.48BCSd, where n = week of lactation, Y = milk yield (kg/d) and BCSd = BCS in week n minus BCS target (2.5) (R^2 = 0.96; mean square prediction error = 0.38 kg/d). More recently, Ellis *et al.* (2006) used a similar approach to adjust static prediction equations of dry matter intake for use in dynamic modelling of dairy cow performance over a whole lactation. The prediction equations used were those of the Agricultural Research Council (1980), the Cornell Net Carbohydrate and Protein System (Fox *et al.*, 2004), and the National Research Council (2001). These were examined with a dataset comprising 777 data points from 21 sets of lactation performance data. By adjusting dry matter intake with a feedback factor, residual sums of squares were reduced on average by 41% for dry matter intake predictions and by 52% for body weight predictions. The feedback factor was based on the difference between initial body energy reserves and current body energy reserves for each week of lactation. It was assumed that cows would attempt to replenish energy reserves to the level at calving, which would be equivalent to BCS 3.5. Perhaps predictions might have been improved still further had the cows' biological target BCS been used, rather than calving BCS which is determined by management policy.

The ability of cows to reach their target BCS is affected by diet composition. With high-energy diets, thin cows can be in positive energy balance and increase BCS, but fat cows will be in negative energy balance and decrease BCS. With low-energy diets, feed intake is limited by physical capacity of the rumen and thin cows cannot increase energy intake to match milk energy output; fat cows mobilise body condition at a faster rate to support milk production and are in negative energy balance longer than with high-energy diets (Jones and Garnsworthy, 1989). High-protein diets result in greater loss of body condition by fat cows, but either increase gain or decrease loss of body condition by thin cows which use excess protein for gluconeogenesis (Garnsworthy and Jones, 1987; Jones and Garnsworthy, 1988). Low-fibre, high-starch diets increase BCS gain in thin cows and decrease BCS loss in fat cows, probably by increasing insulin status (Garnsworthy and Jones, 1993). High-fat diets decrease BCS loss in fat cows, but do not affect BCS change in thin cows (Garnsworthy and Huggett, 1992).

The relationship between BCS at calving and change in BCS during early lactation applies across all feeding systems. Studies reviewed by Garnsworthy (1988) and Broster and Broster (1998) included cows fed on TMR, hay plus concentrates, and self-feed silage. Stockdale (2001) extended the review to include six grazing studies, which confirmed that pasture-fed cows exhibit the same strong relationship.

When the feedback effect of BCS on feed intake was established in the 1980s, the regulatory mechanism was unknown, although lipostatic control of feed intake had been proposed many years earlier (Kennedy, 1953). Subsequently, the main signalling factor was suggested to be leptin, a peptide hormone secreted by adipose tissue and discovered in 1994. Plasma leptin concentrations vary with mass of adipose tissue and leptin has been shown to decrease appetite by direct action on the hypothalamic satiety centre (Vernon *et al.*, 2001). However, the overall regulatory mechanism is complex. In addition to its effects on feed intake, leptin has been found to modulate nutrient transfer and partitioning by interaction with other hormones including insulin, glucagon, glucocorticoids, growth hormone, insulin-like growth factor-I, cytokines and thyroid hormones (Hill, 2004). Other factors secreted by adipose tissue (tumour necrosis factor α and resistin) have also been shown to interact with leptin in regulation of adiposity (Vernon *et al.*, 2001). Meikle *et al.* (2004) found that BCS at parturition affected leptin concentrations. Leptin concentrations during late pregnancy and the first two weeks of lactation were higher in cows with higher BCS. Leptin concentrations decreased at a faster rate postpartum in fat cows (BCS ≥ 3) than in lean cows (BCS < 3), and the leptin nadir was reached 10 days earlier in lean cows than in fat cows. However, although leptin concentrations were positively related to BCS both before and after parturition in fat cows, the relationship was only significant before parturition in lean cows. This is in agreement with the data of Yan *et al*. (2005), mentioned in the previous section, where there was little change in body fat with change in BCS when BCS was below 2.0.

Body condition score, health and reproduction

Cows that are excessively fat at calving are more likely to develop fatty liver and ketosis because high BCS depresses appetite severely and body fat is mobilised too rapidly (Reid *et al*., 1986). Such cows exhibit severe negative energy balance, poor reproductive performance and increased incidence of diseases (Treacher *et al*., 1986). Fatty liver is characterised by accumulation of triglycerides (TAG) in hepatocytes due to overloading of fatty acid oxidation and lipoprotein synthesis systems within the liver. Fatty liver is defined as >20% fat in liver cells observed by microscopy, or >50 g TAG/kg liver tissue by chemical analysis (Newbold, 2005). In a survey of 9 herds in the Netherlands, Jorritsma *et al*. (2001) found that 54% of cows had >50 g TAG/kg liver tissue when sampled between 6 and 17 days postpartum. Causes, prevention and alleviation of fatty liver were reviewed by Newbold (2005), who stated "central to any approach to the prevention of fatty liver is control of body condition: more specifically, the avoidance of fat cows at calving". In terms of BCS, it appears from the data of Treacher *et al*. (1986) and Jorritsma *et al*. (2001) that risk of fatty liver increases considerably when BCS is above 3.5 at calving.

Fatty liver is often associated with ketosis, although fatty liver usually precedes ketosis and ketosis is associated more with carbohydrate metabolism than fat metabolism (Grummer, 1992). In a study of 732 moderate-yielding Norwegian cows, Gillund *et al*. (2001) found that cows calving with a BCS of 3.5 or greater were 2.3 to 2.8 times more likely to experience ketosis compared with a BCS of 3.25 or lower. In an analysis of 3,586 lactations covering a 17-year period at the Langhill Dairy Cattle Research Centre, Rasmussen *et al*. (1999) found that cows with a BCS at calving of 3.5 had double the risk of developing ketosis compared with cows with a BCS at calving of 2.0, all other things being equal.

In addition to fatty liver and ketosis, other disease problems have been linked with BCS. Relationships are variable and inconsistent, but excessive loss of BCS in the dry period or early lactation, low BCS at drying off, and high BCS at calving, have been associated with increased risks of dystocia, retained placenta, metritis, milk fever, mastitis and lameness (see for example: Treacher *et al*., 1986; Gearhart *et al*., 1990; Markusfeld, 1997). Blood biochemistry can be used as an indicator of nutritional status and disease risk; Ward *et al*. (1995) found that ß-hydroxybutyrate (BHBA) and bile acids were higher, and glucose was lower, for the first 40 days of lactation in cows with BCS above 3.0 at calving, compared with cows below 3.0. Although no data on mineral and vitamin status could be found in the literature for fat versus thin cows, it is possible that reduced intake by fat cows could compromise their micro-nutrient reserves.

Even moderate levels of fat mobilisation are associated with negative energy balance and reduced fertility. Several studies have shown that high genetic merit, negative energy balance, body fat mobilisation, high plasma non-esterified fatty acids (NEFA), and low plasma insulin are associated with delayed first ovulation postpartum and reduced pregnancy rates (see reviews by Garnsworthy and Webb, 1999; Butler, 2003; Pryce *et al.*, 2004; Butler, 2005). Butler (2005) reported that cows losing less than 0.5 BCS over the first 30 days postpartum took an average of 30 days from calving to first ovulation; cows losing 0.5 to 1.0 BCS took 36 days; cows losing more than 1.0 BCS took 50 days. Bourchier *et al.* (1987) surveyed 2000 cows in high-yielding herds and found a significant effect of BCS change on conception rate to first service: cows gaining condition during the first 12 weeks of lactation had a 67 % conception rate; cows losing 0.5 to 1.0 BCS had a 55 % conception rate; cows losing more than 1.0 BCS had a 47 % conception rate. A similar relationship was found by Butler (2005), who concluded from several studies that conception rate decreases by 10 % per 0.5 unit BCS loss. In reviewing physiological mechanisms, Butler (2003) reported that negative energy balance is strongly associated with attenuation of LH pulse frequency and low levels of blood glucose, insulin and IGF-I that collectively limit oestrogen production by dominant follicles; with diminished quality of oocytes and capability for embryo development; and with reduced serum progesterone concentrations. This is supported by studies at the University of Nottingham, which showed that dietary manipulation of insulin status affects postpartum anoestrus (Gong *et al.*, 2002) and oocyte quality (Fouladi-Nashta *et al.*, 2005).

Lopez-Gatius *et al.* (2003) performed a meta-analysis of 15 papers corresponding to nearly 8,000 cows to examine relationships between BCS and reproductive performance. Effects of BCS at calving, and at first insemination, on pregnancy rate were highly heterogeneous, which was attributed to variation among farms in voluntary wait period and oestrous detection rate, combined with the dynamic nature of BCS change. Cows not served until their second or third ovulation postpartum, due to either farm policy or undetected oestrus, are more likely to conceive and to have higher BCS than cows served at their first ovulation. On the other hand, effects of BCS on number of days open were consistent among studies. Compared with cows losing 0 to 0.5 BCS, cows losing 0.5 to 1.0 BCS took 3.5 days longer to conceive, and cows losing >1.0 BCS took 10.6 days longer to conceive; cows gaining BCS took 3.7 days less to conceive.

Increased incidence of diseases and reduced fertility in cows that are mobilising body fat could be linked to lymphocyte function and oxidative stress. Lacetera *et al.* (2005) found that BCS at calving affected the ability of cows to mount an immune response; when challenged with mitogens, lymphocytes from thin (BCS 2) cows produced more immunoglobulin M and interferon-γ than fat (BCS 4) cows. Bernabucci *et al.* (2005) measured oxidative stress indicators in cows calving with BCS <2.5 (thin), 2.6-3.0 (medium), or >3.0 (fat). Over the first 30 days of lactation, cows in the fat group lost 0.6 BCS units; cows in the other groups lost 0.3 units. Plasma concentrations of BHBA and NEFA were twice as high in cows from the fat group as in cows from the other groups, and significant correlations were found among BCS loss, BHBA and NEFA. No difference was found in oxidative status between the thin and medium BCS groups. Cows in the fat BCS group, however, had significantly elevated plasma concentrations of reactive oxygen metabolites (ROM) and thiobarbituric acid-reactive substances (TBARS), and significantly lower erythrocyte thiol groups (ESH) and plasma superoxide dismutase (SOD). BHBA and NEFA were positively related to ROM, and NEFA were negatively related to ESH and SOD. None of the cows in this study showed clinical signs of disease or disorders. The ROM and TBARS data suggest that cows with high BCS at calving and high lipid mobilisation are more likely to suffer oxidative stress; the ESH and SOD data suggest that these cows are less able to mount an antioxidant defence. It should be noted that cows in the fat BCS group were not excessively fat; the average BCS at calving for this group was 3.2 ± 0.2, which is within the normally-recommended range and would not be expected to induce clinical signs of fatty liver.

Body condition score and genetic merit

As stated previously, the biological drive for a cow to attain a target BCS appears to be as strong as the drive to attain a genetically-programmed peak milk yield. It also appears that a cow's biological target BCS is determined by genetics. In a classic study reported by Holmes (1988), cows of high genetic merit showed a lower target BCS than cows of low genetic merit; both groups of cows achieved their targets, whether they had a high or low BCS at calving (Figure 3). In a recent study, Roche *et al.* (2006) compared Holstein-Friesian cows of New Zealand origin (NZ) with higher genetic merit cows of North American origin (NA). Cows were managed to calve with similar BCS; 270-day milk yields were 5818 L for NZ cows and 6748 L for

NA cows. There was no effect of genetic merit on rate of BCS loss in early lactation, but NA cows lost BCS for 14 days longer (P<0.01) and reached a lower BCS nadir (P<0.001) than NZ cows. Also, NA cows gained less BCS than NZ cows in later lactation.

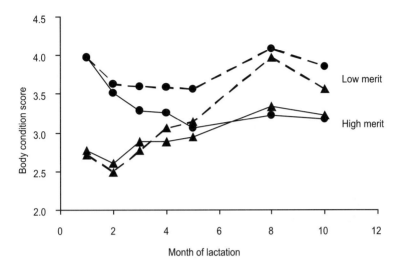

Figure 3. Changes in BCS for cows of high (solid lines) or low (dashed lines) genetic merit, with high (●) or low (▲) BCS at calving. Data are from Holmes (1988) and have been converted to a 1 – 5 BCS scale.

Genetic correlations between BCS and milk yield are always negative (e.g. Veerkamp *et al.*, 2001; Berry *et al.*, 2003; Pryce and Harris, 2006) and the genetic propensity for a modern Holstein cow to lose condition is well known amongst dairy producers. Unfortunately, geneticists do not seem to be able to extract target BCS values from their databases for individual cows because BCS is usually evaluated only once, and at different stages of lactation for different cows (Jones *et al.*, 1999). It is possible, however, to evaluate bulls for changes in average BCS of their daughters at different stages of lactation. Using daughter BCS measurements for six bulls with >1,500 daughters, Jones *et al.* (1999) found significant phenotypic and genetic differences among bulls in the shape of the BCS curves followed by their daughters. Differences were found among bulls in BCS at the beginning and end of lactation, the rate of BCS loss in early lactation, the amount of BCS loss, the stage at which BCS was lowest and the subsequent rate at which BCS was regained during the latter part of the lactation. Three contrasting examples are shown in Figure 4. Daughters of bull A appeared to have a higher target BCS than daughters of bull C. Daughters of bull B experienced relatively little change in BCS throughout lactation. These data suggest that it should be possible to select bulls on the basis of BCS curves of their daughters, but whether genetic BCS curves are related to fertility remains to be seen.

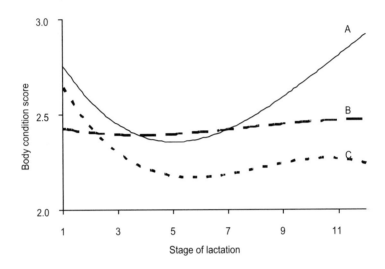

Figure 4. Changes in BCS throughout lactation for daughters of three bulls. Curves are derived from cubic regression coefficients of daughter BCS values. Data are from Jones *et al.* (1999), converted to a 1 – 5 scale.

Dechow *et al.* (2002) examined correlations between BCS and BCS loss in a data set of 310,000 lactation records where multiple BCS evaluations were available for individual cows. Genetics and environment appeared to produce conflicting relationships. Phenotypically, an increase in BCS at calving was associated with more BCS loss in early lactation (correlation 0.54), as expected from the biological principles outlined in this review. Genetically, however, a higher BCS at calving was correlated with less BCS loss during early lactation (correlation -0.15 to -0.48). Management and environmental conditions that increased BCS at calving resulted in more BCS loss in early lactation. However, cows that were genetically inclined to have higher BCS at calving appeared to maintain more BCS in early lactation than genetically thin cows. Therefore, selection for increased BCS at calving would be expected to reduce BCS loss in early lactation and to improve fertility, but to reduce milk yield.

Differences between phenotypic and genetic relationships are seen also for fertility traits and BCS. Pryce *et al.* (2001) studied the effects of BCS change from week 1 to week 10 of lactation on fertility in cows of high and average genetic merit. Phenotypically, an increase of one unit in BCS loss resulted in increases of 21 days to first heat in high-merit cows and 14 days to first heat in average-merit cows; days to first service increased by 14 days per unit BCS loss in high-merit cows, but there was no effect on days to first service in average-merit cows. Genetically, however, BCS at week 10 of lactation was more strongly related to fertility traits than was BCS change because BCS change is influenced greatly by management. In addition, BCS at week 10 had a higher heritability (0.27) than BCS change (0.09). It is likely that BCS at week 10 represents the cow's target BCS, which would have a higher genetic component than BCS change.

These conflicting genetic and phenotypic results emphasise the importance of distinguishing between genetic fatness and phenotypic fatness when comparing studies or making recommendations regarding BCS. Intervention studies, in which cows are matched for breeding value or previous milk yield and in which BCS at calving is manipulated by feeding, will generally reveal phenotypic effects. Large-scale surveys will generally reveal genetic effects, whilst surveys of a small number of farms might include both genetic and phenotypic effects. Genetically thin cows will suffer greater negative energy balance than genetically fat cows if both types have the same BCS at calving. There is a strong case, therefore, for recommending a lower BCS at calving for genetically thin animals.

Body condition score in later lactation and the dry period

The emphasis in the current review, as in most studies, has been on BCS at calving and changes during early lactation. This is because the first 10 to 20 weeks of lactation are the most important for lactation, health and reproduction, and metabolic stress is most likely during this period. There is an abundance of evidence to indicate that a cow has a target BCS that she attempts to reach between 10 and 20 weeks into lactation; her ability to reach that target is governed by feed constraints. In mid- to late-lactation, however, BCS usually increases (e.g. Mao *et al.*, 2004), but is sometimes maintained at target levels (e.g. Yan *et al.*, 2006), and might decrease if feed supply is restricted (e.g. Pryce and Harris, 2006).

Genetic variation is found in the shape of BCS curves, particularly the rate and extent of decline in early lactation (Jones *et al.*, 1999; Mao *et al.*, 2004; Pryce and Harris, 2006), which are clearly related to genetic BCS targets. Genetic and nutritional effects in later lactation are less obvious. In the study of Mao *et al.* (2004), three breeds of cow, fed on two planes of nutrition, reached different BCS nadirs, at different times postpartum. However, the rate of increase in BCS post-nadir was similar for all breeds and feeding systems. On the other hand, rate of increase in BCS post-nadir was influenced by parity; from the first to later parities, BCS nadirs became progressively deeper, but BCS increased post-nadir at faster rates for cows in later parities, especially cows on a low feed level. Chilliard *et al.* (1991) also found no difference in BCS gain between two groups of cows consuming concentrates at 0.27 kg/d or 1.26 kg/d whilst grazing between weeks 20 and 39 of lactation. These results suggest that absolute BCS in later lactation is related to a cow's genetic BCS target in early lactation, but rate of increase in BCS is fixed.

Some studies have observed little or no change in BCS in later lactation, even with different levels of feeding. For example, Yan *et al.* (2006) examined energy partitioning throughout lactation in high-merit Holstein (H) and Norwegian (N) breeds of cow fed on high (H) or low (L) planes of nutrition. From week 15 to week 44 of lactation, HH cows maintained BCS at 2.5; NH cows maintained BCS at 3.1; NL cows maintained BCS at 2.8; in HL cows, BCS decreased from 2.3 to 2.2. These results suggest that BCS targets do not change as lactation progresses in high-merit cows. In later lactation, energy intake was regulated by energy output and the desire to maintain a constant BCS, except in HL cows, where low dietary energy concentration limited energy intake. Similar effects were observed by Chilliard *et al.* (1991) in cows treated with bovine somatotropin (BST). Compared with controls, cows treated with BST lost more BCS in early lactation and maintained this lower BCS until the end of lactation when fed on a high concentrate allowance.

Cows selected under conditions of regular feed restriction appear to respond differently to those selected where feed is not restricted. Pryce and Harris (2006) studied BCS changes in New Zealand cows, which often experience periods of reduced pasture availability in late lactation. Under these conditions, cows that maintained relatively high BCS in early lactation had higher total yields of milk solids because they had body reserves available for mobilisation in late lactation. Roche *et al.* (2006) found that New Zealand Holsteins reached their BCS nadir 14 days earlier than North American Holsteins, and then gained BCS at a faster rate for the rest of lactation, particularly with high concentrate supplementation. These results suggest that New Zealand cows are more sensitive to feed supply and give greater priority to energy reserves when partitioning nutrients.

It is not clear whether BCS usually increases in later lactation because BCS targets vary with stage of lactation, the feedback signal is down-regulated, or different constraints assume priority. Friggens (2003) interpreted increases in BCS during mid- to late-lactation as the cow's investment in future offspring. However, this does not explain increases in BCS observed in non-pregnant cows, nor does it account for the lack of change in BCS observed in some studies. A more likely explanation is that accretion of adipose tissue is passive during mid- to late-lactation. Declining milk yield, coupled with relatively high intake of dry matter, would lead to increases in insulin status. Increasing insulin would encourage deposition of body fat, but feedback from leptin and its associated factors would have a delayed effect on dry matter intake. Chilliard (2001) pointed out that there are several time-scales in ruminant tissue leptin yield and plasma leptin regulation: months for the effect of body fatness; weeks for physiological status or environmental conditions; days for the daily level of intake; and hours or minutes for meal intake or acute metabolic and hormonal regulations.

During the dry period, BCS is more likely to increase than during lactation because plasma insulin is considerably higher in dry cows (Grum *et al.*, 1996). For this reason, producers who wish to increase BCS of cows that are thin at drying off often feed dry cows above their requirements for maintenance and pregnancy. On the other hand, cows with a high BCS at drying off are often fed on a low plane of nutrition so that body fat is mobilised in late gestation. Such practices should be avoided. As shown in previous sections, there is no benefit from higher BCS at calving, which will increase negative energy balance and disease susceptibility. Cows that lose BCS during the dry period are more prone to dystocia (Gearhart *et al.*, 1990; Keady *et al.*, 2005) and are more likely to be culled in their subsequent lactation (Gearhart *et al.*, 1990). The only sensible strategy is to monitor BCS in late lactation and ensure that the cow is dried off with a BCS that is desirable at calving (see next section). Recently there has been interest in reducing the length of the dry period from the traditional 60 days to 30 days or less. Preliminary studies suggest that shortening the dry period improves cow health and reproduction; part of this effect is probably due to reduced BCS gain in the dry period and reduced BCS loss during lactation, as days dry decreased (Rastani and Grummer, 2005).

Body condition score targets for production and fertility

In most countries, increases in milk yield over the past 30 years have been accompanied by reductions in fertility because of unfavourable genetic correlations between milk yield and reproductive traits (Pryce *et al.*, 2004). Poor reproductive performance in high-yielding dairy cows is usually attributed to negative energy balance (Butler, 2003; 2005). For this reason, dairy producers are usually advised to avoid over-fat cows and to feed diets with a high energy concentration. Many papers state that negative energy balance is unavoidable in dairy cows of high genetic merit. As shown in previous sections of the current review, however, this is not true. Cows that calve with a BCS below their target BCS can be in positive energy balance.

Because BCS has a major influence on feed intake and negative energy balance, it is important to evaluate BCS recommendations in relation to genetic targets of cows. If genetic targets decrease with selection for higher milk yield, negative energy balance will become greater if BCS at calving remains high.

According to a brief survey of websites, current UK recommendations for BCS at calving (1-5 scale) are 3.0 (MDC, 2006; DARDNI, 2006) and 2.5 to 3.0 (Defra, 2001). Recommendations in USA and Canada are somewhat higher, but recommendations in New Zealand and Australia are similar to UK values (Table 1). Most recommend that BCS does not fall below 2 to 2.5 at service. Importantly, they also recommend that BCS is the same at drying off and at calving. UK recommendations are 1.3 to 1.8 units (1-5 scale) lower than those made in the 1970s, reflecting either increased awareness of effects of BCS at calving on negative energy balance and fertility, or the difficulty of getting Holstein cows to reach the previous targets.

Table 1. Recommended BCS for dairy cows at drying off, calving and service, published on official web sites accessed in September 2006.

| Country, organisation | BCS at | | Reference |
	Drying off/ calving	Service	
UK, Defra	2.5 – 3.0	2.0 – 3.0	Defra (2001)
UK, MDC	<= 3.0	2.0 – 2.5	MDC (2006)
UK, DARDNI	<= 3.0		DARDNI (2006)
USA, Nebraska	3.5 (3.0 – 4.0)	2.0 (1.5–2.0)	Nebraska (2005)
USA, Penn State	3.25 – 3.5	2.5 – 3.5	Ferguson (2006)
USA, Wisconsin	3.0 – 3.5	2.0	Wattiaux (1999)
Canada, Ontario MAFRA	3.5 (3.0 – 4.0)	2.5 – 3.5	Parker (1996)
New Zealand, Dexcel	2.8 – 3.0[1]		MacDonald and Roche (2004)
Australia, Victoria DPI	3.3 – 3.9[2]		Moran (2006)

[1] Published recommendation: 5–5.5 on 1–10 scale.
[2] Published recommendation: 5–6 on 1–8 scale.

There is evidence from carcass studies that Holstein dairy cows have less external fat and more internal fat than beef breeds (Baber *et al.*, 1984) and, possibly, than Friesians (Kempster *et al.*, 1988). It is likely, therefore, that a modern Holstein cow will have a greater total body fat content than a Friesian cow at the same BCS. In view of the numerical dominance of the Holstein breed, the relevance of BCS could be questioned because BCS assesses subcutaneous fat rather than internal fat. However, strong relationships between BCS and total body fat suggest that BCS is still the best method for monitoring changes in fat reserves.

Recent studies suggest that the lower UK targets are appropriate for optimising production, health and fertility in high-yielding Holstein cows. The relationship between BCS at calving and change in BCS during the first 10-12 weeks of lactation is similar to that seen 20 years ago (Figure 5). BCS at calving predicted to give no change in early lactation has decreased from 2.49 in older studies to 2.10 in recent studies, suggesting that current recommendations are slightly above average biological targets. However, a loss of 0.5 BCS units is considered acceptable and provides a safety margin to allow for variation among cows within a herd. As with any biological parameter, there will be a spread of BCS values and responses among cows. Therefore, it is desirable to assess every cow in a herd at monthly intervals. Unfortunately, few dairy farmers are prepared to make such a commitment. Developments in automatic monitoring of BCS (e.g. Coffey *et al.*, 2003) or a remote BCS service based on digital images (Ferguson *et al.*, 2006) might alleviate the situation and provide early warnings of inappropriate nutrition. In the meantime, attention should be focussed on cows in late lactation and the dry period to ensure that they calve with a BCS of 2.5 to 3.0.

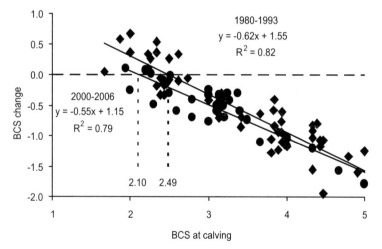

Figure 5. Relationship between BCS at calving and change in BCS over the first 10 – 12 weeks of lactation for studies published 1980 – 1993 (◆) compared with studies published 2000 – 2006 (●). Vertical dotted lines show BCS at calving that result in zero change in BCS, which has decreased from 2.49 in earlier studies to 2.10 in recent studies. Data are group means (converted to a 1 – 5 scale) from Bernabucci *et al.* (2005), Bourchier *et al.* (1987), Garnsworthy and Huggett (1992), Garnsworthy and Jones (1987; 1993), Garnsworthy and Topps (1982), Garnsworthy, Webb, *et al.* (2006: unpublished), Grainger *et al.* (1982), Horan (2005), Jones and Garnsworthy (1988; 1989), Lactera *et al.* (2005), Land and Leaver (1980; 1981), MacMillan *et al.* (1982), Meikle *et al.* (2004), Reist *et al.* (2003), Roche *et al.* (2006), Stockdale (2000; 2004; 2005), Treacher *et al.* (1986), Yan *et al.* (2006).

Conclusions

As stated in the introduction, BCS is a useful management tool for assessing the nutritional status of dairy cows. The numerical scale used is not important within farms or studies, although further comparisons of scales might be useful for comparing studies and for comparing animals across national boundaries. Even though BCS is subjective, consistency can be achieved within and between operators, especially with training. BCS correlates well with body fat content and provides a better indication of energy reserves than live weight.

Changes in BCS during early lactation highlight the role of body fat in controlling feed intake. The strong relationship between BCS at calving and change in BCS provides compelling evidence that cows have a target BCS in early lactation. Cows that are fatter than their target BCS mobilise body fat; cows that are thinner than their target BCS gain body fat. The rate at which a cow changes BCS towards its target is affected by diet composition as well as current BCS; low energy and high protein diets increase BCS loss in cows that are above target BCS; low energy diets reduce BCS gain in cows that are below target BCS.

Recent reports indicate that average target BCS is lower now than it was in the 1980s. This is because cows selected for higher milk yield over the past thirty years are genetically thinner, so they have a stronger drive to mobilise body fat. Consequently, cows of high genetic merit are likely to experience deeper and more prolonged negative energy balance in early lactation. Negative energy balance is undesirable because it reduces reproductive performance and increases susceptibility to diseases. Therefore, short-term financial gains in extra milk production from cows that are fat at calving will be offset by longer-term financial losses through premature culling. Changes in BCS during the dry period are undesirable, so BCS should be monitored and adjusted in late lactation to ensure that cows are dried off with a BCS appropriate for calving.

To reduce the impact of negative energy balance on cow health and performance, BCS at calving should be no more than 0.5 BCS units above a cow's target BCS. Cows of low genetic merit for milk yield (target BCS 2.5-3.0) should calve with BCS of 3.0 or less; cows of high genetic merit for milk yield (target BCS 2.0-2.25) should calve with BCS of 2.75 or less. The most important message for producers is that increasing BCS at calving exacerbates negative energy balance problems instead of overcoming them.

References

Agricultural Research Council (1980). *The Nutrient Requirements of Ruminant Livestock - Technical Review by an Agricultural Research Council Working Party.* Commonwealth Agricultural Bureaux, Slough, UK.

Baber, P.L., Rowlinson, P., Willis, M.B. and Chalmers, A.J. (1984). A comparison of Canadian Holstein x British Friesian and British Friesian steers for beef-production. 2. Carcass characteristics. *Animal Production*, **38**, 407-415.

Bernabucci, U., Ronchi, B., Lacetera, N. and Nardone, A. (2005). Influence of body condition score on relationships between metabolic status and oxidative stress in periparturient dairy cows. *Journal of Dairy Science*, **88**, 2017–2026.

Berry, D.P., Buckley, F., Dillon, P., Evans, R.D., Rath, M. and Veerkamp, R.F. (2003). Genetic parameters for body condition score, body weight, milk yield and fertility estimated using random regression models. *Journal of Dairy Science*, **86**, 3704–3717.

Bourchier, C.P., Garnsworthy, P.C, Hutchinson, J.M. And Benton, T.A. (1987) The relationship between milk yield, body condition and reproductive performance in high-yielding dairy cows. *Animal Production*, **44**, 460.

Broster, W.H. (1971) The effect on milk yield of the cow of the level of feeding before calving. *Dairy Science Abstracts*, **33** 253-270.

Broster, W.H. and Broster, V.J. (1998). Body score of dairy cows. *Journal of Dairy Research*, **65**, 155–173.

Butler, W.R. (2003). Energy balance relationships with follicular development, ovulation and fertility in postpartum dairy cows. *Livestock Production Science*, **83**, 211-218.

Butler, W.R. (2005). Nutrition, negative energy balance and fertility in the postpartum dairy cow. *Cattle Practice*, **13**, 13-18.

Chilliard, Y., Bonnet, M., Delavaud, C., Faulconnier, Y., Leroux, C., Djiane, J., and Bocquier F. (2001). Leptin in ruminants. Gene expression in adipose tissue and mammary gland, and regulation of plasma concentration. *Domestic Animal Endocrinology*, **21**, 271–295.

Chilliard, Y., Cissé, M., Lefaivre, R. and Reyond, B. (1991). Body composition of dairy cows according to lactation stage, somatotropin treatment, and concentrate supplementation. *Journal of Dairy Science*, **74**, 3103–3116.

Coffey, M.P., Mottram, T.B. and McFarlane, N. (2003). A feasibility study on the automatic recording of condition score in dairy cows. *Proceedings of the British Society of Animal Science 2002*, 131.

Cooper, M.D. (1990) Relationship of changes in condition score to cow health in Holsteins. *Journal of Dairy Science*, **73**, 3132–3140.

DARDNI (2006) Farm Managment Notes For July 2006. PA181/A/06. Department of Agriculture and Rural Development Northern Ireland. http://www.dardni.gov.uk/

Dechow, C.D., Rogers, G.W. and Clay, J.S. (2002). Heritability and correlations among body condition score loss, body condition score, production traits and reproductive performance. *Journal of Dairy Science*, **85**, 3062–3070.

Defra (2001). *Condition Scoring of Dairy Cows.* Publication PB6492, Department for Environment, Food & Rural Affairs, London, UK. Available online at http://www.defra.gov.uk/corporate/publications/pubcat/anh.htm

Defra (2003) *Code of Recommendations for the Welfare of Livestock: Cattle.* Publication PB7949, Department for Environment, Food & Rural Affairs, London, UK.

Earle, D.F. (1976). A guide to scoring dairy cow condition. *Journal of Agriculture (Victoria)*, **74**, 228–231.

Ellis, J.L., Qiao, F. and Cant, J.P. (2006) Prediction of dry matter intake throughout lactation in a dynamic model of dairy cow performance. *Journal of Dairy Science*, **89**, 1558–1570.

Ferguson, J.D. (2006) *Implementation of a Body Condition Scoring Program in Dairy Herds.* http://cahpwww.vet.upenn.edu/dairy/bcs.html [accessed 12 September 2006]

Ferguson, J.D., Azzaro, G. and Licitra, G. (2006). Body condition assessment using digital images. *Journal of Dairy Science*, **89**, 3833–3841.

Ferguson, J.D., Galligan, D.T. and Thomsen N. (1994). Principal descriptors of body condition in Holstein dairy cattle. *Journal of Dairy Science*, **77**, 2695–2703.

Fouladi-Nashta, A.A., Gutierrez, C.G., Garnsworthy, P.C. and Webb, R. (2005). Effects of dietary carbohydrate source on oocyte/embryo quality and development in high-yielding, lactating dairy cattle. *Biology of Reproduction Special Issue* 135-136.

Fox, D.G., Tylutki, T.P., Tedeschi, L.O., Van Amburgh, M.E., Chase, L.E., Pell, A.N., Overton, T.R. and Russell. J.B. (2004). The Net Carbohydrate and Protein System for evaluating herd nutrition and nutrient excretion. *Animal Feed Science and Technology*, **112**, 29–78.

Friggens, N.C. (2003). Body lipid reserves and the reproductive cycle: towards a better understanding. *Livestock Production Science*, **83**, 219–236.

Jorritsma, R., Jorritsma, H., Schukken, Y.H., Bartlett, P.C., Wensing, T. and Wentink, G.H. (2001). Prevalence and indicators of post partum fatty infiltration of the liver in nine commercial dairy herds in the Netherlands. *Livestock Producton Science*, **68**, 53-60.

Garnsworthy, P.C. (1988). The effect of energy reserves at calving on performance of dairy cows. In *Nutrition and Lactation in the Dairy Cow* (Ed. P. C. Garnsworthy). pp. 157-170. Butterworths, London, UK.

Garnsworthy, P.C. (1994) Prediction of intake by dairy cows in early lactation from milk yield and body condition. *Proceedings 45th Annual Meeting European Association for Animal Production*, Edinburgh, 123.

Garnsworthy, P.C., Cole, D.J.A., Grantley-Smith, M., Jones, D.W. and Peters, A.R. (1986). The effect of feeding period and trenbolone acetate on the potential of culled dairy cows for beef production. *Animal Production*, **43**, 385-390.

Garnsworthy, P.C. and Huggett, C.D. (1992). The influence of the fat concentration of the diet on the response by dairy-cows to body condition at calving. *Animal Production*, **54**, 7-13.

Garnsworthy, P.C. and Jones, G.P. (1987). The influence of body condition at calving and dietary protein supply on voluntary food intake and performance in dairy cows. *Animal Production*, **44**, 347-353.

Garnsworthy, P.C. and Jones, G.P. (1993). The effects of dietary fibre and starch concentrations on the response by dairy-cows to body condition at calving. *Animal Production*, **57**, 15-21.

Garnsworthy, P.C. and Topps, J.H. (1982). The effect of body condition of dairy cows at calving on their food intake and performance when given complete diets. *Animal Production*, **35**, 113-119.

Garnsworthy, P.C. and Webb, R. (1999) The Influence of nutrition on fertility in dairy cows. In *Recent Advances in Animal Nutrition - 1999* (Eds P.C. Garnsworthy and J. Wiseman), 39-57, Nottingham University Press, Nottingham, UK.

Gearhart, M.A., Curtis, C.R., Erb, H.N., Smith, R.D., Sniffen, C.J. Chase, L.E. and Cooper, M.D. (1990). Relationship of changes in condition score to cow health in Holsteins. *Journal of Dairy Science*, **73**, 3132-3140.

Gillund, P., Reksen, O., Gröhn, Y. T. and Karlberg, K. (2001). Body condition related to ketosis and reproductive performance in Norwegian dairy cows. *Journal of Dairy Science*, **84**, 1390–1396.

Gong, J.G., Lee, W.J., Garnsworthy, P.C. and Webb, R. (2002). Effect of dietary-induced increases in circulating insulin concentrations during the early postpartum period on reproductive function in dairy cows. *Reproduction*, **123**, 419-427.

Grainger, C., Wilhelms, G.D. and McGowan, A.A. (1982). Effect of body condition at calving and level of feeding in early lactation on milk production of dairy cows. *Australian Journal of Experimental Agriculture and Animal Husbandry*, **22**, 9–17.

Gregory, N.G., Robins, J.K., Thomas, D.G. and Purchas, R.W. (1998). Relationship between body condition score and body composition in dairy cows. *New Zealand Journal of Agricultural Research*, **41**, 527–532.

Grum, D.E., Drackley, J.K., Younker, R.S., Lacount, D.W. and Veenhulzen, J.J. (1996). Nutrition during the dry period and hepatic lipid metabolism of periparturient dairy cows. *Journal of Dairy Science*, **79**, 1850–1864.

Grummer, R.R. (1993). Etiology of lipid-related metabolic disorders in periparturient dairy cows. *Journal of Dairy Science*, **76**, 3882–3896.

Hill, R.A. (2004). The role of the leptin axis in modulating energy patitioning and nutrient utilisation in livestock species. In *Recent Advances in Animal Nutrition - 2004* (Eds P.C. Garnsworthy and J. Wiseman), 149-184. Nottingham University Press, Nottingham, UK.

Holmes, C.W. (1988). Genetic merit and efficiency of milk production by the dairy cow. In *Nutrition and Lactation in the Dairy Cow* (Ed. P. C. Garnsworthy). pp. 195-215. Butterworths, London, UK.

Horan, B., Dillon, P., Faverdin, P., Delaby, L., Buckley, F. and Rath, M. (2005). The interaction of strain of Holstein-Friesian cows and pasture-based feed systems on milk yield, body weight, and body condition score. *Journal of Dairy Science*, **88**, 1231–1243.

Jones, G.P. and Garnsworthy, P.C. (1988). The effects of body condition at calving and dietary protein content on dry matter intake and performance in lactating dairy cows given diets of low energy content. *Animal Production*, **47**, 321-333.

Jones, G.P. and Garnsworthy, P.C. (1989). Effects of dietary energy content on the response of dairy cows to body condition at calving. *Animal Production*, **49**, 183-191.

Jones, H.E., White, I.M.S. and Brotherstone, S. (1999). Genetic evaluation of Holstein-Friesian sires for daughter condition-score changes using random regression model. *Animal Science*, **68**, 467–475.

Keady, T.W.J., Mayne, C.S., Kilpatrick, D.J. and McCoy, M.A. (2005). Effect of level and source of nutrients in late gestation on subsequent milk yield and composition and fertility of dairy cows. *Livestock Production Science*, **94**, 237-248.

Kempster, A.J., Cook, G.L. and Southgate, J.R. (1988). Evaluation of British Friesian, Canadian Holstein and beef breed x British Friesian steers slaughtered over a commercial range of fatness from 16-month and 24-month beef-production systems. 2. Carcass characteristics, and rate and efficiency of lean gain. *Animal Production*, **46**, 365-378.

Kennedy, G.C. (1953). The role of depot fat in the hypothalamic control of food intake in the rat. *Proceedings of the Royal Society, Series B*, **139**, 578–592.

Keown, J.F. (2005) *How to Body Condition Score Dairy Animals*. NebGuide No G1583, University of Nebraska – Lincoln, USA. http://www.ianrpubs.unl.edu/epublic/pages/index.jsp [accessed 12 September 2006]

Kristensen, E., Dueholm, L., Vink, D., Andersen, J.E., Jakobsen, E.B., Illum-Nielsen, S., Petersen, F.A. and Enevoldsen, C. (2006). Within- and across-person uniformity of body condition scoring in Danish Holstein cattle. *Journal of Dairy Science*, **89**, 3721–3728.

Lacetera, N., Scalia, D., Bernabucci, U., Ronchi, B., Pirazzi, D.and Nardone A. (2005). Lymphocyte functions in overconditioned cows around parturition. *Journal of Dairy Science*, **88**, 2010–2016.

Land, C. and Leaver, J.D. (1980). The effect of body condition at calving on the milk production and feed intake of dairy cows. *Animal Production*, **30**, 449 (Abstract).

Land, C. and Leaver, J.D. (1981). The effect of body condition at calving on the production of Friesian cows and heifers. *Animal Production*, **32**, 362–363 (Abstract).

Lopez-Gatius, F., Yaniz, J. and Madriles-Helm, D. (2003). Effects of body condition score and score change on the reproductive performance of dairy cows: a meta-analysis. *Theriogenology*, **59**, 801-812.

Lowman, B.G., Scott, N. and Somerville, S. (1973). *Condition Scoring of Cattle*. East of Scotland College of Agriculture, Bulletin No. 6, Edinburgh, UK.

MacDonald, K. and Roche, J. (2004) *Condition Scoring Made Easy*. Dexcel, Hamilton, New Zealand. http://www.dexcel.co.nz/data/usr/ACF6AB.pdf [accessed 12 September 2006]

MacMillan, K.L., Bryant, A.M. and Duganzich, D.M. (1982). Production differences associated with body condition score at calving and production index among cows in commercial herds. In *Proceedings of the Conference on Dairy Production from Pasture*. (Eds K.L. Macmillan and V.K. Taufa) pp. 174–175. Clark and Matheson Ltd, Hamilton, New Zealand [Cited by Stockdale, 2001].

Mao, I.L., Sloniewski, K., Madsen, P. and Jensen, J. (2004). Changes in body condition score and in its genetic variation during lactation. *Livestock Production Science*, **89**, 55–65.

Markusfeld, O., Galon, N. and Ezra, E. (1997). Body condition score, health, yield and fertility in dairy cows. *Veterinary Record*, **141**, 67-72.

MDC (2006) *Economic feeding for high fertility*. Project No. 99/T2/17. Milk

Development Council. http://www.mdc.org.uk/ [accessed 12 September 2006]

Meikle, A., Kulcsar, M., Chilliard, Y., Febel, H., Delavaud, C., Cavestany, D. and Chilibroste, P. (2004). Effects of parity and body condition at parturition on endocrine and reproductive parameters of the cow. *Reproduction*, **127, 727**–737.

Moran, J. (2006) *Weighing and Condition Scoring of Replacement Heifers and Dairy Cows*. Agriculture Note AG0505, Department of Primary Industries, State of Victoria, Australia. http://www.dpi.vic.gov.au/notes/ [accessed 12 September 2006]

Mulvany, P. (1977). *Dairy Cow Condition Scoring*. National Institute for Research in Dairying, Handout No. 4468, Reading, UK.

National Research Council (2001). *Nutrient Requirements of Dairy Cattle*. National Academies Press, Washington DC, USA.

Newbold, J.R. (2005) Liver function in dairy cows. In *Recent Advances in Animal Nutrition - 2005* (Eds P.C. Garnsworthy and J. Wiseman), 257-291. Nottingham University Press, Nottingham, UK.

Otto, K.L., Ferguson, J.D., Fox, D.G. and Sniffen, C.J. (1991). Relationship between body condition score and composition of the ninth to eleventh rib tissue in Holstein dairy cows. *Journal of Dairy Science*, **74**, 852–859.

Parker, R. (1996) *Using Body Condition Scoring in Dairy Herd Management*. Factsheet 94-053, Ontario Ministry of Agriculture, Food and Rural Affairs, Canada. http://www.omafra.gov.on.ca/english/livestock/dairy/facts/94-053.htm [accessed 12 September 2006]

Pryce, J.E., Coffey, M.P. and Simm, G. (2001). The relationship between body condition score and reproductive performance. *Journal of Dairy Science*, **84**, 1508–1515.

Pryce, J.E. and Harris, B.L. (2006). Genetics of body condition score in New Zealand dairy cows. *Journal of Dairy Science*, **89**, 4424–4432.

Pryce, J.E., Royal, M.D., Garnsworthy, P.C. and Mao I.L. (2004) Fertility in the high producing dairy cow. *Livestock Production Science*, **86**, 125-135.

Rasmussen, L.K., Nielsen, B.L., Pryce, J.E., Mottram, T.T. and Veerkamp, R.F. (1999). Risk factors associated with the incidence of ketosis in dairy cows. *Animal Science*, **68**, 379–386.

Rastani, R.R. and Grummer, R.R. (2005) Consequences of shortening the dry period in dairy cows. In *Recent Advances in Animal Nutrition - 2005* (Eds P.C. Garnsworthy and J. Wiseman), 293-314. Nottingham University Press, Nottingham, UK.

Reid, I.M., Roberts, C.J., Treacher, R.J. and Williams, L.A. (1986). Effect of body condition at calving on tissue mobilization, development of fatty liver and blood chemistry of dairy cows. *Animal Production*, **43**, 7–15.

Reist, M., Erdin, D., von Euw, D., Tschuemperlin, K., Leuenberger, H., Delavaud, C., Chilliard, Y., Hammon, H.M., Kuenzi, N. and Blum, J.W. (2003). Concentrate feeding strategy in lactating dairy cows: metabolic and endocrine changes with emphasis on leptin. *Journal of Dairy Science*, **86**, 1690–1706.

Roche, J.R., Berry, D.P. and Kolver, E.S. (2006). Holstein-Friesian strain and feed effects on milk production, body weight, and body condition score profiles in grazing dairy cows. *Journal of Dairy Science*, **89**, 3532–3543.

Roche, J.R., Dillon, P.G., Stockdale, C.R., Baumgard, L.H. and VanBaale, M.J. (2004). Relationships among international body condition scoring systems. *Journal of Dairy Science*, **87**, 3076–3079.

Stockdale, C.R. (2000). Differences in body condition and body size affect the responses of grazing dairy cows to high-energy supplements in early lactation. *Australian Journal of Experimental Agriculture*, **40**, 903–911.

Stockdale, C.R. (2001). Body condition at calving and the performance of dairy cows in early lactation under Australian conditions: a review. *Australian Journal of Experimental Agriculture,* 2001, **41**, 823–839.

Stockdale, C.R. (2004). Effects of level of feeding of concentrates during early lactation on the yield and composition of milk from grazing dairy cows with varying body condition score at calving. *Australian Journal of Experimental Agriculture*, **44**, 1-9.

Stockdale, C.R. (2005). Investigating the interaction between body condition at calving and pre-calving energy and protein nutrition on the early lactation performance of dairy cows. *Australian Journal of Experimental Agriculture*, **45**, 1507-1518.

Treacher, R.J., Reid, I.M. and Roberts, C.J. (1986). Effect of body condition at calving on the health and performance of dairy cows. *Animal Production*, **43**, 1–6.

Veerkamp, R.F., Koenen, E.P.C. and De Jong, G. (2001). Genetic correlations among body condition score, yield, and fertility in first-parity cows estimated by random regression models. *Journal of Dairy Science*, **84**, 2327–2335.

Vernon, R.G., Denis, R.G.P. and Sørensen, A. (2001). Signals of adiposity. *Domestic Animal Endocrinology*, **21**, 197–214.

Ward, W.R., Murray, R.D. White, A.R. and Rees, E.M. (1995). The use of blood biochemistry for determining the nutritional status of dairy cows

In: *Recent Advances in Animal Nutrition – 1995* (Eds P.C. Garnsworthy and D.J.A. Cole), 29-51. Nottingham University Press, Nottingham, UK.

Wattiaux, M.A. (1999) *Body Condition Scores.* Dairy Essentials 12. Babcock Institute for International Dairy Research and Development, University of Wisconsin-Madison, USA. http://www.babcock.wisc.edu/downloads/de/12.en.pdf [accessed 12 September 2006]

Wildman, E.E., Jones, G.M., Wagner, P.E., Boman, R.L., Troutt, H.F. and Lesch, T.N. (1982). A dairy cow body condition scoring system and its relationship to selected production characteristics. *Journal of Dairy Science*, **65**, 495–501.

Wright, I.A. and Russel, A.J.F. (1984). Partition of fat, body composition and body condition score in mature cows. *Animal Production*, **38**, 23–32.

Yan, T., Agnew, R.E. and Mayne, C.S. (2005) Prediction of body weight and composition in lactating dairy cows: Relationship between body condition score and body composition. *Proceedings of the British Society of Animal Science 2002*, 19.

Yan, T., Mayne, C.S., Keady, T.W.J. and Agnew, R.E. (2006). Effects of dairy cow genotype with two planes of nutrition on energy partitioning between milk and body tissue. *Journal of Dairy Science*, **89**, 1031–1042.

5

EXTENDED LACTATIONS IN INTENSIVE AND PASTURE-BASED DAIRYING

K.L. MACMILLAN,[1] C. GRAINGER, [2] M.J. AULDIST [2]

[1] *Department of Veterinary Science, University of Melbourne, Werribee, 3030, Australia;* [2] *Department of Primary Industries, Ellinbank, VIC 3821, Australia*

Introduction

The historical focus for breeding management in most developed dairy industries has been to maintain 12-month calving intervals (CI) so as to maximise milk yield/cow/annum and per cow/lifetime. The calvings within a herd may occur throughout much of the year (year-round calving), or be concentrated into a single period of about 12 weeks (seasonal calving). Year-round calving is most common in industries where most milk is consumed fresh and only the surplus is processed as powder, butter, cheese or casein. Seasonal calving is typical of industries that process most milk into dairy products that are consumed locally or exported.

Since the net price received for milk processed for export is usually less than that received for "liquid" milk, industries with seasonal calving patterns utilise lower cost production systems based on grazing pasture *in situ* with only limited grain supplementation provided during milking. This means that cows in seasonally calving herds may average only around 5000 litres of milk per cow per year in a lactation averaging 290 to 310 days (VandeHaar and St-Pierre, 2006). Cows in confined feeding systems may average from 5,000 to 15,000 litres of milk/cow/year (as a "rolling herd" average), but will have average lactation lengths of over 400 days. VandeHaar and St-Pierre (2006) estimated that the "efficiency" of land use with a seasonal calving, pasture-based system was about 43% compared to 47% for 15,000 litre confined feeding systems without by-product feeds and up to 93% for 15,000 litre systems with by-product feeds.

The calculations of VandeHaar and St-Pierre (2006) did not take into account payment systems that could be based on yield of milk solids and did not consider return on capital. Nonetheless, high levels of feed input to achieve high levels of milk yield had higher net energy efficiency because of the "dilution of maintenance" (VandeHaar and St-Pierre, 2006). However, no consideration was given to increasingly high replacement rates in herds of high producing Holstein cows with reduced fertility (Lucy, 2001; Moore & Thatcher, 2006). Plaizier *et al.* (1997) modelled the effect of declining reproductive performance to show that each one day increase in calving interval, mainly through higher replacement and reduced lifetime milk yield reduced net revenue of a Canadian Holstein herd by \$4.7 CAN/cow/extra day of CI (Plaizier *et al.*, 1997). Since the objective was to achieve a 12-month calving interval, actual calving intervals of from 13 months to 14.9 months represented losses of from \$146 CAN to \$423 CAN/cow.

Effects of declining reproductive performance and survival in Irish dairy cattle, as a consequence of an increasing proportion of Holstein genes, were described by Dillon *et al.* (2006). The financial implications of this decline were measured by Evans *et al.* (2006) in 14 seasonally calving herds. Milk yield/cow had increased by 12% and milk sales/herd (in the absence of quota) had increased by 19% over the 14-year study period. Annual replacement costs had increased by 47% because herd replacement rate had increased from 16% to 27%. These authors estimated that in a quota-free system the potential increase in profitability due to higher production per cow had been halved by the decline in reproductive performance (Evans *et al.*, 2006).

The likely impacts of declining fertility will vary between year-round and seasonal calving systems. In seasonal calving systems, unplanned herd wastage and replacement rate will increase; herd average age and within herd selection rate will decrease. This presumes that it is unprofitable for herds with seasonal calving systems to milk cows through the "dry" period or to carry them for one unproductive season. In contrast, year-round calving herds have greater scope to continue to milk any cow for more than a 12-month CI provided that the income from lower daily milk yield is greater than the marginal feeding costs. This may mean that average yield/cow/year is reduced, but so are the costs of increased replacement rate.

The widely reported declines in fertility for Holstein strains of dairy cows, in dairy industries with year-round calving systems, have not led to many systematic studies on breeding and managing cows for extended lactations. This is in spite of the fact that many herds have CIs averaging 14 months or more, as well as the widespread use of a sustained release formulation of bovine somatotrophin (bST) in cows with longer CIs in American herds.

Extended lactions in high production systems

Holstein cows that produced above herd average milk yields in 19 Israeli herds were enrolled in a study that compared production related effects of delaying the interval from calving to first insemination by 60 days (Arbel *et al.*, 2001). It was assumed that the effect of intentionally extending the voluntary waiting period (VWP) would be "more pronounced in high yielding cows". The results showed that extending VWP by 60 days increased days open and CI by similar extensions in primiparous cows (61 and 59 days respectively; Table 1), but by fewer days in multiparous cows (50 and 47 days respectively; Table 1). The net income/cow/day of CI was increased slightly with the longer VWPs in both parity groups (19 cents and 12 cents, respectively). Lifetime yield was estimated to increase by about 14% even though conception rate to first insemination and wastage rate were not altered by extending the VWP.

Table 1. Effects of extending the voluntary waiting period (VWP) for an extra 60 days in high producing Holstein cows on days open, calving interval (CI) and selected milk yield parameters (Arbel *et al.*, 2001)

Parity	VWP (days)	Days open	CI (days)	Total milk (l/cow)	Milk/CI day[a] (l)	Net income[b] ($/day)	Milk / day2[c] (l)
Primiparous	90	128	405	10678	26.4	3.42	40.8
	150	189	464	12518	27.0	3.61	43.3
Multiparous	60	110	389	12208	31.4	4.34	44.2
	120	160	436	13518	31.0	4.46	44.8

a   milk yield/day of CI
b   net daily return/cow/day of CI
c   milk yield/cow/day for first 150 days of the following lactation

High producing Holsteins were also used in a Cornell University study that compared an extension in the VWP from 60 to 150 days, but with supplementation with bovine somatotrophin (bST) (van Amburgh *et al.*, 1997) from 63 days post-calving. The longer VWP was expected to allow a CI of 16.5 months to be maintained. However, the actual days open in this treatment group was 212 days, corresponding to a CI of 18 months. The figures in Table 2 are based on results for this longer CI and show similar trends to those in Table 1. Milk volume per day of CI was only one litre less for the longer CI and daily protein yields were almost identical. These authors calculated that the longer interval between calvings had beneficial effects on overall health and on days of productive life (+30%) as well as reducing annual culling rate from 34.5% to 25.3%. Cumulatively, these changes improved profitability by $ 0.75/day of productive life, or $ 1191/cow/lifetime. The authors also found that response to bST increased with longer calving intervals.

Table 2. Effects of extending the voluntary waiting period (VWP) by an extra 90 days in high producing Holstein cows receiving bovine somatotrophin (bST) from 63 days post-calving (van Amburgh *et al.*, 1997)

VWP (days)	Lactation (days)	Days open	CI (days)	Total milk (l/cow)	Milk/CI day (l)	Total protein (kg)	Protein/ CI day
60	364	122	401	11583	28.9	371	0.93
150	486	212	547	15255	27.9	504	0.92

Effect of parity with extended calving intervals

An interesting feature of the trials conducted by van Amburgh *et al.* (1997) was the comparison between primiparous and multiparous cows that were not inseminated for over 500 days. Cows in both groups received bST from early lactation. Primiparous cows out-yielded their older contemporaries in the first 486 days of lactation (16,603 vs 15,128 l/cow) because of higher persistency. Daily milk yield at 486 days was 83% of peak yield (38 vs 46 l/cow/day).

Cows of the Swedish Red and White breed were used by Osterman and Bertilsson (2003) in a 3-year study to compare extending the CI from a target of 12 months to one of 18 months in primiparous and multiparous cows that were milked two or three times daily. Energy-corrected milk (ECM)/day of CI was affected by milking frequency (x2 vs x3; $p = 0.05$), but not by CI ($p = 0.73$), and there was no interaction between CI and milking frequency ($p = 0.20$). The results in Table 3 are for cows milked twice daily. Cows with the longer CI had daily ECM yields averaging 94% of contemporaries with the shorter CI. Protein yields averaged 92% of contemporaries. As with Arbel *et al.* (2001), the Swedish study showed that primiparous cows were favoured by the longer CI. Primiparous cows increased daily ECM yield by 1.1 kg, whereas multiparous cows reduced ECM yield by 1.2 kg/d. However, multiparous cows had a greater response to three times daily milking. The authors concluded that: "By combining longer calving intervals with increased milking frequency, the milk production per day from one calving to another might be higher than in a traditional calving interval" (Osterman and Bertilsson, 2003). Alternatively, testing the ability of primiparous cows to tolerate or benefit from an extended lactation could be less risky and prove to be a useful phenotypic assessment of their ability to be milked for longer lactations.

Table 3. Effects of extending calving intervals (CI) from 12 to 18 months on energy-corrected milk yield (ECM) of Swedish Red and White cows (Osterman & Bertilsson, 2003)

CI (days)	Total ECM (l/cow)	ECM/CI day (l)	Total protein (kg)	Protein/CI day (kg)
358	8262	22.7	265	0.74
545	11631	21.3	371	0.68

Effect of genotype on extended lactations

A series of studies in Ireland compared the productive and reproductive capacity of Holstein-Friesians that were typical of Irish commercial cows (HD) with those from New Zealand (NZ) or were genetically of American origin (HP). The NZ cows had been derived from a pasture-based system with seasonally-concentrated calving (also typical of Irish herds), whereas HP Holsteins were derived from high production, intensively managed feedlot systems in which cows calved in most months of each year (Dillon *et al.*, 2006). Results obtained by Horan *et al.* (2005) in comparing strain differences in changes in body condition score (BCS) and in response to grain supplementation with pasture showed the extent of the genetic differences that have developed in the different production environments. A BCS difference of 0.20 between HP and NZ cows at calving increased to 0.29 at first insemination and to 0.45 at drying off (Table 4). HP cows continued to lose BCS throughout lactation and after first insemination, whereas HD cows retained BCS and NZ cows regained some of the BCS lost in early lactation.

The strain differences were also reflected in responses to supplements. Providing additional concentrate supplement to HP cows significantly increased yield with little effect on pasture intake. By contrast, NZ cows had only half the increase in yield and reduced their pasture intake (Table 4).

Table 4. Strain differences in body condition score (BCS) and responses to supplementation among High Production Holsteins (HP), High Durability Irish Friesians (HD) and New Zealand Friesians (NZ) (Horan *et al.*, 2005)

| | *Strain* | | |
	HP	*HD*	*NZ*
Milk yield (kg/cow)	6958	6584	6141
BCS (1 – 5):			
at calving	3.17	3.24	3.37
at 1st service	2.78	2.93	3.07
at drying off	2.68	2.93	3.13
Response to supplements (kg milk/kg DM concentrates)	1.10	1.0	0.55
Pasture substitution rate (kg grass DM/kg DM concentrates)	0.19	0.35	0.51

These strain differences are of relevance to interpreting results obtained by Kolver *et al.* (2006). They compared the productive ability of two of the strains included in the Irish studies that they referred to as OS Holsteins or NZ Friesians. The 56 cows grazed an abundant supply of fresh pasture and received 0, 3 or 6 kg DM of a grain supplement/day until they were producing < 4 kg milk/day, or they were 60 days from calving with a CI of 24 months. Mean calving date for the 56 cows was 28 July 2003. Only 14% (4/29) of the NZ cows were still being milked at final drying off on 6 May 2005, compared with 48% (13/27) of the OS cows. However, 93% of the cows were milked for over 500 days. The summarised results in Table 5 show the differences in milk yield between the two strains. They also show that 300-day yields of milk solids (MS) were similar, except for the lower response of the NZ cows to the higher level of supplement. The most relevant difference in terms of strain effects on genetic potential for completing an extended lactation involving a CI of 2 years is the MS ratio. This reflects yield beyond 300 days compared to yield in the first 300 days. This ratio averaged 0.945 for the OS cows compared to 0.785 for the NZ cows. Feeding grain to the NZ cows did not affect this ratio, but the supplement did contribute to gross obesity to a greater extent than in the OS cows. The equivalent ratios for milk yields were 0.03 to 0.06 less than for MS, but those for protein were from 0.02 to 0.08 higher.

Table 5. Comparative yield, body condition score (BCS) and annualised yields for OS Holsteins and NZ Friesians that had calving intervals of 2 years and were fed fresh pasture with or without grain supplements (Kolver *et al.*, 2006)

Strain		*NZ*			*OS*	
Supplement (kg grain / day)	*0*	*3*	*6*	*0*	*3*	*6*
Days in milk	595	608	567	623	604	630
Milk yield (kg)	8908	10929	9931	10814	13962	15448
Milk protein (kg)	340	411	369	404	522	564
Annualised MS (kg) [a]	381	460	395	441	555	590
Normal lactation MS(kg) [b]	489	551	530	494	556	625
MS ratio [c]	0.79	0.83	0.74	0.89	1.00	0.94
BCS (1-10):						
calving	5.78	5.99	5.81	5.78	5.45	5.89
drying off	7.74	8.53	9.03	6.30	6.10	7.26

[a] annualised milk solids = total protein averaged over 2 years
[b] normal lactation milk solids = milk fat + milk protein produced in first 300 days
[c] MS yield >300days/ MS yield up to 300days

None of the interactions involving strain with diet in relation to this ratio was statistically significant (p>0.17). Kolver *et al.* (2006) concluded that "productive extended lactations of up to 650 days are biologically possible on a range of pasture diets". The OS cows were clearly better suited than the NZ cows because of their ability to produce beyond 300 days. Although reducing the CI to 18 months could also reduce the genotype difference in yield, the OS cows would still have had the greater potential.

Effects of calving interval and level of nutrition in pasture-based systems

Two of the largest studies on extended lactations were conducted at the Ellinbank Dairy Research Centre in Victoria from 2003 to 2006. The first trial involved 125 Holstein cows that were grazed in a single herd with a minimum daily intake of approximately 180 MJ ME/cow/day. They received up to 1.5 tonnes of grain/cow/annum and were divided into 5 groups that were managed to have CIs of 12, 15, 18, 21 or 24 months by varying the date when AI was commenced. The cows with the 12-month CI completed two lactations during the trial.

Cows with CIs of 15 and 18 months had annualised yields of protein and milk fat that were equal to those of cows that had two lactations with a CI of 12 months. Milk yields were only slightly less (Table 6). The longer CIs of 21 and 24 months slightly reduced yields. However, only 83% and 42% of cows in these two groups had lactations for the designated periods of 19 and 22 months, respectively.

Since there was wide individual cow variation in daily yields beyond 300 days, the results indicate that some of the Holstein cows in this study would have had higher annualised yields for milk, protein or milk fat because they had extended lactations, especially with CIs of 15 or 18 months.

The second trial measured effects of level of nutrition on extended lactation yields. 96 cows were each allocated to one of four groups. The first group was fed a pasture and grain diet of about 160 MJ ME/cow/day designed to produce 385 kg MS in a lactation of 300 days (12-month CI). This group calved twice over the 2 years of the trial. Cows in the remaining three groups only calved once. One of these groups received a similar ration to the group with a 12-month CI. The other group received more grain to raise daily intake to 180 MJ ME/cow/day (as in the first trial). The fourth group was fed indoors with a carefully formulated "total mixed ration" (TMR) designed to produce an average yield of 610 kg MS in the first 300 days of lactation.

Table 6. Total (T) and annualised (A) lactation yields for Holstein cows grazing pasture and supplemented with grain with target calving intervals (CIs) ranging from 12 to 24 months (preliminary calculations).

| | | CI (months) | | | | |
		12[b]	*15*	*18*	*21*	*24*
Milk yield (litres/cow)	T	6452	7956	9438	10313	11527
	A	6443	6332	6257	5911	5790
	%[a]	-	98.3	97.1	91.7	89.9
Milk protein (kg/cow)	T	214	269	320	358	399
	A	213	214	212	205	201
	%[a]	-	100.5	99.5	96.2	94.4
Milk fat (kg/cow)	T	284	355	422	470	524
	A	283	284	280	268	264
	%[a]	-	100.4	98.9	94.7	93.2

[a]annualised yield for extended CI / annualised yield for 12 month CI
[b]average of 2 lactations

Only 33% (8/24) of cows on the TMR were in milk for the planned 670 days, as reflected by the lowest average DIM (Table 7). By contrast, 50% (24/48) of cows in the pasture-fed groups were still being milked at 670 days. Consequently, the TMR herd had the lowest MS ratio of 89.1%, compared with 97.6% and 95.7% for the pasture fed cows. A possible reason for the results of the TMR group was that they had regained their calving BCS by the ninth month of lactation and thereafter rapidly increased it. By the thirteenth month of lactation, the average BCS was 8. This was the maximum score of the 1-to-8 scale used in the study. Gradual increases in BCS were not noted in the two pasture-fed groups until the thirteenth or fourteenth months of lactation.

Table 7. Effects of level of nutrition (MJ ME/cow/day) on milk and milk solids (MS) yields in Holstein cows calving once or twice in 2 years and fed on three levels of nutrition (preliminary calculations).

Diet	CI	DIM	Milk yield(kg)	MS yield (kg)	MS Ratio
160 MJ	12	590[a]	10880	822	-
160 MJ	24	637	10091	803	0.98[b]
180 MJ	24	635	11239	919	0.96[c]
TMR	24	608	13212	1087	0.89[c]

[a] 2 lactations
[b] 803 / 822
[c] annualised / planned 300-day yield

The results of this trial showed that high energy rations are not essential for successfully maintaining extended lactations. Pasture-based rations that are high in protein may be preferable and allow most Holstein cows to successfully complete lactations with 18-month CIs and some to complete lactations of over 700 days.

Fertility-related effects of extended lactations

Many studies have reported that reproductive performance of lactating Holstein cows is compromised in early lactation, possibly because of increased "energy deficits" associated with low plasma concentrations of insulin, IGF-1 and glucose as well as increased concentrations of bST (Gutierrez *et al.*, 2006). There are also genotype or strain differences, as reported by Horan *et al.* (2005). Whereas services/cow only varied from 1.8 in NZ cows to 2.0 in HP cows (Table 4), only 59% of HP cows conceived during 6 weeks of AI compared with 66% for HD cows and 73% for NZ cows. By 13 weeks of breeding, only 9% of NZ cows were not pregnant, compared with 15% of HD cows and 21% of HP cows (Table 8).

Table 8. Reproductive performance for Holstein and Friesian cows managed to achieve 12 month or 24 month calving intervals (CI).

		Strain	
	HP[a]	*HD*[a]	*NZ*[a]
21-day insemination Rate (%)	84	90	91
1st insemination conception rate (5)	47	56	60
Services / cow	2.0	1.9	1.8
6-week in-calf rate (%)	59	66	73
13-week in-calf rate (%)	79	85	91

	NZ – 3m[b]	*OS – 3m*[b]	*NZ – 15m*[b]	*OS – 15m*[b]
21-day insemination rate (%)	93	59	86	85
1st insemination conception rate (%)	38	19	59	48
6-week in-calf rate (%)	62	26	79	56
12-week in-calf rate (%)	86	52	97	70
"Phantom" cow (%) [c]	0	11	0	15

[a] see Table 4; Horan *et al.* (2005)
[b] see Table 5; Kolver *et al.* (2006)
[c] non-pregnant inseminated cows failing to return within 24 days

Kolver *et al.* (2006) compared reproductive performance of NZ Friesians and OS Holsteins at 3 months and at 15 months of lactation. Reproductive performance of both strains improved with the breeding program that commenced at 15 months of lactation (Table 8). However, the delay was not sufficient to reduce the fertility difference between the two strains. A major factor contributing to poorer reproductive performance of the OS strain was the high incidence of "Phantom" cows. These are cows that are not confirmed pregnant to a first or second insemination, but do not show oestrus as expected from 18 to 24 days after insemination (Cavalieri *et al.*, 2003). The syndrome has been associated with an increased incidence of late embryonic death occurring between about 21 days and 42 days after insemination. Its estimated occurrence is 13% of Holsteins in Victorian herds, and it has been a major factor contributing to the move from seasonal to bi-seasonal calving.

Numbers of cows were limited in both of the studies summarised in Table 8. Data derived from the InCalf Project conducted in 124 Victorian and Tasmanian herds showed that 3-week insemination rate, conception rate to first insemination and 6 weeks in-calf rate all increased with increasing post-calving interval to insemination up to about 100 days (J. Morton, personal communication). Pino *et al.* (2006) reported that the prevalence of cows affected by the Phantom Cow Syndrome declined from 21% for cows inseminated from 41 to 60 days post-calving to 7% for cows inseminated from 141 to 160 days.

The studies by Arbel *et al* (2001; Table 1), Van Amburgh *et al.* (1997; Table 2) and Osterman and Bertilsson (2003; Table 3) did not reveal marked improvements in reproductive performance of cows that were managed to have extended CIs. An increasing proportion of Victorian herd owners have moved from traditional seasonal calving patterns to bi-seasonal patterns with at least two intensive periods of calving each year. This trend has seen the proportion of herds with seasonal calving patterns decline from 64% in 2004 to 41% in 2006 with a corresponding increase in bi-seasonal calving patterns from 33% to 50% in the same period. One reason frequently given for the change is to reduce the increase in herd wastage rates associated with declining reproductive performance in Holstein cows (Dairy Australia, 2006). Detailed field studies to confirm this outcome have not been conducted. Nonetheless, the change in calving systems will have increased the incidence of extended lactations, particularly involving CIs of 16 to 19 months. Because most Victorian herds are heavily based on "OS" genetics, this change in calving patterns could have occurred without greatly reducing annualised yields of protein.

Milk composition and quality

Although most of the cited studies recorded similar or fewer cases of mastitis among cows with extended lactations, few studies recorded somatic cell counts. In the second Victorian trial (Table 7), the expected late lactation increase was observed in each group. This meant that the control group, which calved twice in 2 years, had two periods when somatic cell counts were elevated.

All the studies reported higher concentrations of fat and protein in milk from cows with extended lactations. Kolver *et al.* (2006) found that protein concentrations in milk produced after 300 days were 5% higher for NZ cows and 8% higher for OS cows (Table 5). Comparable increases in milk fat concentrations were 4% for NZ cows and 5% for OS cows.

Table 9. Cheese yields from milk produced from Holstein cows at 3 or 8 months (12 month CI) and 15 or 20 months (24-month CI) receiving different diets (see Table 7).

| Diet | CI | Cheese yield (kg/100 kg milk) at: | |
		3 or 15 months	*8 or 20 months*
160 MJ	12	9.9	11.5
160 MJ	24	11.7	12.8
180 MJ	24	12.1	13.1
TMR	24	11.8	13.1

Only one trial has provided data on milk processability. The indicative cheese yields obtained from cows included in the second Victorian trial (Table 7) were higher in cows with extended lactations (Table 9) and higher in milk processed in the autumn (8 or 20 months) than in the spring (3 or 15 months). No quality data is currently available. These results suggest that higher returns should be obtained from milk produced by Holstein cows with extended lactations.

Cost-benefit studies on extended lactations

Cost-benefit comparisons involving extended lactations are difficult. Reasons for this difficulty include method of payment. For example, US farmers are paid a price "per 100 pounds of milk" that is marginally adjusted for protein or milk fat concentrations above or below stated limits. Peak yield within a cow's lactation will coincide with peak daily income. In contrast, herd owners in New Zealand and most of Australia receive a payment for milk protein that is 2.5 times greater than for milk fat (6.04 AUD/kg for protein and 2.40 AUD/kg for fat), but have to pay a processing charge and a transport charge that are both based on volume. Under these circumstances, higher income at peak lactation is offset by lower concentrations of milk protein and fat.

Seasonal calving systems are based on the premise that pasture grazed *in situ* is the least expensive source of forage. Consequently, peak herd demand for dry matter is planned to occur during the period of peak pasture growth, usually mid-spring. The fewest number of cows will be milked during the winter when pasture growth in minimal. Under these circumstances, extended lactations will mean more cows will be milked during periods when feed costs are greatest and fewer cows in peak lactation will be milked when feed costs are lowest. Dairy processors have recognised this difference in feed costs and have made seasonal adjustments in payments for milk or MS. For example, protein and milk fat prices paid to Victorian herd owners are 25% higher in June (winter) than in October and November (spring). Extremes of climate can also affect the need to provide shelter to minimise the effects of adverse weather on production.

An additional factor that can affect the cost-benefits derived from extended lactations is the herd's replacement costs. Evans *et al.* (2006) found that a major factor reducing the net income benefits from milking 'HP' cows was their higher replacement rate. This increased from 16% in 1990 to 27% in 2003 mainly because of reduced fertility associated with increased use of American genetics. If levels of reproductive performance are at least maintained in cows managed to have extended lactations, and yield statistics per day of CI are not affected, then replacement rates expressed as per cow/ year or per kg of yield will be reduced. For example, under Victorian conditions, cows managed to achieve CIs of 18 months would produce 20% more milk protein and milk fat with 4 calvings/cow/lifetime than a contemporary that achieved the current industry average of 5 calvings/lifetime with 12-month CIs. If both cows had 5 lactations/lifetime, the cow with the 18-month CI should have lifetime yields of milk fat and milk protein increased by almost 50%.

In addition, health and breeding costs will be reduced with extended lactations. Breeding costs are directly related to CI; fewer calvings should mean lower synchronisation and insemination costs, even if wastage rate remained unchanged. Health costs associated with dystocia, metabolic diseases, mastitis and lameness should also be reduced per cow/lifetime and per unit of yield since they occur most frequently in the period from calving to 3 months of lactation.

Finally, management routines are less complicated with fewer calvings, fewer periods of breeding and fewer groups of cows requiring special attention or feeding. This should mean that less labour would be required to manage a herd that has extended lactations.

The experience of Victorian herd owners who have moved to bi-seasonal calving from seasonal calving is that more AI replacements are produced. This is because AI is used for 12 or 14 weeks/year rather than for 6 weeks. In addition, breeding programs can be confined to 12 to 13 weeks meaning there is less need for calving induction. Later calving cows can also be transferred from calving in one season to calving 6 months later in the alternative season.

Further research

The results from trials that have covered a wide range of yields and several genotypes on different diets have identified an unrealised potential for cows of high genetic merit to sustain extended lactations associated with CIs of 18 months and potentially 24 months. All of the trials used cows whose sires had been progeny tested for yield statistics derived from 305-day lactations. The wide variation among cows beyond 300 days that was partly reflected in their ability to continue lactating suggests that greater use should be made of production data beyond 300 days to identify sires whose daughters may be particularly suited to management systems utilising CIs of 18 to 24 months.

Holsteins seem best suited to being managed for these longer CIs. They have higher plasma concentrations of bST and lower concentrations of insulin, glucose and IGF-1 in early lactation. The cows with the greatest potential for extended lactations may be those that have chronically elevated or depressed concentrations of these hormones so that they continue to divert metabolisable energy to milk synthesis rather than body condition. A third Ellinbank study will specifically focus on quantifying differences in plasma concentrations of hormones and metabolites that may reflect differences in energy partitioning that sustain long lactations. The effects of short periods of restricting feed intake on persistency will also be investigated. Initial attempts to identify phenotypic indicators of ability to milk for extended periods in early lactation have not been successful. Hormonal parameters may be useful in predicting animal suitability, but peak milk yield is not a reliable indicator. An unusual relationship identified by Kolver (personal communication) was the negative correlation ($r = 0.53$) between a cow's breeding value for fertility and its MS yield with a 24-month CI.

The nutritional management of cows during extended lactations will need to be developed. High protein or pasture-based diets would seem most suitable (Table 7). Feeding levels surplus to production needs will lead to fat deposition and to lower milk yields. It may also be preferable to calve cows planned to have extended lactations in lower body condition and to rely on appetite rather than tissue mobilisation to achieve peak yields that may be less than those currently obtained.

The reproductive performance of cows enrolled in AI programs 9 months or more after calving deserves closer study, using records from commercial herds. Synchronisation should be less complicated than with VWPs of around 60 days, but the Phantom Cow Syndrome may still prove problematical. Concern has occasionally been expressed about adverse effects on fertility if VWPs exceed 200 days. However, heifers are allowed to cycle regularly from puberty until insemination at 15 months of age or later and suffer no adverse consequences on fertility. Lactating cows of high genetic merit should be expected to have improved fertility as a consequence of being allowed to cycle for an extended period.

Finally, the potential advantages of extended lactations with longer CIs on lifetime production, reduced annual replacement rate and reduced labour requirements/cow/lactation should be carefully assessed to produce realistic cost-benefit analyses.

References

Arbel, R., Bigun, Y., Ezra, E., Sturman, H. and Hojman, D. (2001). The effect of extended calving intervals in high lactating cows on milk production and profitability. *Journal of Dairy Science*, **84**, 600-608.

Cavalieri, J., Morton, J., Nation, D.P., Hepworth, G., Pino, S., Rabiee, A. and Macmillan, K.L. (2003). Phantom cows: predisposing factors, causes and treatment strategies that have been attempted to reduce the prevalence within herds. *Proceedings of the Dairy Cattle Veterinarians of the New Zealand Veterinary Association* **20**, 365-388.

Dairy Australia (2006). *Dairy 2006: Situation and Outlook*: 8. Calving systems, p.41. Melbourne, Australia.

Dillon, P., Berry, D.P., Evans, R.D., Buckley, F. and Horan, B. (2006). Consequences of genetic selection for increased milk production in European seasonal pasture based systems of milk production. *Livestock Production Science* **99**, 141-158.

Evans, R.D., Wallace, M., Shalloo, L., Garrick, D.J. and Dillon, P. (2006). Financial implications of recent declines in reproduction and survival in Holstein-Friesian cows in spring-calving Irish dairy herds. *Livestock Production Science* **89**, 165-183.

Gutierrez, C.G., Gong, Jin G., Bramley, T.A. and Webb, R. (2006). Selection on predicted breeding value for milk production delays ovulation independently of changes in follicular development, milk production and body weight. *Animal Reproduction Science*, **95**, 193-205.

Horan, B., Mee, J.F., O'Connor, P., Rath, M. and Dillon, P. (2005). The effect of strain of Holstein-Friesian cow and feeding system on postpartum ovarian function, animal production and conception rate to first service. *Theriogenology* **63**, 950-971.

Kolver, E.S., Roche, J.R., Burke, C.R. and Aspin, P.W. (2006). Effect of genotype and diet on milksolids production, body condition and reproduction of cows milked continuously for 600 days. *Proceedings of the New Zealand Society of Animal Production* **66**, 245-251.

Lucy, M.C. (2001). Reproductive loss in high-producing dairy cattle: where will it end? *Journal of Dairy Science* **84E**, E1277-E1293.

Moore, K. and Thatcher, W.W. (2006). Major advances associated with reproduction in dairy cattle. *Journal of Dairy Science* **89**, 1254-1266.

Osterman, S. and Bertilsson, J. (2003). Extended calving interval in combination with milking two or three times per day: effects on milk production and milk composition. *Livestock Production Science* **82**, 139-149.

Pino, C.S., Macmillan, K.L. and Anderson, G.A. (2006). Effects of artificial insemination on the incidence of long return intervals. *Proceedings of the New Zealand Society of Animal Production* **66**, 325-328.

Plaizier, J.C.B., King, G.J., Dekkers, J.C.M. and Lissemore, K. (1997). Estimation of economic values of indices for reproductive performance in dairy herds using computer simulation. *Journal of Dairy Science* **80**, 2775-2783.

Van Amburgh, M.E., Galton, D.M., Bauman, D.E., Everett, R.W. (1997). Management and economics of extended calving intervals with use of bovine somatotropin. *Livestock Production Science* **50**, 15-28.

VandeHaar, M.J. and St-Pierre, N. (2006). Major advances in nutrition: Relevance to the sustainability of the dairy industry. *Journal of Dairy Science* **89**, 1280-1291.

6

ANTIOXIDANTS IN ANIMAL PRODUCTS

GEORGE PAGANGA
AASC Ltd, Unit 5, Stanton Industrial Estate, Stanton Road, Southampton SO15 4HU

Antioxidant defence systems in animals

The existence of an organism in the presence of oxygen is associated with the generation of reactive oxygen species ROS even under physiological conditions. These species are responsible for oxidative damage of biological macromolecules which if unchecked can lead to disease states. Thus, ROS are responsible for some pathobiochemical mechanisms that lead to initiation and propagation of various diseases. The most relevant ROS are peroxyl radicals, nitric oxide radical, superoxide anion radical, singlet oxygen, peroxynitrite and hydrogen peroxide. Of these ROS, superoxide radical anion appears to play a central role, since other reactive intermediates are formed in reactions that start with this species. Superoxide is generated by one-electron reduction of oxygen by xanthine oxidase or NADPH oxidase or indeed by leakage of respiratory chain. Superoxide is rapidly converted to hydrogen peroxide by superoxide dismutase. The hydrogen peroxide is capable of diffusing between living cells. It can react with iron (Fenton reactions) to form hydroxyl radicals. The hydroxyl radical is very reactive, causing immediate reaction at the place where it is produced. It is unlikely that hydroxyl radicals are formed in vivo in animals, since transition metals are well sequestered. However, hydrogen peroxide can react with haem proteins to produce ferryl radicals capable of oxidising bio-macromolecules. An imbalance between antioxidant defence systems and ROS in favour of the latter, can lead to chemical modifications of important biological macromolecules such as DNA, protein and lipids leading to disease states.

- Oxidative damage to DNA is well documented and the measurement of 8-oxo-7,8-dihydro-2/-deoxyguanine (8-oxodG) in urine is used as a marker of ROS induced DNA damage.

- Oxidative damage to lipids is also well documented, with the markers of lipid peroxidation being the peroxides or isoprostanes. These are used as markers of oxidative damage especially in the context of atherosclerosis.
- Protein damage by ROS is important in that it will affect receptors, enzymes and transport proteins. A general assay for protein damage is the carbonyl assay. It is based on the fact that amino acid residues of proteins (particularly proline, lysine, histidine and arginine) are susceptible to attack by ROS producing carbonyl functions. These can then react with 2,4-dinitrophenylhydrazine to produce a chromophore, which is used to quantify the carbonyls.

Antioxidants in animal products

The body's antioxidant defence system is capable of being altered by dietary means. The strategy for balancing antioxidant defence systems and ROS would be to enhance antioxidant capacity by increasing dietary intake of antioxidants. A prerequisite for increased intake of antioxidants is knowledge of the required level and accurate assay of food sources for the desired antioxidants. The potential for the antioxidants vitamins E, C and ß-carotene in disease prevention has been highlighted and is well documented. It is of interest that degenerative diseases of aging such as cardiovascular disease, cancer, cataracts and brain dysfunction are found to have, in many cases, an anti-oxidative origin (Ames, Shigena and Hagen, 1993). A lot of evidence is available to support the notion that dietary antioxidants such as vitamins C and E, and the carotenoids play a major role in minimising oxidative damage. Inadequate fruit and vegetable consumption, for example, increases the rate of most types of cancer about two-fold as evidenced by over 200 epidemiological studies. As a result, fruits and vegetables that contain these antioxidants are taking a greater role in modern recommendations to promote good health and to prevent disease. It has been assumed that diets rich in vitamin E and vitamin C have been shown to be particularly important in protection against heart disease. It has become apparent, however, that these nutrients by themselves cannot account for the beneficial effects that are being observed. The levels of intake of vitamin E so far shown to be maximally protective are not attainable through dietary means alone. The additional role of fruits and vegetables (particularly those high in ß-carotene, vitamin C and fibre), as well as the control of infection, are significant in reducing disease states. The WHO has made recommendations with regard to consumption of fruit and vegetables. The WHO recommendation translates into consumption of 5-9 portions of mixed fruit and vegetables per day as sufficient to satisfy these dietary requirements for maintenance of health. These fruit and vegetables are rich in flavonoids.

Flavonoids are a large class of compounds, ever-present in plants, containing a number of phenolic hydroxyl groups attached to ring structures, bestowing antioxidant activity (Hollman, Tijburg and Yang, 1997). They are multifunctional and can act as reducing agents, hydrogen donating antioxidants, metal chelators and singlet oxygen quenchers. Estimates of daily intake range from about 20mg to 1g (Hertog, Kromhout, Aravanis, Blackburn, Buzina, Fidanza, Giampaoli, Jansen, Monotti, Nedelikovic, Pekkarinen, Simic, Toshima, Feskens, Hollman and Katan, 1995). Table 1 shows some of the dietary sources of flavonoids.

Table 1. Dietary sources of flavonoids

Source	Major component	Flavonoids (mg/100g)
Apples	quercetin, phenolic acids	27 - 298
Oranges	hesperetin, naringenin	50 - 100
Onions	quercetin, kaempferol	100 - 2025
Grapes	kaempferol, anthocyanidins	50 - 490

Flavanols, particularly the catechin family, and the flavonols quercetin, kaempferol and their glycosides, are major constituents of the beverages green tea, black tea and red wine. Quercetin is also a predominant component of onions and apples, and myricetin and quercetin of berries. The flavanones are mainly found in citrus fruits. The requirement and effects of the phenylpropanoids are less appreciated. For example, ferulic acid, p-coumaric acid and caffeic acid are also major constituents of fruit and vegetables and are known to be absorbed from such sources as beer and tomatoes. Little is known about the bio-availability, absorption and metabolism in man of flavonoids. It is likely that different groups of flavonoids have different pharmacokinetic properties. This chapter will focus on analysis of the phenolic constituents of fruit and vegetables.

In determining antioxidants for animal or human feed, it is important to understand the interactions of the antioxidant components resulting in synergism that may be encountered. The chemical properties of polyphenols, in terms of availability of phenolic hydrogen as hydrogen-donating radical scavengers, define their antioxidant activity. The two basic conditions that must be satisfied for a polyphenolic substance to be defined as an antioxidant are:

i)   When present in low concentrations relative to the substrate to be oxidised, they can delay, retard or prevent auto-oxidation or free radical-mediated oxidation (Bors, Heller, Michael and Saran, 1990);

ii)   The resulting radical formed after scavenging must be stable; polyphenols can be stabilised though intramolecular hydrogen bonding or by further oxidation (Agrawal and Schneider, 1983).

Three criteria for effective radical scavenging by the polyphenols (Agrawal and Schneider, 1983; Bors and Saran, 1987)are:

1.   The o-dihydroxy structure in the B ring which confers higher stability to the radical form and participates in electron delocalisation
2.   The 2,3 double bond in conjugation with 4-oxo function in the C ring responsible for electron delocalisation from the B ring
3.   The 3- and 5 -OH groups with 4-oxo function in A and C rings for maximum radical scavenging potential.

Structural evaluation of polyphenols shows clearly that plant phenolics are good sources of antioxidants and that identifying the exact component and concentration of these phenolics within the plant will help to understand the role they play in disease prevention. Chromatographic profiling of the components in plants can provide a means of selecting plant material that has optimal synergy components. HPLC is used for this procedure and a typical component profile can be identified from the standards shown in Figure 1.

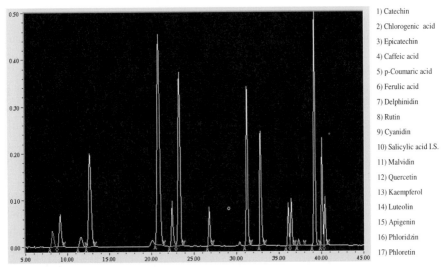

1) Catechin
2) Chlorogenic acid
3) Epicatechin
4) Caffeic acid
5) p-Coumaric acid
6) Ferulic acid
7) Delphinidin
8) Rutin
9) Cyanidin
10) Salicylic acid I.S.
11) Malvidin
12) Quercetin
13) Kaempferol
14) Luteolin
15) Apigenin
16) Phloridzin
17) Phloretin

Figure 1. HPLC chromatogram of plant phenolic components.

After components have been identified, total antioxidant capability of the material can be determined. Several methods for determination of antioxidant activity have been developed. They are useful in getting a global picture of relative antioxidant activities in different food and biological systems. They can determine how antioxidant potential of clinical samples change depending on pathological condition; e.g. normal healthy serum sample versus disease state and supplemented sample will give an indication of deficiencies in antioxidant status. The same criteria can be employed in animal systems. Methods that are available include,

a)   **Total peroxyl radical trapping parameter (TRAP)** (Wayner, Burton and Ingold, 1985): the major problem with this method is that the oxygen electrode used does not maintain stability over the duration of the experiment.

b)   **Ferric reducing ability (FRAP)** (Benzie and Strain, 1996): Simple and cheap, but does not measure -SH group containing antioxidants such as GSH.

c)   **ORAC assay was first developed by Glazer et al. in 1990** (Cao, Alessio and Culter, 1993): Measures net or total resultant antioxidant potential of the many different antioxidant components present in serum samples

d)   **TEAC (Trolox equivalent antioxidant capacity) assay** (Re, Pellegrini, Proteggente, Pannala, Yang and Rice-Evans, 1999): The assay is suitable for food materials such as grape seed extract and can be used to assess antioxidant capacity of juices and powders

The methods of choice are the TEAC or ORAC assays.

TEAC (Trolox equivalent antioxidant capacity) assay

The TEAC method is based on the ability of antioxidant molecules to quench the long-lived ABTS$^{\cdot+}$, a blue-green chromophore with characteristic absorption at 734 nm, compared with that of Trolox, a water-soluble vitamin E analogue. The addition of antioxidants to the preformed radical cation reduces it to ABTS, determining a decolourisation. A stable stock solution of ABTS$^{\cdot+}$ was produced by reacting a 7 mmol/L aqueous solution of ABTS with 2.45 mmol/L potassium persulfate (final concentration) and allowing the mixture to stand in the dark at room temperature for 12–16 h before use (Pellegrini, Del Rio, Colombi, Bianchi and Brighenti, 2003). At the beginning of the analysis day, an ABTS$^{\cdot+}$ working solution was obtained by the dilution in ethanol of the stock solution to an absorbance of 0.70 ± 0.02 AU at 734 nm, verified by a Hewlett-Packard 8453 Diode Array spectrophotometer (HP, Waldbronn, Germany), and used as mobile phase in a flow-injection system, according to Pellegrini, Re, Yang and Rice-

Evans (1999). Results were expressed as TEAC in mmol of Trolox per kg (solid foods and oils) or per L (beverages) of sample. All solid food extracts, obtained by water, acetone and chloroform, can be analysed by this assay.

ORAC (Oxygen Radical Absorbance Capacity) assay

This method can quantitatively measure the total antioxidant capacity as well as qualitatively measure the amount of fast vs. slow acting antioxidants in the sample to be tested. The assay originally measured the effectiveness of various natural antioxidants, present in the sample, in preventing the loss in the fluorescence intensity of the fluorescent marker protein, b-phycoerythrin (beta-PE), during peroxyl radical induced free radical damage. The recent method uses the more stable flourescin as the substrate. Assay results are quantitated by allowing the reaction to reach completion and then integrating the area under the kinetic curve relative to a blank reaction containing no added antioxidants. The area under the curve is proportional to the concentration of *all* the antioxidants present in the sample. Each reaction is calibrated using known standards of Trolox, a water-soluble vitamin E analogue. The results of the assay are reported on the basis of 1 ORAC unit = 1 micro-M Trolox. Thus, the ORAC assay depends on the free radical damage to a fluorescent probe through the change in its fluorescence intensity. The change of fluorescence intensity is an index of the degree of free radical damage. In the presence of antioxidant, the inhibition of free radical damage by an antioxidant, which is reflected in the protection against the change of probe fluorescence in the ORAC assay, is a measure of its antioxidant capacity against the free radical.

ORAC assay requires 60 minutes compared to [Author: insert time required for FRAP or TEAC] FRAP or TEAC to quantitate results. It is very sensitive to changes in temperature and decomposition of AAPH increases with temperature. Therefore temperature must be tightly controlled throughout the long experimental incubation time. Also, the assay requires a fluorescence detector. Examples of antioxidant activities of fruit and vegetables are shown in Table 2.

Table 2. Antioxidant activities of some fruit and vegetables

Fruit/vegetable	Total phenolics (mg GAE/100 g FW)	TEAC (mmol Trolox/100 g FW)	ORAC (mmol Trolox/100 g FW)
Strawberry	330±4 6	2591±68	2437±95
Grapefruit	150±4 52	861±53	1447±67
Broccoli	128±4 45	648±25	1335±62
Onion	88±1 6	532±29	988±30
Tomato	30±1 18	344±7	420±39

Ames *et al.* (1993) investigated responses in serum total antioxidant capacity following consumption of strawberries (240 g), spinach (294 g), red wine (300 ml) or vitamin C (1250 mg) in eight elderly women. Total antioxidant capacity was determined using different methods: oxygen radical absorbance capacity (ORAC) assay, Trolox equivalent antioxidant capacity (TEAC) assay and ferric reducing ability (FRAP) assay. The results showed that the total antioxidant capacity of serum determined as ORAC, TEAC and FRAP, using the area under the curve, increased significantly by 7-25% during the 4-h period following consumption of red wine, strawberries, vitamin C or spinach. The total antioxidant capacity of urine determined as ORAC increased (*P* < 0.05) by 9.6, 27.5, and 44.9% for strawberries, spinach, and vitamin C, respectively, during the 24-h period following these treatments. The plasma vitamin C level after the strawberry drink, and the serum urate level after the strawberry and spinach treatments, also increased significantly. However, the increased vitamin C and urate levels could not fully account for the increased total antioxidant capacity in serum following the consumption of strawberries, spinach or red wine. They concluded that the consumption of strawberries, spinach or red wine, which are rich in antioxidant phenolic compounds, can increase the serum antioxidant capacity in humans. The structural integrity of food plays an important role in protecting the components of the food that have antioxidant capability. The food in its whole form is encased in a protective liposome or cell membrane structures keeping it out of oxygen and thus harm's way. Intact oilseeds are stable protecting the tocopherols contained in them, but once the seeds are crashed, resistance to oxidation is decreased. Heat has been of particular interest feed manufacturers. Not all heat is bad as was seen in a study by Stahl and Sies (1992). They showed that heat treatment of tomato juice increased lycopene absorption compare with the same dose of raw tomato juice. It has to be remembered that antioxidants exact their effect at low concentrations and do not need to be present in high concentrations in food. Some losses will be tolerated as long as they are kept to a minimum.

Dietary modification of the immune system

It should be noted that a wide variety of methods are available to assess the function of various components of the immune system and to detect nutrient-immune system interactions. The immune system is very complex and requires more than one assay for a meaningful assessment.

Vitamin A is effectively used in the treatment of measles in children. It is an example of the enhancement of immune system by nutritional means as was seen in trials with the vitamin in developing countries that has become accepted in medical practice. Mortality from measles was decreased in supplemented children compared to placebo controls. On the other hand, it is well known for example that natural killer cells are able to kill tumour cells, but no evidence has yet been found to suggest that enhancement of natural killer cells by dietary intervention will reduce the risk of certain tumours. Numerous studies have shown that dietary factors can be linked to increased risk of heart disease. Atherosclerosis is a major cause of mortality from heart disease. It is an inflammatory disease of the arteries resulting from the deposition of fatty plaques. The immune system is involved in the pathogenesis of atherosclerosis through interaction of the monocytes and macrophages with the arteriole wall. In autoimmune disease for example, it has been shown that fish oils containing n-3 PUFA have significant clinical, immunological and biochemical effects in a number of animal models. Population studies have also indicated that diets high in n-3 PUFA may inhibit autoimmune disease for example Greenland Inuits have high n-3 PUFA and low rates of autoimmune and inflammatory disease (Bang, Dyerberg and Sinclair, 1980; Kromann and Green, 1980; Cleland, James, Keen, Danda, Caughey and Proudman, 2005).

In general, the life style of an animal should enable its immune system to operate at its genetically determined optimal level of activity. Thus, a well balance diet should be able to support an effective immune system. More meaningful work has to be done to provide evidence of the level of antioxidants needed to maintain health and well being of the animal. It is necessary to refine and validate methods that are already available for measurement of oxidative damage in animals in a cheap non-invasive manner. This will enable the real measurement of variables related to oxidative damage to be obtained and to be used in assessing the best possible antioxidant composition. Although synthetic antioxidants have a role in protecting feed ingredients, naturally-derived antioxidants go further than that; they also provide much needed antioxidant benefit to the animal. For example, in pigs that are growing at such a high rate as to induce arthritic joints, a case could be made for increasing the antioxidant capacity of such animals.

Antioxidants are needed to detoxify ROS, which are detrimental to the animal's well being. To this end, antioxidants work synergistically by reducing a very reactive oxygen species to a relatively less reactive one. Synergism comes from the Greek word *"synergos"* meaning working together. It refers to the interaction between two or more antioxidants whose combined effect is greater than that of the individual components added together (a type of "when one plus one is greater than two" effect). In toxicology, synergism refers to the effect caused when exposure to two or more chemicals at a time results in health effects that are greater than the sum of the effects of the individual chemicals, i.e. synergism occurs when both chemicals have an effect individually and a more than additive effect when together.

The effect of tomato flavonoid concentrations can be used to explain synergism in biological systems. Ferulic acid, p-coumaric acid and caffeic acid have varying concentrations in the fruit depending on harvesting, handling etc. (Figure 2). p-Coumaric acid has the highest TEAC value, 2.22mmol/L, ferulic 1.90 and caffeic acid 1.26 mmol/L. It would be expected that the tomato extract with the highest level of p-coumaric acid and caffeic acid (Tomato B) would have the best antioxidant protection in copper induced LDL oxidation systems. This is not the case as Tomato C gave the best results when copper induced LDL oxidation was subjected to protection by these components. The results indicate the importance of synergism in antioxidant systems. Furthermore, halving the concentration of antioxidants does not necessarily mean that activity is halved. Activity may be reduced more than the theoretical value; this is important for inclusion levels of antioxidants for feed manufacturers. It should be noted that levels of α-tocopherol increase by approximately 1.7 times their original value on supplementation. Typical human plasma and LDL α-tocopherol values are show in Table 3.

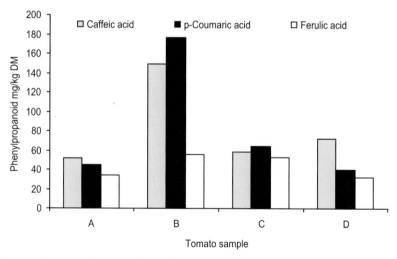

Figure 2. Phenylpropanoid concentration of four tomato samples.

Compelling chemical, biochemical, clinical and epidemiological evidence supports the contention that antioxidants play a vital role in prevention or delayed onset of certain diseases. Antioxidants are considered to exert their effects by attenuating oxidative events that contribute to the pathophysiology of these diseases. Thus supplementation of animal feed with the appropriate antioxidant will help to improve the health of the animal. Since absorption of

Table 3. Typical human plasma and LDL α-tocopherol concentrations

	α-Tocopherol (μmol/L)	
	Plasma	*LDL*
	34.7	12.7
	31.7	17.3
	41.2	11.2
	32.7	11.4
	39.2	20.4
	40.6	17.6
	44.3	19.0
	32.1	8.7
	33.7	14.4
	43.9	15.9
	28.2	15.2
	28.3	14.7
	20.5	14.1
	29.9	13.2
	24.6	11.4
	31.1	15.1
	24.6	8.8
	19.7	10.4
	25.5	13.2
Sum	606.6	264.6
Mean	31.9	13.9
Range	19.7-44.3	8.8-20.43

α-tocopherol is of interest in both animals and humans and a tocopherol binding protein is responsible for uptake of vitamin E in animals, it follows that if there is a deficiency in tocopherol-binding protein then some disease state would result. There is evidence in cocker spaniels that have a degenerative eye disease due to a deficiency in tocopherol binding protein. The disease is eradicated if high doses of vitamin E are introduced. These are absorbed via a passive pathway. In animal feeds tocopherol acetate is a major ingredient. Its uptake is dependent on conversion to tocopherol by gut esterases. This introduces a rate-limiting step in uptake of tocopherol either by passive or active pathway. Thus, you can increase the tocopherol acetate as much as you want, but uptake depends on conversion of tocopherol acetate to tocopherol. Synthetic antioxidants, such as BHT, BHA and ethoxyquin, are primarily used for protection of the feed and not for the biological benefit of animals. Figure 3 illustrates the ideal function of antioxidants.

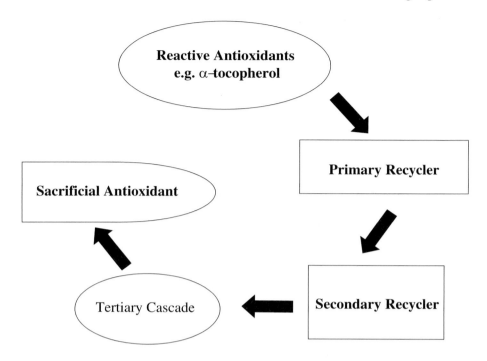

Figure 3. Ideal function of antioxidants

Conclusions

In conclusion, healthy nutrition requires appropriate dietary intake of energy in the form of macronutrients as well as an adequate intake of essential nutrients. Requirements for different nutrients are related to the animal's energy requirements, age, height, physiological condition, etc. It is impossible to establish an animal's precise nutrient requirements, so it is also impossible to establish precise requirements for antioxidants. Healthy nutrition is only possible by combining different foods to maintain the required balanced diet and this is also the case for antioxidants. Ideally, an animal's lifestyle should enable its immune system to operate at its genetically-determined optimal level. However, in today's environment, this is unattainable and the concept of promoting health or treating disease by nutritional means shows great promise.

References

Agrawal, P.K. and Schneider, H.J. (1983). Deprotonation-induced ^{13}C-NMR shifts in phenols and flavonoids. *Tetrahedron Letters*, **24**, 177-180.

Ames, B. M., Shigena, M. K. and Hagen, T. M. (1993). Oxidants, antioxidants and the degenerative diseases of aging. *Proc. Natl. Acad. Sci.*, **90**, 7915-7922.

Bang, H.O., Dyerberg, J. and Sinclair, H.M. (1980). The composition of Eskimo food in north western Greenland. *Am J Clin Nutr*, **33**, 2657-2661.

Benzie, I.F.F. and Strain, J.J. (1996). The ferric reducing ability of plasma (FRAP) as a measure of ''antioxidant power'': The FRAP assay. *Anal. Biochem.*, **239**, 70-76.

Bors, W., Heller, W., Michael, C. and Saran, M. (1990). Flavonoids as antioxidants: Determination of radical scavenging efficiencies. *Methods Enzymol.*, **186**, 343-355.

Bors, W. and Saran, M. (1987). Radical scavenging by flavonoid antioxidants. *Free Rad. Res. Commun.*, **2**, 289-294.

Cao, G., Alessio, H. M. and Culter, R. (1993). Oxygen-radical absorbance capacity assay for antioxidants. *Free Radical Biol. Med.*, **14**, 303-311.

Cleland, L.G., James, M.J., Keen, H., Danda, D., Caughey, G. and Proudman, S.M. (2005). Fish oil: an example of an anti-inflammatory food. *Asia Pac J Clin Nutr*, Suppl, S66-S71.

Hertog, M.G.L., Kromhout, D., Aravanis, C., Blackburn, H., Buzina, R., Fidanza, F., Giampaoli, S., Jansen, A., Monotti, A., Nedelikovic, S., Pekkarinen, M., Simic, B.S., Toshima, H., Feskens, E.J.M., Hollman, P.C.H. and Katan, M.B. (1995). Flavonoid intake and long-term risk of coronary disease and cancer in the Seven Countries Study. *Arch. Intern. Med.*, **155**, 381-386.

Hollman, P.C.H., Tijburg, L.B.M. and Yang, C.S. (1997). Bioavailability of flavonoids from tea. *Crit. Rev. Food Sci. Nutr.*, **37**, 719-738.

Kromann, N. and Green, A. (1980). Epidemiological studies in the Upernavik district, Greenland. *Acta Med Scand*, **208**, 401-406.

Pellegrini, N., Del Rio, D., Colombi, B., Bianchi, M. and Brighenti, F. (2003). Application of the 2, 2'-azobis(3-ethylenebenzothiazoline-6-sulfonic acid) radical cation assay to a flow injection system for the evaluation of antioxidant activity of some pure compounds and beverages. *J. Agric. Food Chem.* **51**, 260-264.

Pellegrini, N., Re, R., Yang, M. and Rice-Evans, C. A. (1999). Screening of dietary carotenoids and carotenoid-rich fruit extracts for antioxidant activities applying the 2, 2'-azobis(3-ethylenebenzothiazoline-6-sulfonic) acid radical cation decolorization assay. *Methods Enzymol.* **299**, 379-389.

Re, R., Pellegrini, N., Proteggente, A., Pannala, A., Yang, M. and Rice-Evans, C. (1999). Antioxidant activity applying an improved ABTS radical cation decolorization assay. *Free Radic. Biol. Med.*, **26**, 1231-1237.

Stahl, W. and Sies, H. (1992). Uptake of lycopene and its geometrical isomers is greater from heat processed than from unprocessed tomato juice in humans. *J. Nutr.*, **122**, 2161-2166.

Wayner, D.D., Burton, G.W. and Ingold, K.U. (1985). Quantitative measurement of the total, peroxyl radical-trapping antioxidant capability of human blood plasma by controlled peroxidation. The important contribution made by plasma proteins. *FEBS Lett.*, **187**, 33–37.

7

MEAT AS A COMPONENT OF A HEALTHY DIET – ARE THERE ANY RISKS OR BENEFITS IF MEAT IS AVOIDED IN THE DIET?

H.-K. BIESALSKI

Universität Hohenheim, Institut für Biologische Chemie und Ernährungswissenschaft, Garbenstrasse 30, 70593 Stuttgart, Germany

Introduction

Meat is frequently associated with a "negative" health image due to its "high" fat content and, in the case of red meat, is seen as a cancer-promoting food. Therefore a low meat intake, especially red meat, is recommended to avoid the risk of cancer, obesity and metabolic syndrome. However, this recommendation overlooks the fact, that meat is an important source for some micronutrients, such as iron, selenium, vitamins A, B12 and Folic acid. These micronutrients are either not present in plant derived food or have poor bioavailability. In addition, meat as a protein rich and carbohydrate "low" product contributes to a low glycemic index, which is assumed to be "beneficial" with respect to obesity, diabetes development and cancer (insulin resistance hypothesis). Taken together, these factors indicate that meat is an important nutrient for human health and development. As an essential part of a mixed diet, meat ensures adequate delivery of essential micronutrients and amino acids and is involved in regulatory processes of energy metabolism. The following article will review the role of meat as a source of micronutrients, especially for groups at risk for low intake or higher need and the importance of the individual micronutrients for maintaining health.

Is there any benefit, if meat is avoided in human nutrition? Does meat promote or prevent cancer? It is frequently argued that a diet which contains only "traces" of meat or excludes meat completely might prevent colon cancer. Based on a couple of studies and with respect to the cancer preventive effects of selected nutrients present in meat, this hypothesis seems more and more unlikely.

Proteins

It has been assumed, based on per capita protein intake and colon cancer risk, that total protein, is related to colon cancer risk (Youngman & Cambell, 1998). However the majority of epidemiological cohort and case control studies could not confirm these assumptions. Only for protein derived from red meat is there some evidence that risk increases if red meat is consumed twice a day and more (MacIntosh & Le Leu, 2001) or processed (boiled or fried). Whether the non-fat matrix of meat, i.e. the amino acid composition or the amount of heme iron, plays a role in carcinogenesis is not understood. McIntosh and coworkers observed a non-significant increase from 33% to 59% in the incidence of DMH-induced (differential methylation hybridization) intestinal tumours in mature rats when barbecued beef was substituted for whey protein concentrate against a high fat (20%) diet background (MacIntosh, Royle, & Le Leu, 1998). Whether the concentration of protein in a diet determines the risk for cancer is controversial (MacIntosh et al., 2001). In contrast, the type of protein seems more important with respect to carcinogenesis. A high methionine diet, determined by type of protein as well as quantity ingested, has been reported to lead to increased circulating insulin which has been assumed to contribute to colon carcinogenesis (McKeoween-Eyssen, 1994). From epidemiological studies there is accumulating evidence to support the insulin resistance (IR) hypothesis to explain the risk from colon cancer. It was hypothesised that IR leads to increased initiation and promotion of colon cancer by elevating serum insulin as a growth factor or raised glucose and triglycerides as fuels (McKeoween-Eyssen, 1994). Bruce, Wolever, and Giacca (2000) summarise different explanations that strengthen the hypothesis: colon cancer patients frequently have evidence of glucose intolerance and insulin resistance (IR); cohorts of type 2 diabetes have been found to have an excess mortality due to colon cancer; cohort and case control studies have revealed a clear association of early colon cancer, colon cancer and colonic polyps with increased levels of fasting insulin, triglycerides, VLDL (very low density lipoproteins) and abdominal obesity; subjects who developed colonic polyps consumed more carbohydrates with a higher glycemic index than controls; recent case control studies have also shown an association between plasma insulin like growth factor I (IGF-I), which is often increased in insulin resistant individuals, and IGF-binding protein (IGF-BP) levels with risk for colon cancer. From a couple of animal experiments there is evidence that IR leads to an increased colon cancer risk.

Diets with a high glycemic index are thought to be associated with or to favour insulin resistance (Frost, Leeds, & Trew, 1998). Red meat has a low glycemic index, however, and may not contribute to the metabolic syndrome as long as its fat/energy content does not contribute primarily to daily energy intake. Koohestani, Tran, and Lee (1997) showed that a high fat diet promotes aberrant crypt formation (ACF) in IR rats as an important step in colon carcinogenesis. Based on their results they conclude that: diets high in energy, saturated fat, and glycemic carbohydrate and low in ù3-fatty acids could deleteriously affect cell signalling in colonic cells in ways that lead to IR and colon cancer. Dietary intervention that reduces IR may also reduce colon cancer risk. So far, low fat meat seems not to contribute to colon cancer.

Fat

Several epidemiological early case control and cohort studies suggested a positive correlation between fat intake and incidences of breast-, colon- and prostate cancer (Schottenfeld & Fraumeni, 1996; Potter, Slattery, & Bostick, 1993). However, more recent cohort, large case control and pooled analysis of 13 case control studies failed to detect an association between fat intake and colon cancer (Howe, Aronson, & Benito, 1997; Giovannucci, Rimm, & Stampher, 1994). The relation between dietary fat intake and breast cancer has been examined in a couple of prospective studies. In a pooled analysis, no overall association was seen for total fat intake over the range 15% to > 45% of energy from fat (Hunter, Spiegelman, & Adami, 1996). In contrast, among the small number of women consuming less than 15% of energy from fat, breast cancer risk was elevated twofold. With respect to prostate cancer, the few existing studies show a relative consistency in supporting an association between consumption of fat-containing animal products and cancer incidence. However the majority of the studies were not adjusted for total energy intake. Studies adjusting for energy intake did not find an increased risk (Kolonel, 2001). Meat intake, however, correlates more or less with prostate cancer risk. 16 out of 22 case control or cohort studies showed an increased risk above a risk ratio of 1.3. A recent prospective study (Michaud, Augustsson, & Rimm, 2001) documented an elevated risk (RR, relative risk) of prostate cancer (RR 1.47) from red meat consumption (>5/ week). Meat consumption up to 2-4 times a week had a RR below 1.0 (0.96) demonstrating that moderate red meat consumption, as usually recommended, does not contribute to prostate cancer risk.

Despite the long history of studies on fat and cancer, there remains some controversy. It is more or less generally suggested that animal fat rich in saturated fat is more closely related to cancerogenesis and plant-derived mostly unsaturated fat (PUFA) is more protective. In animal models, the tumour promoting effect of fat intake has been observed primarily for PUFA (Hopkins & Carroll, 1979; Hopkins, Kennedy, & Carroll, 1981). A couple of studies show that polyunsaturated *ù*6 fatty acids (linoleic acid) enhance cancer development in rodents (Carroll, 1991; Fay, Freedman, & Clifford, 1997). The prostaglandin E2 (PGE2) seems to be involved in colon carcinogenesis and is formed from ω6 fatty acids (arachidonic acid). EP1 (PGE2-receptor) k.o. mice showed resistance to AOM induction of neoplastic colon lesions (Watanabe, Kawamori, & Natatsugi, 1999). ω3 fatty acids (linolenic acid), however, suppress colon carcinogenesis by inhibiting the arachidonic pathway (Takahashi, Fukutake, & Isoi, 1997).

The suggestion that consumption of red meat as a source of dietary fat increases risk of colon cancer is based on the rather simple fat-colon cancer hypothesis, which is based on the premise that dietary fat promotes excretion of bile acids that can be converted to carcinogens (Reddy, 1981). The controversial results from different studies and the fact that meta analyses show that fat might have a rather minor role, if any, in cancerogenesis of the colon or in other cancer sites might be explained in different ways. The fat content of red meat varies widely and shows different fatty acid patterns. Palmitic acid but not stearic acid present in different amounts in red meat has been shown to be a strong mitogen of adenoma cells in culture (Friedman, Isaksson, & Rafter, 1989). Fat derived from red meat might be less absorbed, due to either its composition (stearic acid) or due to matrix (muscle) interactions. Polymorphisms of genes involved in the expression of cleavage and re-esterification of triglycerides may also play important roles regarding individual susceptibility. Finally, components not belonging to lipids might contribute to carcinogenesis, such as HCAs (heterocyclic amines) or at least the iron content of meat. Dietary iron enhances lipid peroxidation in the mouse colon (Younes, Trepkau, & Siegers, 1990) and increases the incidence of DMH-induced colorectal tumours in mice and rats (Siegers, Bumann, Baretton, & Younes, 1988; Nelson, Yoo, & Tanure, 1989). Indeed, studies in humans point to a relationship between body iron stores and incidence of colon tumours (Stevens, Jones, & Micozzi, 1988; Knekt, Reunanen, & Takkunen, 1994a). Finally, carcinogens and promoters, e.g. HCAs, are formed when meat is fried or cooked and may contribute more or less to individual cancer risk, especially in colorectal, breast and prostate cancers.

Processed meat and genetic polymorphisms

HCAs are converted to their hydroxyamino derivatives by cytochrome P450s, especially CYP 1A2, and are further activated by esterification enzymes acetyltransferase and sulfotransferase. The reactive ultimate forms produce DNA adducts with guanines at their C8 position, resulting in base substitution and at least mutation. Similarly, oxidative modification of DNA via reactive oxygen species (ROS) results in formation of 8-oxo-deoxy-guanin with subsequent base substitution and mutation.

Epidemiological studies revealed some positive (Zheng, Gustaffson, & Sinha, 1998) and some negative (Augustsson, Skog, Jägerstad, Dickman, & Steineck, 1999) links between cancer risk and intake of well-done meat or fish. Some studies that have examined intensity of cooking have tended to show positive associations with breast cancer (Knekt, Steineck, & Järvinen, 1994b); others have not (Ambrosone, Freudenheim, & Sinha, 1998). The latter investigated the role of genetic polymorphisms of enzymes involved in DNA adduct formation of HCAs, which could play a critical role in individual cancer susceptibility. HCAs require enzymatic activation to bind to DNA and to initiate carcinogenesis. N-acetyltransferase (NAT2) may play a role, its rate determined by a polymorphic gene. The results of Ambrosone, et al., (1998) were recently confirmed by studies of Delfino, Sinha, and Smith (2001) who did not find a correlation between NAT2 and breast cancer, nor any association between intake of red meat or degree of cooking and breast cancer.

Genetic polymorphisms including environmental aspects (gene-environment interactions) may also play a critical role in colorectal cancer with respect to red meat intake. Le Marchand (1999) investigated the colorectal cancer rates in Japanese immigrants in Hawaii. The colorectal cancer incidence of these groups (214.000 immigrants between 1886 and 1924) was initially very low and is now the highest in the world. The fast acetylator genotype (NAT2), without the polymorphism is present in 90% of Japanese compared with 45% of Caucasians; the frequency of CYP1A2 phenotype is similar in both groups. Consumption of –well-done meat together with a specific genotype of NAT2 and CYP1A2 may increase colorectal cancer risk substantially. Among the Japanese migrants who ate well-done red meat, those without the polymorphisms in both NAT2 and CYP1A2 had a 3.6 times greater risk of developing colon cancer than those with the polymorphisms. Another family of genes might determine individual susceptibility: glutathione transferase M1 (GSTM1) and T1 (GSTT1). Both code for cytosolic enzyme glutathione S-transferase which are involved in phase 2 metabolism especially in polycyclic aromatic hydrocarbon metabolism. The results of the few studies dealing with genetic polymorphisms of GST are inconsistent. Two studies suggest increased colon cancer risk in subjects with high meat intake and GST nonnull genotype, contrary to the underlying hypothesis. One study suggests a strong inverse relation between colorectal adenomas and broccoli consumption, particularly in subjects who are GSTM1 null (review, see Cotton,

Sharp, Little, & Brockton, 2000). As long as genotypically defined cohorts are not studied with respect to their susceptibility against meat intake (in different forms) the risk of red meat cannot be clearly identified. White meat and fish seem to be without risk; red meat only in a form where cytotoxic by-products such as HCA are formed.

Formation of HCAs can be significantly reduced by inexpensive and practical measures, such as avoidance of exposure of meat surfaces to flames, use of aluminium foil to wrap meat before oven roasting and by microwave cooking. Another protecting approach is the combination with protective bioactive constituents derived from plant food. For example, diallyl sulphide an organosulphur compound in garlic, blocks HCA carcinogenesis (Hasegawa, Hirose, & Kato, 1995; Morie, Sugie, Rahman, & Suzui, 1999). Nevertheless, even if there are some induction or promotion factors present in meat, diet composition may determine whether anti-carcinogenic factors from plants neutralise any harmful factors in meat. In addition, meat contains bioactive constituents known to be protective against cancer formation.

Protecting factors in meat with respect to cancer

FOLATE

Meat is an important source for methyl donors, such as folate and vitamin B12, and transfer factors methionine and choline. Folate and methionine as methyl donors influencing methyl group availability have also been associated with colon cancer incidence. It is frequently argued that the increased risk of different types of cancer resulting from low intake of fruit and vegetables is a result of a folate deficient diet, because fruit and vegetables are important sources of folate. Although this is true, it must be remembered that bioavailability of folate from meat and liver is much better than from fruits and vegetables. A few studies measured folate directly and it was claimed that a low folate intake has been related to an increased occurrence of colon adenomas (Giovannucci, Stampfer, & Colditz, 1993a; Benito, Stiggelbout, & Bosch, 1991) and cancer (Freudenheim, Graham, & Marshall, 1991; Lashner, Heidenreich, & Su, 1989). Zhang, Hunter and Hankinson (1999) studied the effect of alcohol and folate on breast cancer. The increased cancer risk associated with alcohol consumption (>15g/day) was reduced in women who consumed at least 300µg folate/day. The major source of folate was supplements. Even though an intake of 300µg/day does not reach the RDA (400µg/day), this study shows that increasing folate intake might be beneficial with respect to cancer. Indeed, increasing folate intake via supplementation, a form which has a very good bioavailability compared to vegetable-derived folic acid, decreases the risk of colon cancer significantly (Giovannucci, Stampfer, & Colditz, 1993b). The decreased risk however was not evident before 15 years, documenting that protective factors, if they indeed exist as single bioactive constituents, need to be present in the diet for a long time period. On the other hand, their absence or a low intake might also contribute to an increase cancer risk after a long time period. In rodents, diets deficient of methyl donors or transfer factors (folate, B12, methionine, choline) induce tumours at different sites (Shivapurkar & Poirer, 1983; Wainfan, Dizik, & Stender, 1989; Cravo, Maso, & Dayal, 1992). A methyl deficient diet lowers the concentration of the methyl donor S-adenosylmethionine, which leads to a reduction in methylation of DNA cytosine. Tumour supressor genes are inactivated by methylation of normally unmethylated sites. DNA hypomethylation due to a diet low in methyl donors (e.g. low in meat) may contribute to a loss of protooncogene expression (Nyce, Weinhouse, & Magee, 1983). Indeed, throughout the different stages of colonic neoplastic transformation, genomic hypomethylation (Goelz, Vogelstein, & Hamilton, 1985), methylation of usually unmethylated sites (Makos, Nelkin, & Lerman, 1992) and abnormal elevated DNA methyl transferase activity (Issa, Vertino, & Wu, 1993) are described.

An additional aspect, also involved in methylation reactions, which might contribute to individual colon cancer risk, is a genetic polymorphism of a key enzyme of folate metabolism: the methylenetetrahydrofolate-reductase (MTHFR). This enzyme converts 5,10- methylenetetrahydrofolate to 5-methyltetrahydrofolate, the major circulatory form of folate in the body and primary methyl donor for methylation of homocysteine to methionine. This pathway is a critical key in the methylation process of DNA. As described above, alterations in the methylation process can result in abnormal expression of oncogenes and tumour suppressor genes (Baylin, Makos, & We, 1991). The polymorphism of the human MTHFR gene (alanine to valine substitution, coding for a thermolabile enzyme with reduced activity) results in elevated plasma homocysteine levels. Homozygous individuals have 30% normal enzyme activity, heterozygous 65%. Up to now, there are controversial results in correlating this polymorphism with individual colon cancer risk. However, supplementation of folate or a diet rich in folate with optimum bioavailability, lowers homocystein and might therefore influence individual risk (Bronstrup, Hages, Prinz-Langenohl, & Pietrzik, 1998).

VITAMIN A

The German society for Nutrition recommends an increase in vitamin A intake of 40% for pregnant women and of 90% for breastfeeding women. Pregnant women and those who want to become pregnant are asked to avoid liver for scientifically very weakly proved reasons, therefore the provitamin A-carotenoid ß-carotene remains the essential vitamin A source. The most important sources of vitamin A are oranges and dark-green vegetables followed by enriched juices, which represent between 20 and 40% of the daily supply. In Germany, mean intake is about 1.5 and 2 mg of ß-carotene a day. If one supposes a conversion rate for ß-carotene for juices of 4:1, for fruit and vegetables of 12:1 to 26:1, this supply leads to a vitamin A supply of 10 to 15% of the recommendation. Because liver consumption of the population per head per year amounts to less than 500 g, ß-carotene is an important vitamin A source for young women, especially pregnant women and breastfeeding women.

Studies in Great Britain showed that in the middle and working classes, vitamin A supply can be regarded as insufficient. The American Association for Paediatrics called vitamin A one of the most critical vitamins during pregnancy and the breastfeeding period, especially in terms of the function and maturation of the lung. If the vitamin A supply of the mother is low, the supply to the foetus and concentrations in breast milk, which cannot be compensated by post-natal supplementation, are also low. At the same time, one has to keep in mind that there is a relationship between folic acid, vitamin A and iron status and low birth weight. This applies especially to premature babies, which show a direct correlation between vitamin A supply and occurrence of complications such as respiratory distress syndrome as one of the most frequent and serious complications.

In summary, the major source of vitamin A is liver, which contributes approximately 75% to the human vitamin A intake. Concerning a sufficient vitamin A supply, the provitamin A, ß-carotene, is of minor importance. Its conversion efficacy seems to be nearer to 1:12 and not 1:6 as frequently mentioned.

Is supply of vitamin A involved in the individual lung cancer risk? On the basis of a few reports, it is assumed that a "local" vitamin-A-deficiency exists in meta- and dysplastic-areas. Measurements of vitamin-A concentrations in metaplastic areas of the respiratory epithelium and the cervix epithelium proved that vitamin A was no longer to be found, in contrast to the surrounding healthy tissues.

At the moment it is difficult to distinguish between cause and effect. Studies carried-out by Edes and co-workers (Edes, 1991) hint at an induction of metaplasia caused by a vitamin-A-deficit. These studies showed that a depletion of vitamin-A-ester stores in different tissues (Edes, 1991) is caused by toxins that are present in cigarette-smoke (predominantly polyhalogenated compounds).

Epidemiological evidence supports the assumption that the development of obstructive respiratory diseases (COPD) plays an important role in cancer mortality of smokers. It was shown that the relative risk for smokers to be affected by lung cancer, when they suffered from obstructive ventilation disorder (FEV 1% < 60 respectively 70) (Skillud, Offord, & Miller, 1987), was significantly higher than that of comparative groups with normal lung-function-parameters.

A survey of dietary habits within the "National Health and Nutritional Examination Survey" showed an inverse correlation (Morabia, Sorenson, Kumanyika, Abbey, Cohen, & Chee, 1989) between vitamin-A-supply, as the only one of 12 examined dietary components, and obstructive respiratory diseases (COPD). COPD increase lung cancer risk significantly. If a diminished supply of vitamin A increases the appearance of obstructive respiratory diseases, a marginal or local vitamin-A-deficit could be responsible for the observed changes of the respiratory mucosa. Such a deficit results in loss of cilia, an increase in secreting cells and formation of squamous metaplasia (Stofft, Biesalski, Zschaebitz, & Weiser, 1992; Chytil, 1985; Biesalski, Wellner, Stofft, & Baessler, 1985).

Such changes (decrease of ciliated cells with simultaneous increase of the secretion) are noted among smokers (Gouveia, Mathe, & Hercend, 1982; Mathe, Gouveia, Hercend, Gros, & Dorval, 1983) and cause a reduction in mucociliary-clearance. This reduction in mucociliary-clearance, associated with an increased adsorption of the respiratory syncytial virus (RSV) (Donelly, 1996), could explain the extraordinarily high morbidity and mortality for respiratory infections of children with vitamin A deficiency in developing countries (Sommer, 1993).

There is sound evidence from experimental studies that alteration of the respiratory mucosa, caused by the vitamin A deficiency, can be re-differentiated into its functional original epithelium, *in vivo* as well as *in vitro*, following vitamin A supply (Biesalski et al., 1985; McDowell, Keenan, & Huang, 1984a; McDowell, Keenan, & Huang 1984b; McDowell, Ben, Coleman, Chang, Newkirk, & De Luca, 1987a; McDowell, Ben, Newkirk, Chang, & De Luca 1987b; Rutten, Wilmer, & Beems, 1988a, b). Squamous metaplasia of the bronchial mucosa, which occurs in smokers in spite of a sufficient supply with vitamin A as an effect of inhalative noxae, could also be reversed through systemic application of high retinoid-concentrations *in vitro* (Lasnitzki & Bollag, 1982; 1987) and in humans *in vivo* (Gouveia et al., 1982; Mathe et al., 1983).

SELENIUM

Selenium is found largely in grains, fish and meats and enters the food chain through plants at geographically variable rates dependent on selenium concentration of the soil. The best known biochemical role for selenium is as part of the active site of the enzyme glutathione peroxidase (GPx). The metabolic function of this enzyme is vital for cells, as it is part of a mechanism responsible for metabolism and detoxification of oxygen. It is assumed that GPx can protect DNA from oxidative damage and consequently from mutation leading to neoplastic transformation of cells (Combs & Clark, 1985). At relatively high levels, selenium protects against the action of certain carcinogens in various animal models (Halliwell & Gutteridge, 1989). In *in vitro* and *in vivo* studies, organic and inorganic selenium has been demonstrated to inhibit proliferation of normal and malignant cells and inhibit tumor growth (Griffin, 1982; Redman, Xu, & Peng, 1997). Apoptosis may result from competition of selenium for s-adenosyl-methionine with ornithine decarboxylase (ODC). ODC acitivity is indeed critically involved in cancerogenesis. From geographical studies it is documented that in areas with sufficient selenium concentrations in the diet (depending on selenium concentrations of the soil), there is an inverse relationship between selenium status and cancer (Schrauzer, White, & Schneider, 1977; Clark, Cantor, & Allaway, 1991). Epidemiological studies showed inverse associations of selenium intake or plasma levels and cancers of different sites (prostate, colon, skin etc.). In a recent, double blind, placebo controlled cancer prevention trial 200µg selenium (approximately 3 times RDA) was given daily to patients with histories of basal and squamous skin carcinoma (Clark et al., 1996). Selenium supplementation did not influence the primary endpoint prevention of recurrent skin cancers, but surprisingly was inversely associated with incidence of and mortality from total prostate, lung and colorectal cancers. Recently Yoshizawa, Willet, & Morris (1998) reported a strong inverse association of toenail concentration of selenium and prostate cancer risk (65% reduced risk in the highest quintile). Toenail concentration reflects long term intake of selenium and is consequently influenced by bioavailability. From intervention trials and from epidemiological studies there is now evidence indicating "that substantial increases in the consumption of selenium by men taking 80-90µg/day or more may have striking impact on prostate cancer rates" (Giovannucci, 1998). Recent surveys indicate that average intake of selenium may be as low as 30-40µg/day (Rayman, 1997). Intake data, however, do not really reflect bioavailability. Consequently, diet has a strong influence on total selenium supply to tissues. Especially in areas with low soil selenium, dietary sources containing substantial amounts of selenium with good bioavailability should be recommended. In the US Selenium is supplied mainly by cereals, breads, meats and meat products. Beef alone is estimated to contribute approximately 17% of total selenium in the American diet. Two recent studies in humans showed that meat was as good a source of selenium as wheat (Van der Torre, van Dokkum, & Schaafsma, 1991) and that SeMet was absorbed more rapidly than selenite in selenium deficient men (Xia, Zhao, & Zhu, 1992). In a recent study the bioavailability of selenium in rats was estimated from various portions of fully cooked commercial cuts of beef, including liver, striploin, round, shoulder and brisket (Shi and Spallholz, 1994). The bioavailability from the beef diets was compared with that of selenium as selenite or L-selenomethionine (SeMet). Liver GPx recovery (after depletion), muscle tissue depostion and plasma levels were taken as markers of bioavailability. Liver GPx-recovery was highest from SeMet > beef muscle > selenite = beef liver. Muscle deposition was highest from SeMet > beef muscle > selenite = beef liver. From these results the authors concluded that bioavailability of selenium from beef is higher than, or at least equal to, that of selenite, and slightly lower than that of SeMet. In summary, meat is an important source for bioavailable selenium.

ZINC

Zinc is a component of some metalloenzymes and is important for cell growth and replication, osteogenesis and immunity. It may further contribute to the overall antioxidative defence. The primary dietary sources of zinc are red meat, sea food, poultry, grains, dairy, legumes and vegetables (Groff & Grooper, 2000). Lower zinc levels were described in cancer patients (Mellow, Layne, & Lipman, 1983; Rogers, Thomas, & Davis, 1993); others did not find this association (Kok, Van Duijn, & Hofman, 1988; Kabuto, Imai, & Yonezawa, 1994). There is good evidence that zinc may contribute to prostate cancer incidence. Total zinc levels in the prostate are 10 times higher than in other soft tissues (Mawson & Fischer, 1952). Uptake of zinc via a membrane transporter into prostatic epithelial cells is under the control of hormones (testosterone, prolactin) (Costello, Liu, & Zou, 1999). Physiological concentrations of zinc inhibit growth of androgen-sensitive and androgen-independent prostate cancer cell lines via cell cycle arrest, apoptosis and necrosis (Iguchi, Hamatake, & Ishida, 1998; Liang, Liu, & Zou, 1999). Epidemiological findings are not consistent and a few studies estimating the effect of supplementation on prostate cancer risk are more or less controversial (for review, see Platz & Helzlsouer, 2001). One important reason for this inconsistency might be the high variability of zinc content of different sources, especially meat and sea food. Furthermore, zinc has a much better bioavailability from meat than from vegetables (Groff & Grooper, 2000) and other factors, present in the diet may increase (citric acid, histidine, cystein) or decrease (phytate, oxalate) the absorption of zinc (Groff & Grooper, 2000).

Consequently, the use of food questionnaires might not be a suitable approach to measure zinc intake. Adequate biomarkers, at present not available, may help to estimate individual zinc status and consequently individual risk. At present there is no clear cut evidence for a preventive effect of zinc on prostate cancer from epidemiological studies. Some small case control studies indicate low plasma zinc or low prostatic zinc levels in patients with prostate cancer compared with healthy controls (for review, see Platz & Helzlsouer, 2001). An optimum zinc intake can be recommended not only with respect to prevention of prostate cancer, and intakes below RDA should be avoided. One factor contributing to low intake might be a decline in red meat consumption which has been reported in New Zealand (Laugesen & Swimburn, 2000), as well as in the UK (Whitehead, 1995), USA (Popkin, Haines, & Reidy, 1989) and Canada (Zafiriou, 1985), concomitant with an increase in intakes of unrefined cereals, nuts and legumes. Red meat is a rich source of readily available zinc, whereas cereals contain different levels of phytic acid, a potent inhibitor of zinc absorption. Indeed, the recommendation to decrease or even avoid meat intake may result in a low zinc status as recently documented in women from New Zealand (Gibson, Heath, & Limbaga, 2001). In a cross sectional study of 330 women, the authors assessed the interrelationship of dietary intake, biochemical zinc status and anthropometric indices. Changes in food selection patterns (reduction of red meat) were suggested to be responsible for the lower biochemical zinc nutrition. This study is an example that a mixed and balanced diet, including meat and meat products, is the best way to ensure sufficient intake of all essential and potentially cancer preventive components.

Meat consumption, especially red meat, is not carcinogenic per se, even if it contains components which, based on epidemiological and animal experiments, are assumed to contribute to cancer formation. On the other hand, a lot of studies exist which demonstrate a reduced cancer risk in persons with a high intake of fruit and vegetables. As a basis for the preventive effect, protecting factors such as carotenoids, flavonoids and further phytochemicals are discussed. Within these protecting factors derived from fruit and vegetables, folic acid, selenium, zinc and other components are claimed to be preventive candidates. Why should theses compounds be less effective if they reach the body via meat, which is an important source for these compounds? The balance of promoting and protecting factors within the diet is important for protection against cancer. Furthermore, the IR-hypothesis shows that nutritional behaviour leading to a metabolic syndrome (high energy, high glycemic carbohydrates) might favour colon cancer or even cancers from other sites. The "goals for nutrition in the year 2000" (Willett, 2000) give very good and comprehensive advice: "Current nutritional recommendations for the prevention of cancer include increased consumption of fruit and vegetables; reduced consumption of red meat and animal fat; and avoidance of excessive alcohol. For many individuals a daily multivitamin that contains folic acid may also be part of a reasonable cancer prevention strategy."

To improve the "preventive capacity" of an individual, a balanced diet, rich in fruit and vegetables, including meat and meat products in moderate quantities, normal body weight and a reasonable amount of exercise represent the best choice.

The importance of meat as a source for micronutrients

The reason why meat is an essential source for some micronutrients is the fact that meat is either the only source or has a much higher bioavailability for some micronutrients.

Two important micronutrients occur only in meat: vitamins A and B12. Both cannot be compensated for by plant-derived provitamins. Provitamin B12 does not exist and the provitamin A, ß-carotene, has to be taken in high amounts due to a poor conversion rate (1:12).

Iron has a higher bioavailability when derived from meat as heme iron than plant-derived iron. Similarly folic acid has a nearly ten-fold higher bioavailability from meat (especially liver) and eggs than from vegetables. Consequently a low intake of meat (including liver) is associated with a risk of deficiencies in selected micronutrients.

WHO NEEDS MEAT – OR: ARE THERE GROUPS AT RISK FROM A LOW INTAKE OF MEAT DERIVED MICRONUTRIENTS?

Elderly people are generally considered at risk to develop vitamin and trace element deficiencies, especially vitamins A, D, E, and folate as well as iron and calcium (Martins, Dantas, Guimar, & Amorin, 2002; Bates et al., 2002; Anderson, 2001; Viteri & Gonzalez, 2002). The multifactorial causes of this health hazard comprise quantitative and qualitative decreased food intake, reduced energy expenditure due to sedentary life style and loss of metabolically active body cell mass, and development of chronic age-associated disorders.

It was generally assumed that impaired bioavailability of micronutrients was a common problem among elderly. However, the digestive and absorptive capacity of the digestive tract is well retained during ageing; if decreased absorption of macronutrients occurs, it is the result of disease rather than ageing itself (Black, 2001). An exception to this rule is the impaired bioavailability of dietary iron due to gastric mucosal atrophy, the occurrence of which is age-related and in many cases could be regarded as a disorder rather than a disease. Nevertheless, the frequently occurring atrophic gastritis in elderly, which also affects vitamin B12 absorption, should be one reason to recommend meat intake in this risk group.

Adequate nutrition during pregnancy plays an important role in the well-being of mother and child and influences the health of the offspring during childhood and adulthood. Nutritional requirements are increased during pregnancy, but will generally be met by dietary intake and adaptive physiological changes (Draper, Lewis, Malhotra, & Wheeler, 1993). However, the micronutrient status of vitamin D, folic acid, iron, and zinc may become compromised without supplementation (Draper et al., 1993; Fogelholm, 1999; Saletti, Lindgren, Johansson, & Cederholm, 2000) especially when meat is avoided, which can be frequently seen in women of child-bearing age. Folic acid supplementation is generally recommended to decrease the risk of serious births defects. Especially in multiparious women, the essential fatty acid status may become impaired and negatively affect the neurological and cognitive development of the offspring (Lowik, van den Berg, Schrijver, Odink, Wedel, & van Houten, 1992; Reynolds, 2002).

The micronutrient intake of vegans is easily imbalanced with respect to recommended dietary allowances. Intake of vitamin B12, riboflavin, and selenium often is inadequate. Even the use of dietary supplements often does not meet the recommended intake of vitamin B12 and selenium (Boelsma, Hendriks, & Roza, 2001; Andersson et al., 1986).

Although it seems obvious that subjects on a weight reduction diet are at risk to develop micronutrient deficiencies, the scientific evidence for this is weak. Most reports include less than fifty subjects and deal with the combination of energy restriction and increased physical activity, and hence are difficult to interpret (Philipsen-Geerling & Brummer, 2000). The micronutrients at risk appear to be iron, magnesium, zinc, fat soluble vitamins and essential fatty acids. Although a nutritionally adequate low-fat diet seems feasible in a motivated, free-living population (Gassull & Cabre, 2001), data exist which show that a high protein intake even when associated with a higher fat intake might favour weight loss.

A recent meta-analysis of studies dealing with dietary weight loss showed that protein rich diets low in carbohydrates and a moderate or high fat content resulted in better weight loss than diets low in fat and protein and rich in carbohydrates (Bravata et al., 2003). Several factors are suggested to contribute to this increased weight loss: better satiety, higher energy expenditure (thermogenesis), greater loss of fat cell mass.

Energy restricted diets and traditional cholesterol lowering diets are typically focussed on the reduction of total fat intake while simultaneously increasing the proportion of polyunsaturated fatty acids (PUFAs). However these PUFAs usually contain high concentrations of n-6 fatty acids and low amounts of n-3 fatty acids. This may have an adverse effect not only on reducing the risk for obesity-related metabolic disorders such as vascular disease and heart rhythm disturbances, but also on the regulation of the intermediary metabolism of brain monoamines such as serotonin, which may lead to impaired mood status and depression (Alonso-Aperte & Varela-Moreiras, 2000).

It is well known that malnutrition is far more common among institutionalized and chronic hospitalized elderly compared to free-living subjects in the community and that the prevalence of malnutrition is associated with the severity of morbidity, functional impairments and mental state (Bates, Mansoor, van der Pols, Prentice, Cole, & Finch, 1997; Selhub, Jacques, Bostom, Wilsin, & Rosenberg, 2000; Rasmussen, Ovesen, Bûlow, Knudsen, Laurberg, & Perrild, 2000; Koehler, Baumgarter, Garry, Allen, Stabler, & Rimm, 2001). The deficiency affects a broad spectrum of micronutrients, such as the B vitamins, especially B1, B6, folate and B12, vitamins C, D and E, essential fatty acids and selenium (Brubacher, Moser, & Jordan, 2000; Bates, Prentice, Cole, van der Pols, Doyle, Finch, Smithers, & Clarke, 1999). Thiamine and folate status need special attention in this respect, as a deficiency of these nutrients is associated with depression and impaired cognition and dementia (Block, Norkus, Hudes, Mandel & Helzlsouer, 2001; Report on Health and Social Subjects No. 49, 1998). Intervention trials with micronutrient supplementation consisting of zinc and selenium, vitamin C, beta-carotene and alpha-tocopherol were associated with a reduction of infectious events, probably due to the micronutrients administration rather than the supplementation of vitamins (Gey, Brubacher, & Staehelin, 1987; Gey, 1993).

Chronic use of drugs may lead to micronutrient deficiency by decreasing food intake, mainly due to impaired appetite or reduced motility of the upper gastrointestinal-tract, or by decreasing the bioavailability of micronutrients, for example cholestyramine which impairs absorption of fatty acids and fat-soluble vitamins, or by interfering with metabolism. A number of micronutrients, such as zinc and magnesium, play a role in phase I oxidation reactions involved in drug metabolism. Typical examples are increased folate requirements with chronic use of sulphasalazine, methotrexate, or valproic acid. However, a relevant interaction between drugs and specific micronutrients only occurs in case of prolonged use of specific drugs in high doses in susceptible subjects.

Selected meat derived micronutrients

Meat is an excellence source for various micronutrients: Low-fat pork meat contains 1.8 mg iron, 2.6 mg zinc, pig liver contains 360 mg magnesium, 20 mg iron and 60 µg selenium per 100 g. Meat and liver (100 g/day) can provide up to 50% of RDA for iron, zinc, selenium, Vitamins B12, B1, B2, B6 and 100% of vitamin A.

VITAMIN A

Vitamin A is essential for growth and development of cells and tissues. In its active form, retinoic acid (RA), it controls regular differentiation as a ligand for retinoic acid receptors (RAR, RXR) and is involved in integration (gap junction formation) of cell formations (Kurokowa, DiRenzo, & Boehm, 1994). Vitamin A plays a substantial role, especially in the respiratory epithelium and the lung. During moderate vitamin A -deficiency, incidence of diseases of the respiratory tract is considerably increased and repeated respiratory infections can be influenced therapeutically by moderate vitamin A - supplementation (Pinnock, Douglas, & Badcock, 1986; Sommer, 1993; West, Pokhrel, & Katz, 1991). In addition to the importance of the vitamin for lung function, vitamin A is also responsible for development of many tissues and cells as well as for embryonic lung development. Recent studies proved that the control occurs by different expressions of retinoid receptors.

The influence of vitamin A on maturation and differentiation of the lung

The alveolar cells of type II are especially prepared to synthesize and secrete surfactant (Zachman, 1989). RA is able to stop, concentration-dependently (Metzler & Snyder, 1993) expression of surfactant-protein A (SP-A) in human foetal lung explants. Insulin, TGF-ß and high concentrations of glucocorticoids can also down-regulate the SP-A-mRNA-expression (Weaver & Whitsett, 1991), but lower concentrations of glucocorticoids stimulate expression of these genes (Odom, Snyder, Boggaram, & Mendelson, 1988). In contrast, SP-B-mRNA-expression is increased in human foetal lung explants both by hyperoxia (rats) (Metzler & Snyder, 1993) and by dexamethason (human foetal lung explant). Consequently, formation of some surfactant-proteins is regulated differently and selectively by RA together with glucocorticoids.

Prostaglandins of type PGE2 are able to increase surfactant-synthesis. Under the influence of EGF (epidermal growth factor), formation of prostaglandin rises, especially of PGE2. On the other hand, expression of the

EGF-receptor is increased by RA. EGF increases proliferation of lung tissues and this leads to amplified formation of surfactant phospholipids (Sundell, Gray, Serenius, Escobedo, & Stahlman, 1980). RA and EGF both lead to an increase (40%, 80%) in PGE2-secretion in foetal lung cells of rat *in vitro* (Haigh, D'Souza, & Micklewright, 1989). Combination of RA and EGF though leads to a more than a six-fold increase in PGE2-secretion. Consequently, RA can interfere with lung development by its modulating effect on EGF-expression and subsequent PGE2-induced surfactant formation. A sufficient and continuous availability (either on the blood pathway or by local storage sides) is pivotal, especially for a time-dependent regulation of lung-development and related formation of the active metabolite retinoic acid.

Vitamin A -kinetics during foetal lung development

Local extra-hepatic stores are present in fibroblast-like cells close to alveolar cells, in type-II-cells as well as in respiratory epithelium retinyl-esters. The importance of these retinyl-esters as "acute reserve" during development of the lung becomes apparent during the late phase of gestation and the beginning of lung maturation. During this period, a rapid emptying of the retinyl-ester stores in the lung of rat embryos occurs (Geevarghese & Chytil, 1994). This depletion is the result of an increased demand in the process of lung development, because retinoic acid is "instantly" needed for the process of cellular differentiation (e.g. proximalization) and metabolic work (surfactant).

Prenatal lung development is also influenced by glucocorticoids. Steroid hormones have a similar effect on lung development to vitamin A, i.e. these two factors complement each other. This is not surprising, because the receptors for steroids and retinoids belong to the same multireceptor-complex. The mode of action of glucocorticoids does not only operate at the level of gene-expression, but seems to have an impact in a much earlier phase of vitamin release. Application of dexamethason leads to an increase in maternal and foetal retinol-binding protein. Thus, vitamin A supply is improved via the regular hepatic export pathway. Such an increase in vitamin A concentration in systemic circulation obviously diminishes morbidity and mortality of prematures due to bronchopulmonal dysplasia (Shenai, Kennedy, Chytil, & Stahlman, 1987; Shenai, Rush, Stahlman, & Chytil, 1990). Dexamethason respectively glucocorticoids not only lead to improvement in total vitamin A supply through a change in release from the liver, but they also influence, as recently described (Geevarghese & Chytil, 1994), metabolism of vitamin A esters, which are stored in the lung. After administration of dexamethason, as well as after administration of steroids, a significant reduction in retinyl-esters can be detected in the maturing lung, together with a moderate increase in retinol, the hydrolyzation product of retinyl-ester. This observation may explain the therapeutic success of steroids, and also their failure during therapy of lung-distress syndrome in prematures. As far as an insufficient supply is concerned, inappropriate retinyl-ester stores, caused by a shortage of supply to the fetal lung during late pregnancy, the regulatory effect of glucocorticoids on vitamin A -metabolism of lung cells cannot take place.

Very low plasma vitamin-A levels (Shenai, Chytil, Jhaveri, & Stahlman, 1981) are recurrently found in prematures, especially in cases with lung-distress-syndrome. This can be attributed, amongst other things, to the relative immaturity of the liver for synthesis of retinol-binding proteins. The neonate is almost exclusively dependent on the mother for its supply, this includes the lung retinyl-esters which are either absorbed by the cells directly (from chylomicrons) or by esterification of retinol after uptake into the cells. These lung retinyl-ester stores can only be sufficiently filled if the mother provides an appropriate vitamin A supply, especially during the late pregnancy.

The influence of an insufficient vitamin A -supply on post-natal development of the lung

A disease seen recurrently in connection with vitamin A -supply is the bronchopulmonary dysplasia (BDP). The pathogenesis of BDP depends on a multitude of factors. Some of the observed morphological changes are very similar to those seen in vitamin A deficiency of humans and animals. In particular, there is focal loss of ciliated cells with keratinizing metaplasia and necrosis of the bronchial mucosa as well as an increase of mucous secreting cells (Stahlmann, 1984; Stofft et al., 1992).

Because focal keratinizing metaplasia may occur as a consequence of vitamin A deficiency, impairment of differentiation is probably at the level of gene expression. Since vitamin A regulates expression of different cytokeratins, and therefore influences terminal differentiation, it seems obvious to assume common mechanisms. Consequently, prematures, especially neonates, are dependent on a sufficient supply of vitamin A to ensure regulation of cellular differentiation of respiratory epithelium and lung epithelium. The earlier a child is born before due date, the lower are its serum retinol levels (Mupanemunda, Lee, Fraher, Koura, & Chance, 1994). Since further decreases in serum retinol level and RBP level occur post-natally, the plasma value at birth is considered to be a critical parameter regarding lung development.

It has been shown repeatedly that serum retinol level and RBP level in prematures are significantly lower than in neonates (Shah and Rajalekshmi,

1984). Significantly lower retinol levels can be found in the liver of prematures compared with neonates (Shenai, Chytil, & Stahlman, 1985). Plasma values lower than 20 µg/dl are not rare in this case and they should be taken as an indicator of a vitamin A deficit.

Reduced plasma levels during the first months of life have a considerable influence on overall development as well as on susceptibility of infants to infections. With reduced plasma retinol levels, repeated infections are more often described (Barretto, Santos, & Assis, 1994; Filteau, Morris, & Abbott, 1993; Pinnock et al., 1986) and they are counted among the main complications of poor vitamin A supply in developing countries. In addition, serum vitamin A level continues to drop during infectious diseases, particularly diseases of the respiratory tract (Neuzil, Gruber, Chytil, Stahlman, Engelhardt, & Graham, 1994). On one hand, this can be explained by an increased metabolic demand and, on the other hand, by an increased renal elimination of retinol and of RBP during acute infections (Stephensen, Alvarez, Kohatsu, Hardmeier, Kennedy, & Gammon Jr., 1994).

The suggestion that liver should be avoided as a component of a healthy diet is primarily based on questionable contaminants suspected in liver (e.g. hormones, xenobiotics, metals etc.). If ß-carotene from vegetables were the only source of vitamin A, more than 500 g mixed and ß-carotene rich vegetables must be eaten per day to reach the recommended 1 mg retinol. Concerning contaminants, it has not been evaluated whether this amount of vegetables contains more contaminants than a portion of liver. A small portion of liver (100 g) twice a month is neither toxic nor teratogenic and contributes to a sufficient supply of vitamin A for the body.

IRON

Iron supports oxidative metabolism. It is essential for gas exchange at the tissue and cellular levels through hemoglobin oxygenation in red cells and myoglobin in skeletal muscle (Beard, Dawson, & Pinero, 1996). Moreover, iron-containing enzymes are involved in cellular energy metabolism and in host-defence responses (Beard et al., 1996; Griffiths, 1996). These various roles are due to the biological catalytic activity of iron. Like many other transition elements, iron posses unfilled atomic orbitals that allow it to co-ordinate electron donors and to participate in redox processes (Griffiths, 1996; Fraga & Oteiz, 2002).

Iron is one of the most abundant elements in the Earth's crust. Paradoxically, iron deficiency is the most common and widespread nutritional disorder in the world (DeMaeyer & Adiels-Tegman, 1985). Due to biological losses, such as cyclical monthly bleeding of fertile-aged women, excessive infestation with blood-feeding parasites, or poor bioavailability of iron from plant-based diets, it is estimated that as many as 4-5 billion people, 66-80% of the world's population, may be iron deficient (DeMaeyer & Adiels-Tegman, 1985; World Health Organization, 1992). At any given time, 2 billion people – over 30% of the world's population – are anaemic, mainly due to iron deficiency, and in developing countries this is frequently exacerbated by malaria and worm infections (World Health Organization, 1992).

There is a particular risk of iron deficiency for women and girls of child-bearing age, because of menstrual losses. In a recent Irish food consumption survey, almost half of women aged 18-50 years had inadequate iron intakes when compared with national average requirements (Beard et al., 1996). In the British National Diet and Nutrition Survey, iron intakes were found to be low in girls (aged 7-18 years), with iron intakes decreasing with age. Adolescent females (15-18 year) were found to have extremely low intakes of iron when compared to UK dietary reference values. Depending on composition of the individual diet, bioavailability of iron can differ 5 to 10-fold. Bioavailability depends on the presence or absence of different ligands (phytates from cereal products, tannins from coffee and tea, and oxalates from vegetables) which form complexes with iron and zinc to block their absorption. A diet which is primarily composed of vegetables, rice, beans and maize is associated with poor iron bioavailability, which explains the high incidence of anaemia in developing countries. 100g pork meat added to the vegetarian diet described above increases iron absorption 3.6 fold.

FOLIC ACID

In European countries the average folate intake in adults was found to be remarkably similar, around 300 μg/day in adult males and 250 μg/day in adult women (De Bree, van Dusseldorp, Brouwer, van het Hof, & Steegers-Theunissen, 1997). This is at about the recommended intake level, but lower than that recommended for pregnant women and women planning a pregnancy. For these groups an intake of >400 μg/day is considered protective against neural tube defects. More than 90% of women of childbearing age have dietary folate intakes below this optimal level. However, it must be realised that it is difficult to assess dietary folate intake because databases often do not have complete and updated information for folate content of many foods.

The link between poor folic acid status and neural tube defects is well documented but poorly characterized. Poor status is also linked to risen plasma homocysteine, a risk indicator for cardiovascular diseases and poor status may also increase the risk of neurological disorders and cancers. Supplementation with folate (100% bioavailability) reduces risk of neural tube defects up to 70%. Regarding bioavalability, liver might be also a good source.

VITAMIN B12

Vitamin B12 is found only in animal products. In a recent UK study of 250 vegetarian and 250 vegan men, approximately one quarter of vegetarians and more than half of vegans had sub-optimal intakes of vitamin B12. Plasma vitamin B12 levels were low in the vegetarians and extremely low in the vegan group, with more than a quarter below the threshold level where neurological signs may develop (130 ng/L) (Lloyd-Wright, Allen, Key, & Sanders, 2001). The elderly are also at risk of vitamin B12 deficiency, due to physiological changes resulting in reduced absorption. In the UK, vitamin B12 status in some people aged 65 and over was inadequate. There was no difference in mean levels between men and women. However, vitamin B12 intakes were adequate when compared with UK dietary reference values (Finch et al., 1998).

SELENIUM

Selenium is often considered as belonging to the group of antioxidant nutrients, since it is incorporated into the enzyme glutathion peroxidase, which acts as a cellular protector against free radical oxidative damage. A secondary end-point analysis of a randomised placebo-controlled skin cancer prevention trial suggested that supplemental selenium might reduce incidence of and mortality from cancers at several sites (Clark et al., 1996). However, the efficacy of selenium as a cancer preventive agent should await the results of large on-going controlled studies. Like many other nutrients, selenium is necessary for a well-functioning immune system, and has been suggested as particularly efficacious in HIV and AIDS. However, a systematic review found no evidence for a clinically-relevant function of selenium in that context (Ozsoy & Ernst, 1999).

Although selenium is widely distributed in the environment, the selenium content of animal-derived foods is greatly affected by soil on which crops grow or animals graze. Recent evidence suggests that selenium intakes in most parts of Europe are falling and are low when compared with recommended intakes (Rayman, 1997; Rayman, 2000). Declining intakes in the last three decades have been attributed mainly to a change in the source of wheat for bread and cereal products, from predominantly North American to European origin (from a high to low selenium content). These are reflected in decreasing plasma or serum selenium levels. Due to its antioxidant effects, selenium may be protective against chronic degenerative diseases. In the UK, selenium intakes were low in the majority of the elderly (aged 65 and over) in the British National Diet and Nutrition Survey when compared with UK dietary reference values (Thane & Bates, 2001). Selenium intakes decreased with increasing age in this population subgroup. Sufficient zinc intake is important for proper function of the immune system.

ZINC

Zinc deficient individuals demonstrate slower wound healing and are more prone to infections. However, studies of the effect of zinc supplementation aimed at the healing rate of venous leg ulcers have been inconclusive. A Cochrane review concluded that oral zinc did not appear to aid the healing of leg ulcers, and that there was only weak evidence that zinc was of benefit in patients with venous leg ulcers and low serum zinc (Wilkinson & Hawke, 2002). Zinc has been found to inhibit rhinovirus replication *in vitro*. Some studies have demonstrated that zinc may beneficially affect cold symptoms; however a meta-analysis of randomised controlled trials concluded that evidence for the effectiveness of zinc in reducing the duration of common cold symptoms is lacking (Jackson, Lesho, & Peterson, 2000). Finally, in settings with high rates of stunting and low plasma zinc concentrations, zinc supplementation may improve children's growth (Brown, Peerson, & Allen, 1998). So far, studies with supplementation did not reveal consistent results. However, a low intake of zinc is associated with a weakened immune system. T-cell count, T-cell proliferation and function and NK-cell activity are reduced. Reduced zinc status is especially evident in the elderly (Lukito, Wattanapenpaiboon, Savige, Hutchinson, & Wahlqvist, 2004). In elderly people, a higher protein intake (together with slight exercise) stops sarkopenia, a progressive loss of lean body mass. During pregnancy and lactation a higher zinc requirement is documented as well as during chronic inflammatory diseases (Rink & Gabriel, 2000).

Conclusion

Meat as a component of a mixed and healthy diet contains important and essential micronutrients. Adequate meat intake ensures normal function of the immune system, the mucous membranes and the general metabolism of substrates. A sufficient intake ensures that during times of higher requirement, e.g. diseases and pregnancy, this need is adequately covered. Consequently, meat should be recommended, especially in risk groups (elderly, pregnant women, growing children).

References

Alonso-Aperte, E., & Varela-Moreiras, G. (2000). Drugs-nutrient interactions: a potential problem during adolescence. *European Journal of Clinical Nutrition, 54 Suppl 1*, S69-74.

Ambrosone, C. B., Freudenheim, J. L., & Sinha, R. (1998). Breast cancer risk, meat consumption and acetyltransferase (NAT2) genetic polymorphisms. *Journal of Cancer, 75*, 825-830.

Anderson, A. S. (2001). Symposium on 'nutritional adaptation to preganancy and lactation'. Pregnancy as a time for dietary change? In *the Proceedings of the Nutrition Society, 60*, 497-504.

Andersson, H., Bosaeus, I., Brummer, R. J., Fasth, S., Hultén, L., Magnusson, O., & Strauss, B. (1986). Nutritional and metabolic consequences of extensive bowel resection. *Digestive Diseases, 4*, 193-202.

Augustsson, K., Skog, K., Jägerstad, M., Dickman, P. W., & Steineck, G. (1999). Dietary heterocyclic amines and cancer of the colon, rectum, bladder and kidney: a population based study *Lancet, 353,* 703-707.

Barreto, M. I., Santos, I. M. P., & Assis, A. M. O. (1994). Effect of vitamin A supplementation on diarrhoea and acute lower-respiratory-tract infections in young children in Brazil. *Lancet, 344,* 228-231.

Bates, C. J., Mansoor, M. A., van der Pols, J., Prentice, A., Cole, T. J., & Finch, S. (1997). Plasma total homocysteine in a representative sample of 972 British men and women aged 65 and over. *The European Journal of Clinical Nutrition, 51*, 691-697.

Bates, C. J., Prentice, A., Cole, T. J., van der Pols, J. C., Doyle, W., Finch, S., Smithers, G., & Clarke, P. C. (1999). Micronutrients: Highlights and Research Challenges from the 1994/5 National Diet and Nutrition Survey of People Aged 65 Years and Over. *The British Journal of Nutrition, 82*, 7-15.

Bates, C. J., Benton, D., Biesalski, H. K., Staehelin, H. B., van Staveren, W., Stehle, P., Suter, P. M., & Wolfram, G. (2002). Nutrition and aging: a consensus statement. *The Journal of Nutrition, Health & Aging, 6*, 103-116.

Baylin, S. B., Makos, M., & We, J. (1991). Abnormal patterns of DNA methylation in human neoplasia: Potential consequences for tumor progression. *Cancer Cells*, 3, 382-390.

Beard, J. L., Dawson, H., & Pinero, D. J. (1996). Iron metabolism: a comprehensive review. *Nutrition Reviews, 54(10)*, 295-317.

Benito, E., Stiggelbout, A., & Bosch, F. X. (1991). Nutritional factors in colorectal cancer risk: a case control study in Majorca. *The International Journal of Cancer*, 49, 161-167.

Biesalski, H. K., Wellner, U., Stofft, E., & Baessler, K. H. (1985). Vitamin A deficiency and sensory function. *Acta Vitaminologica et Enzymologica*, 7 Suppl, 45-54.

Black, R. E. (2001). Micronutrients in pregnancy. *The British Journal of Nutrition, 85 (Suppl 2)*, S193-197.

Block, G., Norkus, E., Hudes, M., Mandel, S., & Helzlsouer, K. (2001). Which plasma antioxidants are most related to fruit and vegetable consumption? *The American Jounal of Epidemiology*, 154, 1113-1118.

Boelsma, E., Hendriks, H. F., & Roza, L. (2001). Nutritional skin care: health effects of micronutrients and fatty acids. *The American Journal of Clinical Nutrition*, 73, 853-864.

Bravata, D. M., Sanders, L., Huang, J., Krumholz, H. M., Olkini, I., Gardner, C. D., & Bravata, D. M. (2003). Efficacy and safety of low-carbohydrate diets: a systematic review. *The Journal of the American Medical Association, 289(4)*, 1837-1850.

Bronstrup, A., Hages, M., Prinz-Langenohl, R., & Pietrzik, K. (1998). Effects of folic acid and combinations of folic acid and vitamin B-12 on plasma homocysteine concentrations in healthy, young women. *The American Journal of Clinical Nutrition*, 68, 1104-1110.

Brown, K. H., Peerson, J. M., & Allen, L. H. (1998). Effect of zinc supplementation on children's growth: a meta-analysis of intervention trials. *Bibliotheca Nutritio et Dieta*, 54, 76-83.

Brubacher, D., Moser, U., & Jordan, P. (2000). Vitamin C concentrations in plasma as a function of intake: a meta-analysis. *The International Journal for Vitamin and Nutrition Research*, 70, 226-237.

Bruce, W. R., Wolever, T. M. S., & Giacca, A. (2000). Mechanism linking diet and colorectal cancer: The possible role of insulin resistance. *Nutrition and Cancer* 37, 19-26.

Carroll, K. K. (1991). Dietary fats and cancer. *The American Journal of Clinical Nutrition*, 53, 1064-1067.

Chytil, F. (1985). Function of vitamin A in the respiratory tract. *Acta Vitaminologica et Enzymologica*, 7, 27-31.

Clark, L. C., Cantor, K. P., & Allaway, W. H. (1991). Selenium in forage crops and cancer mortality in US countries. *Archives of Environmental Health, 46,* 37-42.

Clark, L. C., Combs, G. F., Turnbull, B. W., Slate, E. H., Chalker, D. K., Chow, J., Davis, L. S., Glover, R. A., Graham, G. F., Gross, E. G., Krongrad, A., Lesher, J. L., Park, H. K., Sanders, B. B., Smith, C. L., & Taylor, J. R. (1996). For the Nutritional Prevention of Cancer Study Group. Effects of selenium supplementation for cancer prevention in patients with carcinoma of the skin. *Journal of the American Medical Association, 276,* 1957-1963.

Combs, G. F., & Clark, L. C. (1985). Can dietary selenium modify cancer risk? *Nutrition Reviews, 43,* 325-331.

Costello, L. C., Liu, Y., & Zou, J. (1999). Evidence for a zinc uptake transporter in human prostate cancer cells which is regulated by prolactin and testosterone. *The Journal of Biological Chemistry, 274,* 17499-17504.

Cotton, S. C., Sharp, L., Little, J., & Brockton, N. (2000). Glutathione S transferase polymorphisms and colorectal cancer: A HuGE review. *American Journal of Epidemiology, 151,* 7-32.

Cravo, M. L., Maso, J. B., & Dayal, Y. (1992). Folate deficiency enhances the development of colonic neoplasia of dimethylhydrazine treated rats. *Cancer Research,* 52, 5002-5006.

De Bree, A., van Dusseldorp, M., Brouwer, I. A., van het Hof, K. H., & Steegers-Theunissen, R. P.M. (2001). Folate intake in Europe: recommended, actual and desired intake. *The European Journal of Clinical Nutrition, 51,* 643-660.

Delfino, R. J., Sinha, R., & Smith, C. (2001). Breast cancer, heterocyclic aromatic amines from meat and N-acetyltransferase 2 genotyp. *Carcinogenesis, 21,* 607-615.

DeMaeyer, E. M., & Adiels-Tegman, M. (1985). The prevalence of anaemia in the world. *World Health Statistics Quarterly, 38,* 302-316.

Donelly, B. I. (1996). Vitamin A and respiratory syncytial virus infection. *Archives of Pediatrics and Adolescent Medicine, 150,* 882-892.

Draper, A., Lewis, J., Malhotra, N., & Wheeler, E. (1993). The energy and nutrient intakes of different types of vegetarian: a case for supplements? *The British Journal of Nutrition, 69,* 3-19.

Edes, T. E. (1991). Exposure to the carcinogen benzopyrene depletes tissue vitamin A. *Nutrition and Cancer;* 15, 159-166.

Fay, M. P., Freedman, L. S., & Clifford, C. K. (1997). Effects of different types and amounts of fat on the development of mammary tumors in rodents: A review: *Cancer Research,* 57, 3979-3988.

Filteau, S. M., Morris, S. S., & Abbott, R. A. (1993). Influence of morbidity on serum retinol of children in a community-based study in northern Ghana. *The American Journal of Clinical Nutrition, 58,* 192-197.

Finch, S., Doyle, W., Lowe, C., Bates, C. J., Prentice, A., Smithers, G., & Clarke, P. (1998). National Diet and Nutrition Survey: People Aged 65 Years or Over. Volume 1, *Report of the Diet and Nutrition Survey.* The Stationery Office, London

Fogelholm, M. (1999). Micronutrients: interaction between physical activity, intakes and requirements. *Public Health Nutrition, 2,* 349-356.

Fraga, G. C., & Oteiz, P.I. (2002). Iron toxicity and antioxidant nutrients. *Toxicology, 180,* 23-32.

Freudenheim, J. L., Graham, S., & Marshall, J. R. (1991). Folate intake and carcinogenesis of the colon and rectum. *International Journal of Epidemiology, 20,* 368-374.

Friedman, E., Isaksson, P., & Rafter, J. (1989). Fecal diglycerides as selective endogenous mitogens for premalignant and malignant human colonic epithelial cells. *Cancer Research, 49,* 544-554.

Frost, G., Leeds, A., & Trew, R. (1998). Insulin sensitivity in women at risk of coronary heart disease and the effect of a low glycemic diet. *Metabolism, 47,* 1245-51.

Gassull, M. A. & Cabre, E. (2001). Nutrition in inflammatory bowel disease. *Current Opinion in Clinical Nutrition and Metabolic Care, 4,* 561-569.

Geevarghese, S. K., & Chytil, F. (1994). Depletion of retinyl esters in the lungs coincides with lung prenatal morphological maturation. *Biochemical and Biophysical Research Communications, 200,* 529-535.

Gey, K. F. (1993). Prospects for the prevention of free radical disease, regarding cancer and cardiovascular disease. *British Medical Bulletin, 49,* 679-699.

Gey, K. F., Brubacher, G. B., & Staehelin, H. B. (1987). Plasma levels of antioxidant vitamins in relation to ischemic heart disease and cancer. *The American Journal of Clinical Nutrition, 45,* 1368-1377.

Gibson, R. S., Heath, A. L., & Limbaga, M. L. (2001). Are changes in food consumption patterns associated with lower biochemical zinc status among women from Dunedin, New Zealand? *The British Journal of Nutrition, 86,* 71-80.

Giovannucci, E. (1998). Selenium and risk of prostate cancer. *Lancet, 352,* 755-756.

Giovannucci, E., Rimm, R. B., & Stampher, M. J. (1994). Intake of fat, meat, and fibre in relation to risk of colon cancer in man. *Cancer Research, 54,* 2390-2397.

Giovannucci, E., Stampfer, M. J., & Colditz, G. A. (1993a). Folate, methionine, and alcohol intake and risk of colorectal adenoma. *Journal of the National Cancer Institute, 85*, 875-884.

Giovannucci, E., Stampfer, M. J., & Colditz, G. A. (1993b). Multivitamin use, folate, and colon cancer in women in the Nurse's health study. *Annals of Internal Medicine, 129,* 517-524.

Goelz, S. E., Vogelstein, B., & Hamilton, F. R. (1985). Hypomethylation of DNA from benign and malignant human colon neoplasma. *Science, 228,* 187-190.

Gouveia, J., Mathe, G., & Hercend, T. (1982). Degree of bronchial metaplasia in heavy smokers and its regression after treatment with retinoid. *Lancet, 1(8274),* 710-712.

Griffin, A. C. (1982). The chemopreventive role of selenium in carcinogenesis. In M. S. Arnott & J. Van Eys (Eds.), *Molecular interrelations of nutrition and cancer* (pp. 401-408). New York Raven Press.

Griffiths, E. (1996). Iron in biological systems. In J. J. Bullen, & E. Griffiths (Eds.), *Iron and Infection. Molecular, Physiological and Clinical Aspects. 2nd ed.* New York.

Groff, J. L., & Grooper, S. S. (2000). Advanced nutrition and human metabolism. Belmont, CA. Wadsworth.

Haigh, R., D'Souza, S. W.,& Micklewright, L. (1989). Human amniotic fluid urogastrone (epidermal growth factor) and fetal lung phospholipids. *British Journal of Obstetrics and Gynaecology, 96,* 171-178.

Halliwell, B., & Gutteridge, J. M. (1989). *Free radicals in biology and medicine.* New York, Oxford University Press.

Hasegawa, R., Hirose, M., & Kato, T. (1995). Inhibitory effect of chlorophillin on PhIP induced mammary carcinogenesis in female F344 rats. *Carcinogenesis, 16,* 2243-2246.

Hopkins, G. J., & Carroll, K. K. (1979). Relationship between amount and type of dietary fat in promotion of mammary carcinogenesis induced by 7,12-dimethylbenz[a]anthracene. *Journal of the National Cancer Institute, 62,* 1009-1012.

Hopkins, G. J., Kennedy, T. G., & Carroll, K. K. (1981). Polyunsaturated fatty acids as promotors of mammary carcinogenesis induced Sprageu Dawley rats by 7,12-dimethylbenz[a]anthracene. *Journal of the National Cancer Institute, 66,* 517-522.

Howe, G. R., Aronson, K. J., & Benito, E. (1997). The relationship between dietary fat intake and risk of colorectal cancer: Evidence from the combined analysis of 13 case control studies. *Cancer causes control, 8,* 215-228.

Hunter, D. J., Spiegelman, D., & Adami, H. O. (1996). Cohort studies of fat intake and the risk of breast cancer: a pooled analysis. *The New England Journal of Medicine, 334,* 356-361.

Iguchi, K., Hamatake, M., & Ishida, R. (1998). Induction fo necrosis by zinc in prostate carcinoma cells and identification of proteins increased in association with this induction. *European Journal of Biochemistry, 253,* 766-770.

Issa, J. P., Vertino, P. M., & Wu, J. (1993). Increased cytosine DNA methyltransferase activity during colon cancer progression. *Journal of the National Cancer Institute, 85,* 1235-1240.

Jackson, J. L., Lesho, E., & Peterson, C. (2000). Zinc and the common cold: a meta-analysis revisited. *The Journal of Nutrition, 130,* 1512S-1515S.

Kabuto, M., Imai, H., & Yonezawa, C. (1994). Prediagnostic serum selenium and zinc levels and subsequent risk of lung and stomach cancer in Japan. *Cancer Epidemiology, Biomarkers & Prevention, 3,* 465-469.

Knekt, P., Reunanen, A., & Takkunen, H. (1994a). Body iron stores and the risk of cancer. *International Journal of Cancer, 56,* 379-382.

Knekt, P., Steineck, G., & Järvinen, R. (1994b). Intake of fried meat and risk of cancer: a follow up study in Finland. *International Journal of Cancer, 59,* 756-760.

Koehler, K. M., Baumgarter, R. N., Garry, P. J., Allen, R. H., Stabler, S. P., & Rimm, E. B. (2001). Association of folate intake and serum homocysteine in elderly persons according to vitamin supplementation and alcohol use. *The American Journal of Clinical Nutrition, 73,* 501-502.

Kok, F. J., Van Duijn, C. M., & Hofman, A. (1988). Serum cooper and zinc and the risk of death from cancer and cardiovascular disease. *American Journal of Epidemiology, 128,* 352-359

Kolonel, L. N. (2001). Fat, meat and prostate cancer. *Epidemiologic Reviews, 23,* 72-81.

Koohestani, N., Tran, T. T., & Lee, W. (1997). Insulin resistance and promotion of aberrant crypt foci in the colons of rats on a high fat diet. *Nutrition and Cancer, 29,* 69-76.

Kurokowa, R., DiRenzo, J., & Boehm, M. (1994). Regulation of retinoid signalling by receptor polarity and allosteric control of ligand binding. *Nature, 371,* 528-531.

Lashner, B. A., Heidenreich, P. A., & Su, G. L. (1989). Effect of folate supplementation on the incidence of dysplasia and cancer in chronic ulcerative colitis. *Gastroenterology, 97,* 255-259.

Laugesen, M., & Swimburn, G. (2000). The New Zealand food supply and diet-trends 1961-1995 and comparison with other OECD countries. *New Zealand Medical Journal, 113,* 311-315.

Lasnitzki, I., & Bollag, W., (1982). Prevention and reversal by a retinoid of 3,4-benzpyrene and cigarette smoke condensate-induced hyperplasia of rodent respiratory epithelia in organ culture. *Cancer Treatment Reports, 66,* 1375-1380.

Lasnitzki, I., & Bollag, W., (1987). Prevention and reversal by non-polar carotenoid (Ro 150778) of 3,4-benzpyrene and cigarette smoke condensate-induced hyperplasia of rodent respiratory epithelia grown in vitro. *European Journal of Cancer & Clinical Oncology, 23,* 861-865.

Le Marchand, L. (1999). Combined influence of genetic and dietary factors on colorectal cancer incidence in Japanese Americans. *Journal of the National Cancer Institute. Monographs, 26,* 101-105.

Liang, J. Y., Liu, Y. Y., & Zou, J. (1999). Inhibitory effect of zinc on human prostatic carcinoma cell growth. *Prostate, 40,* 200-207.

Lloyd-Wright, Z., Allen, N., Key, T., & Sanders, T. (2000). How prevalent is vitamin B12 deficiency among British vegetarians and vegans? *Proceedings of the Nutritional Society, 60,* 1-16.

Lowik, M. R., van den Berg, H., Schrijver, J., Odink, J., Wedel, M., & van Houten, P. (1992). Marginal nutritional status among institutionalized elderly women as compared to those living more independently (Dutch Nutrition Surveillance System). *Journal of the American College of Nutrition, 11,* 673-681.

Lukito, W., Wattanapenpaiboon, N., Savige, G. S., Hutchinson, P., & Wahlqvist, M. L. (2004). Nutritional indicators, peripheral blood lymphocyte subsets and survival in an institutionalised elderly population. *Asia Pacific Journal of Clinical Nutrition, 13(1),* 107-112.

MacIntosh, G. H., & Le Leu, R. K. (2001). The influence of dietary proteins on colon cancer risks. *Nutrition Research, 21,* 1053-1066.

MacIntosh, G. H., Royle, P. J., & Le Leu, R. K. (1998). Whey protein as functional food ingredients? *International Dairy Journal, 8,* 425-438.

Makos, M., Nelkin, B. D., & Lerman, M. I. (1992). Distinct hypermethylation patterns occur at altered chromosome loci in human lung and colon cancer. In *Proceedings of the National Academy of Sciences of the United States of America, 89,* 1929-1933.

Martins, I., Dantas, A., Guiomar, S., & Amorin, J. A. (2002). Vitamin and mineral intakes in the elderly. *The Journal of Nutrition, Health & Aging, 6,* 63-65.

Mathe, G., Gouveia, J., Hercend, T., Gros, F., & Dorval, T. (1983). Detection of precancerous bronchus metaplasia in heavy smokers and its regression following retinoid treatment. In F. Meyskens (Ed.), *Modulation and mediation of cancer by vitamins* (pp. 317-321). Basel:

Karger.

Mawson, C. A., & Fisher, M. I. (1952). The occurrence of zinc in the human prostate gland. *The Canadian Journal of Medical Science, 30,* 336-339.

McDowell, E. M., Ben, T., Coleman, B., Chang, S., Newkirk, C., & De Luca, L. M. (1987a). Effects of retinoic acid on the growth and morphology of hamster tracheal epithelial cells in primary culture. *Virchows Archiv. B, Cell Pathology Including Molecular Pathology,* 54, 38-51.

McDowell, E. M., Ben, T., Newkirk, C., Chang, S., & De Luca, M. (1987b). Differentiation of tracheal mucociliary epithelium in primary cell culture recapstulates normal fetal development and regeneration following injury in hamsters. *American Journal of Pathology, 129,* 511-522.

McDowell, E. M., Keenan, K. P., & Huang, M. (1984a). Effects of vitamin A-deprivation on hamster tracheal epithelium. A quantitative morphologic study. *Virchows Archiv. B, Cell Pathology Including Molecular Pathology, 45,* 197-219.

McDowell, E. M., Keenan, K. P., & Huang, M. (1984b). Restoration of mucociliary tracheal epithelium following deprivation of vitamin A. A quantitative morphological study. *Virchows Archiv. B, Cell Pathology Including Molecular Pathology, 45,* 221-240.

McKeoween-Eyssen, G. (1994). Epidemiology of colorectal cancer revisited: is serum triglycrides and/or plasma glucose associated with risk? *Cancer Epidemiology, Biomarkers & Prevention, 3,* 687-695.

Mellow, M. H., Layne, E. A., & Lipman, T. O. (1983). Plasma zinc and vitamin A in human squamous carcinoma of the oesophagus. *Cancer, 51,* 1615-1620.

Metzler, M. D., & Snyder, J. M. (1993). Retinoic acid differentially regulates expression of surfactant-associated proteins in human fetal lung. *Endocrinology; 133,* 1990-1998.

Michaud, D. S., Augustsson, K., & Rimm, E. B. (2001). A prospective study on intake of animal products and risk of prostate cancer. *Cancer Causes and Control, 12,* 557-567.

Morabia, A., Sorenson, A., Kumanyika, H., Abbey, H., Cohen, B. H., & Chee, E. (1989). Vitamin A, cigarette smoking, and airway obstruction. *The American Review of Respiratory Disease, 140,* 1312-1316.

Morie, H., Sugie, S., Rahman, W., & Suzui, N. (1999). Chemoprevention of 2-amino-1-methyl-6-phenylimidazo[4,5-b]pyridine-induced mammary carcinogenesis in rats. *Cancer Letters, 143,* 195-198.

Mupanemunda, R. H., Lee, D. S. C., Fraher, L. J., Koura, I. R., & Chance, G. W. (1994). Postnatal changes in serum retinol status in very low birth weight infants. *Early Human Development, 38,* 45-54.

Nelson, R. L., Yoo, S. J., & Tanure, J. C. (1989). The effect of iron on experimental colorectal carcinogenesis. *Anticancer Research, 9*, 1477-1482.

Neuzil, K. M., Gruber, W. C., Chytil, F., Stahlman, M. T., Engelhardt, B., & Graham, B. S. (1994). Serum vitamin A levels in respiratory syncytial virus infection. *The Journal of Pediatrics, 124*, 433-436.

Nyce, J., Weinhouse, S., & Magee, P. N. (1983). 5-methylcytosine depletion during tumor development: an extension of the miscoding concept. *British Journal of Cancer, 48*, 463-475.

Odom, M. J., Snyder, J. M., Boggaram, V., & Mendelson, C. R. (1988). Glucocorticoid regulation of the major surfactant associated protein (SP-A) and its messenger ribonucleic acid and of morphological development of human fetal lung in vitro. *Endocrinology, 123*, 1712-1720.

Ozsoy, M., & Ernst, E. (1999). How effective are complementary therapies for HIV and AIDS; a systematic review. *International Journal of STD & AIDS*,10, 629-635.

Philipsen-Geerling, B. J., & Brummer, R. J. M. (2000). Nutrition in Crohn's disease. *Current Opinion in Clinical Nutrition and Metabolic Care, 3*, 305-309.

Pinnock, C. B., Douglas, R. M., & Badcock, N. R. (1986). Vitamin a status in children who are prone to respiratory tract infections. *Australian Paediatric Journal, 22*, 95-99.

Platz, E. A. & Helzlsouer, K. J. (2001). Selenium, zinc and prostate cancer. *Epidemiologic Reviews, 23(1)*, 93-101.

Popkin, B. M., Haines, P. S., & Reidy, K. C. (1989). Food consumption trends of US women: patterns and determinants between 1977-1985. *Journal of Clinical Nutrition, 49*, 1307-1319.

Potter, J. D., Slattery, M. L., & Bostick, R. M. (1993). Colon cancer: a review of the epidemiology. *Epidemiologic Reviews, 15*, 299-545.

Rasmussen, L. B., Ovesen, L., Bûlow, I., Knudsen, N., Laurberg, P., & Perrild, H. (2000). Folate intakes, lifestyle factors, and homocysteine concentrations in younger and older women. *The American Journal of Clinical Nutrition, 72*, 1156-1163.

Rayman, M. P. (1997). Dietary selenium: time to act. *British Medical Journal, 314*, 387-388.

Rayman, M. P. (2000). The importance of selenium to human health. *Lancet, 356*, 233-241.

Reddy, B. S. (1981). Diet and excretion of bile acids. *Cancer Research, 41*, 3766-3768.

Redman, C., Xu, M. J., & Peng, Y. M. (1997). Involvement of polyamines in selenomethionine induced apoptosis and mitotic alterations in human tumor cells. *Carcinogenesis, 18,* 1195-1202.

Reynolds, E. H. (2002). Folic acid, ageing, depression, and dementia. *British Medical Journal, 324,* 1512-1515.

Rink, L., & Gabriel, P. (2000). Zinc and immune system. In t*he Proceedings of the Nutrition Society,* 59(4), 541-52.

Rogers, M. A. M., Thomas, D. B., & Davis, S. (1993). A case control study of element levels and cancer of the upper aerodigestive tract. *Cancer Epidemiology, Biomarkers & Prevention, 2,* 305-312.

Rutten, A. A., Wilmer, J. W., & Beems, R. B. (1988a). Effects of all-trans retinol and cigarette smoke condensate on hamster tracheal epithelium in organ culture. I. A cell proliferation study. *Virchows Archiv B, Cell Pathology Including Molecular Pathology,* 55, 167-175.

Rutten, A. A., Wilmer, J. W., & Beems, R. B. (1988b). Effects of all-trans retinol and cigarette smoke condensate on hamster tracheal epithelium in organ culture. II A histomorphological study. *Virchows Archiv B, Cell Pathology Including Molecular Pathology,* 55, 177-186.

Saletti, A., Lindgren, E. Y., Johansson, L., & Cederholm, T. (2000). Nutritional status according to mini nutritional assessment in an institutionalized elderly population in Sweden. *Gerontology, 46,* 139-145.

Schottenfeld, D., & Fraumeni, J. F. (1996). *Cancer epidemiology and prevention* (pp. 1-1521). Oxford University press: New York.

Schrauzer, G. N., White, D. A., & Schneider, C. J., (1977). Cancer mortality correllation studies. III. *Bioinorganic Chemistry, 7,* 23-34.

Selhub, J., Jacques, P. F., Bostom, A. G., Wilson, P. W., & Rosenberg, I. H. (2000). Relationship between plasma homocysteine and vitamin status in the Framingham study population. Impact of folic acid fortification. *Public Health Reviews, 28,* 117-145.

Shah, R. S., & Rajalekshmi, R. (1984). Vitamin A status of the newborn in relation to gestational age, body weight, and maternal nutritional status. *American Journal of Clinical Nutrition, 40,* 794-800.

Shenai, J. P., Chytil, F., Jhaveri, A., & Stahlman, M. T. (1981). Plasma vitamin A and retinol-binding protein in premature and term neonates. *Journal of Pediatrics, 99,* 302-305.

Shenai, J. P., Kennedy, K. A., Chytil, F., & Stahlman, M. T. (1987). Clinical trial of vitamin A supplementation in infants susceptible to bronchopulmonary dysplasia. *Journal of Pediatrics, 111,* 269-277.

Shenai, J. P., Rush, M. G., Stahlman, M. T., & Chytil, F. (1990). Plasma retinol-binding protein response to vitamin A administration in infants susceptible to bronchopulmonary dysplasia. *Journal of Pediatrics, 116,* 607-614.

Shenai, J. P., Chytil, F., & Stahlman, M. T. (1985). Liver vitamin A reserves of very low birth weight neonates. *Pediatrics Research, 19,* 892-893.

Shi, B. B., & Spallholz, J. E. (1994). Selenium from beef is highly bioavailable as assessed by liver glutathione peroxidase acitivity and tissue selenium. *British Medical Journal, 72,* 873-81.

Shivapurkar, N., & Poirer, L.A. (1983). Tissue levels of S-adenosylmethionine and S-adenosylhomocysteine in rats fed methyl deficient diets for one to five weeks. *Carcinogenesis, 4,* 1052-7.

Siegers, C. P., Bumann, D., Baretton, G., & Younes, M. (1988). Dietary iron enhances the tumor rate in DMH-induced colon carcinogenesis in mouse colon. *Cancer Letters, 41,* 251-6.

Skillud, D. M., Offord, K. P., & Miller, R. D. (1987). Higher risk of lung cancer in chronic obstructive pulmonary disease. A prospective matched controlled study. *Annals of Internal Medicine, 105,* 503-507.

Sommer, A. (1993). Vitamin A supplementation and childhood morbidity. *Lancet, 342,* 1420-1224.

Stahlman, M. T. (1984). Chronic lung disease following hyaline membrane disease. In L. Stern, & P. Vert (Eds.), *Neonatal Medicine* (pp. 454-473). New York; Masson.

Stephensen, C. B., Alvarez, J. O., Kohatsu, J., Hardmeier, R., Kennedy, J. I., & Gammon Jr., R. B. (1994). Vitamin A is excreted in the urine during acute infection. *American Journal of Clinical Nutrition, 60,* 388-392.

Stevens, R. G., Jones, D. Y., & Micozzi, M. S. (1988). Body iron stores and the risk of cancer. *N Engl J Med 319,* 1047-52.

Stofft, E., Biesalski, H. K., Zschaebitz, A., & Weiser, H. (1992). Morphological changes in the tracheal epithelium of guinea pigs in conditions of „marginal „ vitamin A deficiency. *International Journal of Nutrition Research, 62,* 134-142.

Sundell, H. W., Gray, M. E., Serenius, F. S., Escobedo, M. B., & Stahlman, M. T. (1980). Effects of epidermal growth factor on lung maturation in fetal lambs. *Am J Pathol, 100,* 707-725.

Takahashi, M., Fukutake, M., & Isoi, T. (1997). Supression of azoxymethane-induced rat colon carcinoma development by a fish oil component docosahexaenoic acid (DHA). *Carcinogenesis, 18,* 1337-42.

Thane, C. T., & Bates, C. J. (2001). Intake and sources of selenium in British elderly people. In *Proceedings of the Nutrition Society, 60,* 60A.

van der Torre, H. W., van Dokkum, W., & Schaafsma, G. (1991). Effect of various levels of selenium in wheat and meat on blood selenium status indices and on selenium balance in Dutch men. *British Journal of Nutrition, 65,* 69-80.

Viteri, F. E., & Gonzalez, H. (2002). Adverse outcomes of poor micronutrient status in childhood and adolescence. *Nutrition Reviews, 60,* 77-83.

Wainfan, E., Dizik, M., & Stender, M. (1989). Rapid appearance of hypomethylated DNA in livers of rats fed cancer promoting, methyl deficient diets. *Cancer Research, 49,* 4094-4097.

Watanabe, K., Kawamori, T., & Natatsugi, S. (1999). Role of the prostaglandin E receptor subtype EP1 in colon carcinogenesis. *Cancer Research, 59,* 5093-96.

Weaver, T. E., & Whitsett, J. A. (1991). Function and regulation of expression of pulmonary surfactant-associated proteins. *Biochemical Journal, 273,* 249-264.

West, K. P., Pokhrel, R. P., & Katz, J. (1991). Efficacy of vitamin A in reducing preschool child mortality in Nepal. *Lancet, 338,* 67-71.

Whitehead, R. G. (1995). Lowered energy intake and dietary macronutrient balance: potential consequences for micronutrient status. *Nutrition Reviews, 53,* S2-S8.

Wilkinson, E. A. J., & Hawke, C. I. (2002). Oral zinc for arterial and venous leg ulcers (Cochrane Review). In *The Cochrane Library, Issue 2,.* Oxford: Update Software

Willett, W. C. (1999). Goals for nutrition in the year 2000. *CA: a Cancer Journal for Clinicians, 49,* 331-352.

World Health Organization (1992). *Iron Deficiency Anemia. Assessment, Prevention and Control. A guide for programme managers.* United Nations Children Fund, United Nations University and World Health Organization. WHO/NHD/01.3.

Xia, Y., Zhao, X., & Zhu, L. (1992). Metabolism of selenate and selenomethionine by selenium deficient population of men in China. *Journal of Nutritional Biochemistry, 3,* 202-210.

Yoshizawa, K., Willet, W. C., & Morris, S. J. (1998). Study of prediagnostic selenium level in toenails and the risk of advanced prostate cancer. *Journal of National Cancer Institute, 90,* 1219-24.

Younes, M., Trepkau, H. D., & Siegers, C. P. (1990). Enhancement of dietary iron peroxidation in mouse colon. *Research Commununications of Chemical Pathology and Pharmacolology, 70,* 349-354.

Youngman, L. D., & Cambell, T. C. (1998). The sustained development of preneoplastic lesions depends on high protein intake. *Nutrition and Cancer, 18,* 131-142

Zachman, R. D. (1989) Retinol (vitamin A) and the neonate: special problems of the human premature infant. *American Journal of Clinical Nutrition, 50,* 413-424.

Zafiriou, M. (1985) Changing meat consumption patterns in Canada. *Food Marketing commentary, 7,* 20-36

Zhang, S., Hunter, D. J., & Hankinson, S. E. (1999). A prospective study of folate intake and the risk of breast cancer. *The Journal of the American Medical Association, 281*, 1632-1637.

Zheng, W., Gustaffson, D. R., & Sinha, R. (1998). Well done meat intake and the risk of breast cancer. *Journal of the National Cancer Institute, 90*, 1724-1729.

8

INTERPRETATION AND APPLICATION OF EC RULINGS

JUDITH NELSON – *Head of Feed Sector, AIC*
HELEN D RAINE – *Technology and Regulatory Affairs Director, ABNA Ltd*
TIM OLIVER – *Legislation & Raw Materials Assessment Manager, ABN*
P O Box 250, Oundle Road, Peterborough PE2 9PW, UK

Introduction

This chapter discusses those pieces of legislation having a significant impact on the UK feed industry both now and over the next few years. The legislation considered covers a wide range of issues including labelling, composition, production and supply of non-medicated, medicated and organic feedingstuffs. Reference is also made to environmental issues such as the need to control the amount of nitrogen and phosphorus in animal feeds as well as the legal definition of by-products from a range of manufacturing processes. All of this legislation emanates from Brussels.

Feed labelling

This section concerns two main issues which are the:

- Response to the European Court of Justice (ECJ) ruling on percentage ingredient declaration in compound feedingstuffs;
- Commission proposal to recast all EU feed labelling legislation.

ECJ RULING

On 6th December 2005 the ECJ handed down its ruling on the percentage declaration of ingredients case. The key features of the ruling on Directive 2002/2/EC amending Directive 79/373/EEC on the circulation of compound feedingstuffs were:

i.   Article 1(1)b of the amending Directive (concerning the disclosure of *exact* percentages to customers on request) was invalid;

ii.   Article 1(4) (concerning the requirement to list the feed materials with an indication, in descending order, of the percentages by weight present in the compound feed subject to a ± 15% tolerance) was valid.

The ruling has to be reflected in national and EU legislation as required by EU law. For its part, the Food Standards Agency (FSA) commenced consultation on the Feeding Stuffs (England) (Amendment) Regulations 2006 in March 2006. Separate but parallel legislation will apply in Scotland, Wales and Northern Ireland. There was a twelve-week consultation period in which stakeholders, including AIC, were invited to comment on the draft regulations reintroducing the percentage ingredient declaration within a tolerance of ± 15%.

The UK Government, like the EU feed industry, maintains its opposition to this provision. In its response to the consultation, AIC has reiterated the arguments used over the years to the percentage ingredient declaration. Percentage ingredient declarations do not contribute to food or feed safety, are disproportionate and require feed manufacturers to reveal their intellectual property. It should also be noted that it is only this single provision within the legislation which is of concern to the feed industry; the rest of the legislation requiring the declaration of individual ingredients in descending order by weight is not an issue. Also, percentage ingredient declaration is not a requirement of EU food legislation.

To date, the Feeding Stuffs (England) (Amendment) Regulations 2006 have not been finalised. The FSA has not advised an exact date on which the legislation is likely to come into force, but this is expected to be in autumn 2006.

AIC has alerted both the FSA and Local Authorities Co-ordinators of Regulatory Services (LACORS) to the problems of confusion associated with the percentage ingredient declaration within a ± 15% tolerance as follows:

•   It would give the purchaser a feeling that a precise percentage declaration was being provided, whereas this was not necessarily the case e.g. wheat formulated at 35% could be declared as 40%;

•   The ranking order of percentage ingredient declarations could legally be changed;

•   It does not contribute to either feed or food safety;

•   Despite the tolerance, it reveals a company's intellectual property, particularly for the lower inclusion materials.

As a result of the above concerns and the need for feed manufacturers to comply with the ECJ ruling, AIC has had extensive discussions with the FSA and LACORS. AIC's view is that by operating a banding system member companies will meet the spirit of the forthcoming legislation. Furthermore, unlike the actual legal requirement for individual percentage declaration within a ± 15% tolerance, it is not misleading. The proposed approach is as follows:

0-10%	operationally being:	0-9.99%
10% - 25%		10% - 24.99%
25% - 40%		25% - 39.99%
> 40%		40% and above.

It is of course left to individual companies to decide whether or not they wish to apply the banding approach. A specimen label illustrating the banding approach is attached as *Annex 1*.

On 27th June 2006 the Commission published a proposal for a European Parliament and Council Decision correcting Directive 79/373/EEC on the circulation of compound feedingstuffs in line with the ECJ Judgement. This has provided the EU feed industry, led by FEFAC, with an opportunity to try to influence discussions on the draft proposal at European Parliament level. A series of meetings with MEPs, including a number from the UK, has been arranged.

The arguments which AIC used with the FSA against the percentage ingredient declaration will be reiterated.

RECASTING OF EU FEED LABELLING LEGISLATION

In October 2005 the Commission announced a period of consultation on the scope and content of the future legislative proposal to replace the four existing Directives on labelling and authorisation of certain feedingstuffs. The Directives concerned are on compound feedingstuffs, dietetic feedingstuffs, feed materials and certain products used in animal nutrition (i.e. bio-proteins). The new regulation will apply across all sectors covering both producers and suppliers of feed materials as well as compound feedingstuffs manufacturers. The objectives are to ensure food and feed safety and to tighten labelling and traceability requirements for animal feed.

AIC submitted a detailed response to the Commission's questionnaire at the beginning of 2006. However, completion of this entailed a "tick box" approach which is not a totally satisfactory means of conducting a major review of EU feed labelling requirements. Thus, in preparation for the forthcoming negotiations on the Commission's proposal, an AIC Working Group is to meet in September:

- To identify the superfluous labelling requirements in the four Directives being reviewed;
- To consider the current derogations and establish those which the industry cannot do without.

The Commission has provisionally scheduled discussions on the proposal to recast the feed labelling legislation for the autumn of 2007. The EU feed industry would prefer the debate to take place earlier as this would provide a further opportunity to seek amendment to the percentage ingredient declaration requirement if the current attempts are unsuccessful.

Feed Hygiene Regulation

Regulation 183/2005 on feed hygiene was brought into operation on 1st January 2006. This Regulation replaced Directive 95/69/EC laying down the conditions and arrangements for approving and registering certain establishments and intermediaries operating in the animal feed sector. Under Regulation 183/2005 virtually all businesses involved in making, storing, transporting or marketing feeds and feed products have to be approved or registered and have to comply with certain standards concerning facilities, storage, and record-keeping. This includes farms and food manufacturers selling co-products for feed. In addition, all except primary producers have to ensure that controls are put in place under HACCP Principles. The Regulation exempts from its scope farms selling small quantities of feed to other local farms although they will continue to be subject to existing feed safety legislation.

The Regulation also requires that feed businesses will only be permitted to import feed from non-EU country establishments if these establishments comply with the requirements of the regulation. Whilst the conditions relating to imports came into force from 1 January 2006, the lists of compliant countries do not yet exist. The transitional arrangements laid down in 183/2005 apply and require third country establishments to have a representative in the EU. These controls are a continuation of some of the provisions already in operation and thus are not new. The drawing up of the lists of third country establishments is a matter for the European Commission and it has not yet provided a timetable for the completion of this work.

AIC updated both UFAS (the Universal Feed Assurance Scheme) and FEMAS (Feed Materials Assurance Scheme) to include any relevant new provisions being introduced by 183/2005. AIC assurance schemes take into consideration all relevant EU legislation as, amongst other things, this helps companies within the feed industry comply with the law and provides evidence of compliance to their customers.

Two provisions within Regulation 183/2005 are worthy of specific mention. The first concerns financial guarantees. During negotiations on the draft Regulation a provision that would have made it mandatory for businesses to have financial guarantees to cover the withdrawal of feed, and food and animals produced therefrom, was removed. Both the EU feed industry and the UK Government were opposed to financial guarantees. The FSA has advised that the European insurance industry indicated that it did not have the capacity to provide such cover and costs were likely to be prohibitively expensive. Such guarantees will only be introduced, if appropriate, after a Commission feasibility study has been conducted.

The second provision concerns the discussions in Brussels on guides to good practice. The Commission is, in the first instance, to encourage the development of Community Guides to Good Practice in the feed sector and for the application of HACCP principles. Compliance with these codes of practice is not mandatory. EU feed organisations have submitted their codes of practice to the Commission. For its part, FEFAC has submitted the European Feed Manufacturers Code (EFMC). For each of these guides the Commission and member states have reviewed the text and commented on those provisions it considered should be changed before they could be accepted as "Community Guides

Undesirable Substances

THE FEED (SPECIFIED UNDESIRABLE SUBSTANCES) (ENGLAND) REGULATIONS 2006

The FSA is seeking comments on some draft regulations to transpose into domestic law in England three Commission Directives which amend Directive 2002/32/EC on undesirable substances in animal feedingstuffs. These measures amend or extend the existing maximum permitted levels for certain undesirable substances in feed, as follows:

- Camphechlor, a pesticide now banned in the EU but which persists in the environment;

- Lead, fluorine and cadmium, which are natural environmental contaminants;
- Dioxin-like PCBs, which are brought within the scope of the existing MPLs for dioxins because of their potential to contribute to the dioxin loading of food and feed.

Separate but parallel legislation is being introduced into Scotland, Wales and Northern Ireland.

In view of the new MPLs for cadmium and lead in mineral feedingstuffs, manufacturers of these products should check the levels of these contaminants in key ingredients in case it is necessary to declare some of their blends as premixtures rather than as mineral feedingstuffs. This is due to the high concentration of trace element salts.

Some feed companies have, through AIC, participated in FSA-sponsored sampling and analysis of dioxins and PCBs in a range of feed products. Data from the 2004 research project are available from the FSA Library in hard or electronic format. The overall results confirmed compliance with the statutory maximum limits for dioxins.

Data from the 2006 project are not yet available to the public, but should be obtainable from the FSA's London Library in September. The FSA hope, but cannot guarantee, that it will be available also via the Agency website at some point. Both reports may be obtained from the FSA's Information Centre (tel: 020 7276 8181 / 8182 or email: infocentre@foodstandards.gsi.gov.uk).

MYCOTOXINS

In July 2006 the Commission published its final draft of the suggested guidance levels for mycotoxins in cereals and cereal products for feed. This is an EU Commission recommendation rather than a regulation and is intended to guide member states in their approach to mycotoxins in the feed sector.

The draft document gives no specific guidance on when the recommendations would be adopted, with the exception of fumonisim B1 and B2 which are predominantly a maize issue where it is suggested that the levels should be in operation by October 2007.

Another aspect of the recommendation is that much more monitoring of mycotoxin levels should take place both by member states and the industry. Additionally, the Commission will review the situation in 2009 and it does not rule out the possibility of turning the guidance levels into a regulation, as is now the case with limits for grain destined for food use.

The guidance values being proposed are set out in *Annex 2*. It she noted that the reference to cereal products includes not only feed mater. listed under existing legislation but also other feed materials derived from cereal, such as cereal forages, e.g. whole crop cereals. Thus this draft recommendation also places obligations on farmers who feed cereals directly to their own livestock or who sell cereals or cereal forage to others.

HGCA CONTAMINANTS MONITORING PROGRAMME

AIC, together with NABIM representing the millers and MAGB representing the maltsters is participating in a 3-year contaminants monitoring programme which commenced in early 2006. This is an UK-wide project funded by HGCA to coordinate monitoring of grain and grain-derived co-products for potential contaminants. It involves analysis of both harvest and stored samples. The results from the 2005 stored harvest samples were recently circulated to AIC members. These results provide a valuable means by which the feed industry can assess its compliance with relevant undesirable substance legislation as well as meeting its due diligence requirements.

The feed industry also took part in an HGCA funded project entitled "Monitoring the wholesomeness of grain and grain-derived co-products destined for animal feed", which was published in December 2005. Again, the results of this project are available for quality control purposes by feed companies. The results obtained so far in both projects indicate a satisfactory position for the feed industry.

Additives Regulation:

AUTHORISATION AND RE-EVALUATION OF EXISTING FEED ADDITIVES

Regulation 1831/2003 on feed additives has now been in operation for almost 2 years. This legislation both strengthens and streamlines the EU's controls on safety evaluation and marketing authorisation of feed additives.

A very important feature of 1831/2003 is the re-evaluation of all existing feed additives. This exercise is being carried out in two stages. In order to ensure continued authorisation of existing feed additives, companies marketing them or other interested parties had to notify the Commission and the European Food Safety Authority (EFSA) by November 2004 with details of the current authorisation of the additives. On completion of this exercise, the Commission issued the Community Register of Feed Additives which is now available from the Commission's website.

The second stage concerning reauthorisation of all existing additives must be completed by 2010. In support of reauthorisation, the companies marketing the additives, or other interested parties, have to submit dossiers supporting reauthorisation based on safety, quality and efficacy. If an existing authorisation is the subject of an expiry date, a relevant dossier must be submitted at least 1 year before that date. The problem for the feed additive and feed industries throughout the EU is lack of a final text of the guidelines for reauthorisation of additives. The latest advice from the FSA is that the draft guidelines should be available for discussion at working group level during the course of the next few months with a view to the guidelines being adopted early in 2007. Indications are that the deadline for re-evaluation of all existing feed additives will not be extended.

The EFSA has also commenced consultation on the environmental impact of feed additives. This is with a view to producing Europe-wide guidelines on carrying out risk assessments. The move reflects concerns that feed additives, which are typically used over a long period of time, may contaminate groundwater or soil. This development could have a serious impact on the use of some feed additives such as copper and zinc.

IODINE – REDUCED FEEDING LEVELS FOR DAIRY COWS:

In the summer of 2005 member states agreed to reduce the statutory maximum content of iodine in complete feeds/diets for poultry layers and dairy cows from 10 mg/kg to 5 mg/kg. The UK government did not support the lowering of the level for iodine in dairy cows and succeeded in securing an agreement that the new level would not be brought into operation for 12 months. This delay was obtained because UK officials accepted the briefing from AIC and veterinary experts, who had expressed concern that the reduction to 5 mg/kg could result in iodine deficiency in some animals where there was insufficient available iodine in pastures. The 12-month period was to be used to collect further data forpresentation to the EFSA to see if a revision of its Opinion was justified.

Unfortunately, the further data provided by AIC to the FSA were not sufficient to persuade EFSA to revise its published Opinion on iodine supplementation of feed, nor to support maintenance of the 10 mg/kg maximum permitted level (MPL) of iodine in feed for dairy cows. The new MPL will be introduced on 9 September 2006.

GM Food and Feed Controls

The authorisation procedures and labelling requirements for genetically modified food and feed are laid down in Regulation 1829/2003. This legislation, which was brought into operation in April 2004, introduced labelling for GM animal feed and a harmonised procedure for scientific assessment and authorisation of GMOs and GM food and feed. There are currently two issues arising from this legislation of interest to the feed industry which are:

UNAUTHORISED PIONEER MAIZE EVENT

In 2006 a new GMO event was introduced on the US maize seed market, marketed by Pioneer and DOW, registered as DAS-59122-7. Pioneer introduced a request for authorisation for import and processing of this event in the EU in January 2005. The product has yet to be authorised in the EU; meanwhile maize containing the DAS-59122-7 event represents 1% of the current US maize area, i.e. 400,000 hectares.

Given the importance of maize gluten feed as a feed material, the EU feed industry has been developing an action plan in conjunction with Pioneer, the US National Corn Growers Association and the US Corn Refiners Association. The aim is to avoid the non-EU approved event being exported to the EU. The action plan is composed of two major elements:

- Measures to prevent the non-EU approved event ending up in maize by-products designed for export to the EU; this includes measures to inform farmers about the EU status of the event DAS-59122-7 and a request to deliver their harvest to dedicated silos;
- Monitoring Measures – this includes systematic analysis of each barge of maize gluten feed at the loading point. If a barge tests positive for the event, then it would be directed first of all to the US domestic market and, to a limited extent, to non-EU markets. The analysis would be carried out by independent accredited agencies and the results would be provided on a certificate issued by the accredited agency.

It is important to note that the situation with DAS-59122-7 is different from the BT10 case. Whereas DAS-59122-7 has been evaluated and authorised for use and processing in eight countries including Japan and Korea and is authorised for planting in the US and Canada, BT10 was not approved in the US.

FEFAC together with COCERAL representing the importers and Pioneer have met with Commission officials. Officials are understood to be eager to facilitate co-ordination of national control approaches.

COMMISSION REPORT ON GM FOOD AND FEED REGULATIONS:

The report on the operation of Regulation 1829/2003 is expected this autumn. The Commission has not, so far, divulged the content of the report. It is anticipated that there will be some issues for clarification on the operation of the Regulation. A ruling is also awaited from the WTO which was expected to influence the release of the Commission's report.

The FSA has also advised that there has been criticism in some Member States on the approval of some events by clearance at Standing Committee level. The Commission is able, under current rules, to have such lines authorised in the absence of a qualified majority vote. There has also been some concern at the clearance procedures in operation at EFSA. Consequently the process is to become more open, with EFSA being more transparent about its consideration of the views of both Member States and independent assessors. The new procedure is to be set out on the EFSA website.

Rapid Alert System for Food and Feed (RASFF)

A rapid alert system for food has been operating within the Commission since 1979. However under the general food law (Regulation 178/2002) the Rapid Alert System for Food and Feed was brought into operation. RASFF is primarily a tool for exchange of information between food and feed central competent authorities in member states in cases where a risk to human health has been identified and measures have been taken such as withholding, recalling, seizure or rejection of products concerned. It is a quick information exchange that allows member states to identify immediately whether they are also affected by a problem, and to take appropriate measures, thereby ensuring coherent and simultaneous actions and consumer safety. RASFF notifications are published weekly on the Commission website.

The 2005 report is now available. The total number of notifications for feed in 2005 was 85, making up 3.0% of all RASFF notifications. This figure represents a moderate increase compared to the previous year: 65 notifications (2.5% of the total) in 2004. The main problems were related to microbiological contamination of feed (49 notifications), mostly salmonella in feed materials and dog chews. Other identified problems were the presence of fragments of bone (18 notifications) mainly in sugar beet pulp and the detection of unauthorised feed additive organic selenium in several products (5 notifications). The problems identified with bone fragments might have persuaded the Commission to accept the need to refine the EU TSE legislation to permit the feeding of tuber and root crops with bone spicules, subject to a favourable risk assessment, as commented on later in this paper.

Another example of the impact of RASFF notifications is the consultation on a Commission Decision on special conditions governing import of zinc sulphate from China. This legislation has been drawn up in response to findings of high levels of cadmium in zinc sulphate from China. The draft Decision requires future consignments of zinc sulphate from China for use in animal feed to be accompanied by an official certificate guaranteeing compliance with EU feed legislation.

The draft Commission Decision is under discussion at Standing Committee level in Brussels.

Veterinary Medicines Regulations 2006:

During the major review of UK veterinary medicines legislation in 2004/ 2005 it was decided to provide a "One Stop Shop" as far as possible so that all the legislative provisions in respect of veterinary medicines are included in a single set of regulations – the Veterinary Medicines Regulations 2005. To maintain the clarity of the new regulations the Veterinary Medicines Directorate (VMD) agreed to revoke and remake them each year. The VMD commenced consultation on the draft Veterinary Medicines Regulations 2006 and the Veterinary Medicines Guidance Notes in March 2006.

In response to this consultation, AIC set up an ad-hoc working group to review the implications of the proposed legislation to the feed industry. The group identified the following points of concern:

- The need to clarify the definitions of "wholesale" and "retail" and the consequent effect of these definitions on the operation of the legislation. On this point the VMD undertook to clarify the chart on "who can sell what to whom" which is attached to Veterinary Medicines Guidance Note 22 – Medicated Feedingstuffs and Specified Feed Additives;
- Definition of "premixture" – there are two definitions for a "premixture" in the Veterinary Medicines Regulations one of which is the EU definition under the Additives Regulation (1831/2003). This fact in itself causes confusion. In addition the definition of premixture causes difficulties when labelling medicated complementary feedingstuffs

such as a balancer meal for pigs. The problems caused in this instance have been overcome by an 'agreement' reached between the Animal Medicines Inspectorate and AIC. A copy of the guidance is attached at *Annex 3* for information;

• The change in legal status of in-feed wormers (formerly MFSX products) to veterinary medicinal products requiring authorisation for incorporation by a Suitably Qualified Person (SQP) - AIC considers that suitably trained people within feed mills should be eligible for this activity. This matter needs further discussion with the VMD;

• Prescriptions – AIC asked the VMD to accept electronic and faxed copies rather than the original prescription as it would save time, money and paper and this request was accepted.

The Veterinary Medicines Regulations 2006 are currently being finalised and will be brought into operation from 1st October 2006. A copy of the Regulations will be published on the VMD website on 2nd October. The AMI will take a proportionate view when enforcing these Regulations immediately after their publication.

TSE Legislation:

There have been developments both at national and EU level as follows:

THE TSE REGULATIONS 2006

In March the TSE Regulations 2006 were brought into operation and reflect changes to EU legislation. With regard to feed controls, the legislation:

• Provides officials with the scope to permit the feeding of tuber and root crops where bone spicules have been detected in official control samples, subject to a favourable risk assessment;

• Permits the use of non-ruminant blood products (and bloodmeal for farmed fish only) for non-ruminant feed use subject to the same authorisation/registration requirements that apply for the use of fishmeal.

Defra updated the guidance note on the TSE Regulations which is available from the BSE website. The note is intended to be used as guidance:

• For industry – on the requirements of the BSE related feed ban as it affects the manufacture, storage, transport and use of animal feedingstuffs, and for those with enforcement responsibilities for the feed ban;

• For enforcement authorities – to co-ordinate policy at a local level.

THE EU TSE ROADMAP

The Commission issued its TSE Roadmap in 2005. Of particular interest to the UK feed industry was the discussion in the document on the fishmeal tolerance principle. The UK Government went into the TSE Roadmap process with two negotiating positions on fishmeal. The established UK position on fishmeal is that the ban of its use in ruminant feed is unjustified on food safety grounds and should be lifted. Future discussion on the overall question of fishmeal in ruminant feed is awaited in the European Parliament, however, and thus the UK Government's secondary aim for the Roadmap process is for introduction of a fishmeal tolerance principle allowing for residual traces of fishmeal in ruminant feed. This line was fully supported by AIC as it would enable the use of shared equipment i.e. a single production line with appropriate controls.

The fishmeal tolerance principle is in the proposal adopted by the European Parliament in May 2006 to amend Regulation 999/2001 which lays down rules for the prevention, control and eradication of certain TSEs. It is hoped that the Agriculture Council will accept this amendment proposal at the end of October 2006. The provision on the fishmeal tolerance principle also requires the Commission to prepare a report before implemention "covering sourcing, processing, control and traceability of feedingstuffs of animal origin".

AIC is involved in discussions with Government officials on the detailed implementation of the fishmeal tolerance principle.

Organic Production Regulation:

REGULATION 2091/92 ON ORGANIC PRODUCTION

Regulation 2091/92 sets out the current controls for the organic production method for feedingstuffs, compound feedingstuffs and feed materials. Defra has recently set up an Organic Feed Group to discuss the implications of the EU Organic Production Regulations for the feed sector. An issue discussed at recent meetings has been the difficult feed materials supply situation exacerbated by the increase in demand for organic products and the commencement of the staged transition period towards 100% organic feed material usage. The transition period laying down a maximum non-organic feed allowance under Regulation 2092/91 is as follows:

- For herbivores:
    5% until 31st December;

- For other species, primarily pigs and poultry:
    15% from 25th August 2005 to 31st December 2007;
    10% from 1st January 2008 to 31st December 2009; and
    5% from 1st January 2010 to 31st December 2011

These percentages are to be calculated on an annual dry matter basis of ingredients from agricultural origin. The maximum daily non-organic allowance is 25% dry matter. The list of permitted non-organic ingredients is set out in Annex IIC of Regulation 2091/91. This list is, however, subject to review by the Commission.

PROPOSAL TO AMEND REGULATION 2092/91

At the beginning of 2006 the Commission commenced consultation on a new draft regulation on organic production. The Commission's intention is that the proposed new rules will be simpler, and will allow a certain amount of flexibility to take account of regional differences in climate and conditions.
    Important features of the new regulation include provision for:

- the production of organic compound feed which has to be kept separate in time or space from the production of processed non organic feed – AIC very much welcomes this provision which it most definitely hopes will be retained in the finalised regulation.;
- production rules for aquaculture animals which are not in Regulation 2092/91.

The implications of this proposed regulation are being assessed on behalf of the feed industry by an Organic Farming Working Group recently established by AIC.

Environmental Legislation

There are numerous measures applying across industry but, as far as agriculture is concerned, the key measures are the Pollution and Prevention

Control Regulations, Waste Management (England and Wales) Regulations 2006, Water Framework Directive (achieve 'good' ecological and chemical status in all rivers and ground water by 2015), EC Drinking Water Directive 1998, Nitrates Directive and cross compliance requirements.

AIC has supplied Catchment Sensitive Farming and Nutrient Management Divisions in Defra with comprehensive information confirming that the UK feed and livestock industries have made significant progress in reducing nitrogen and phosphorus inputs since 2000. The main contribution from the feed industry has been to minimise the levels of P and N in feed by, amongst other things, formulating to digestible nutrients and use of enzymes. Defra has been advised that the feed industry has more control on the amounts of N and P fed to monogastric animals where complete feedingstuffs are supplied. However, it has less control in the ruminant sector, where the farmer could feed a combination of forage and other crops, feed mixed on farm, purchased complementary dairy feedingstuffs and minerals for top dressing. In these circumstances the message was that farmers needed to look at the whole diet and to get expert advice on formulations in order to control input and output.

In discussions with Defra, it has been acknowledged that industry has already achieved much. One of the aims of AIC and other interested organisations is to promote the good work that has already been done.

Classification of Feed Products Derived from Manufacturing Processes

Over the last few years discussions have been held between AIC and officials from the Environment Agency (EA), Defra and the FSA on the legal classification of by-products / co-products from manufacturing processes. These discussions can be divided into the following two sections:

FOOD AND DRINK SECTOR

In October 2005 and further to information being provided by AIC and other interested organisations the Environment Agency issued a legal guidance note on the use of materials resulting from the manufacture or sale of food / drink for human consumption as animal feed (with or without further processing). In writing the guidance note, the EA ensured that it was compatible with the aims of the Waste Framework Directive. A copy of the guidance note is attached as Annex 4.

BIO-FUELS FROM AGRICULTURAL CROP PROCESSING

Over the last few months, AIC has been in discussion with the EA, Defra and the FSA on the need to clarify the implications of the Waste Framework Directive on the position of various products of other industrial processes including bio-fuel production which are used as feed materials but in danger of being re-classified as 'waste'. One prime example is US maize gluten feed, an important feed material within the EU, which is principally a by-product of starch recovery and further processing into a variety of industrial starches including glucose syrups for use in food and bio-ethanol. AIC has submitted an explanatory paper to government outlining the issues and highlighting numerous legal inconsistencies including the fact that maize gluten, amongst other examples, is an approved feed material.

Of concern to EA lawyers was the need to look at legal precedence. Indeed the ECJ has given a number of rulings in this area. Also issues such as "certainty of use" enter the debate. The EA was also concerned that waste could be channelled into the feed supply chain in order to avoid the waste legislation and circumnavigate some of the costs of disposal. Both the FSA and AIC have emphasised to the EA the comprehensive legal framework covering feed material products from industrial processes in terms of food and feed safety. Also, in the view of AIC there is genuine food / feed safety concern that products which are "waste" and therefore unsuitable for feeding could enter the food chain; such an event would undermine all the work that had been carried out over the last few years both in relationship to the development of food and feed safety legislation at EU level as well as the industry codes of practice.

Some clarification has already been received. Defra has confirmed in respect of virgin material, such as oilseed rape and sugar beet processed for biofuel, that the remaining meal fractions are being classed as non-waste. The EA's Waste Policy and Legal Division have supported this advice. The outstanding questions relate to products from more complex processing chains.

Discussions with the EA, FSA, Defra and AIC are continuing.

Conclusion

The legislation covering the production, supply and composition of feedingstuffs, whether feed materials or manufactured products, is very complex and comprehensive. Inevitably the legislation poses many challenges to feed business operators some of which can threaten their very existence.

Thanks must be extended to the Chairmen and members of the AIC committees and working groups who work so hard to identify the threats, opportunities and shortcomings in order to help shape   the UK, and to a lesser extent the EU, feed industry's policies on all this legislation.

References

Regulation (EC) No. 183/2005 of the European Parliament and of the Council laying down requirements for feed hygiene (OJ No L35 page 1, 8 February 2005).

The Feeding Stuffs (England) Regulations 2005 (SI 2005 No. 3281).

The Feeding Stuffs (Safety Requirements for Feed for Food-Producing Animals) Regulations 2004 (SI 2004 No. 3254).

The Feeding Stuffs, the Feeding Stuffs (Sampling and Analysis) and the Feeding Stuffs (Enforcement) (Amendment) (England) Regulations 2004 (SI 2004 No. 1301)

The Veterinary Medicines Regulations 2005 (SI 2005 No. 2745).

Regulation (EC) No 882/2004 of the European Parliament and of the Council on official controls performed to ensure the verification of compliance with feed and food law, animal health and welfare rules (OJ No L191 page 1, 28 May 2004).

Regulation (EC) No 1829/2003 of the European Parliament and of the Council on genetically modified food and feed (OJ No L268 page 1, 18 October 2003).

Regulation (EC) No 1830/2003 of the European Parliament and of the Council concerning the traceability and labelling of genetically modified organisms and the traceability of food and feed products produced from genetically modified organisms and amending Directive 2001/18/EC (OJ No L268 page 24, 18 October 2003).

Regulation (EC) No 1831/2003 of the European Parliament and of the Council on additives for use in animal nutrition (OJ No L268 page 29, 18 October 2003).

The Feeding Stuffs, the Feeding Stuffs (Sampling and Analysis) and the Feeding Stuffs (Enforcement) (Amendment) (England) Regulations 2003 (SI 2003 No. 1503).

Community Register of Feed Additives pursuant to Regulation (EC) No 1831/2003 (reference the Europa website link of: http://ec.europa.eu/food/food/animalnutrition/feedadditives/authoadditives_en.htm)

Commission Regulation (EC) No 1234/2003 amending Annexes I, IV and XI to Regulation (EC) No 999/2001 of the European Parliament and of the Council and Regulation (EC) No 1326/2001 as regards transmissible spongiform encephalopathies and animal feeding (OJ No L173 page 6, 11 July 2003).

Regulation (EEC) No 2092/91 on organic production of agricultural products and indications referring thereto on agricultural products and foodstuffs (OJ No L198 page 1, 22 July 1991).

Commission Regulation (EC) No 223/2003 on labelling requirements related to the organic production method for feedingstuffs, compound feedingstuffs and feed materials and amending Council Regulation (EEC) No 2092/91 (OJ No L031 page 3, 6 February 2003).

Commission Directive 2003/126/EC on the analytical method for the determination of constituents of animal origin for the official control of feedingstuffs (OJ No L339 page 78, 24 December 2003).

Directive 2002/32/EC of the European Parliament and of the Council on undesirable substances in animal feed (OJ No L140 page 10, 30 May 2002).

Commission Directive 2003/57/EC amending Directive 2002/32/EC of the European Parliament and of the Council on undesirable substances in animal feed (OJ No L151 page 38, 19 June 2003).

Commission Directive 2003/100/EC amending Annex I to Directive 2002/32/EC of the European Parliament and of the Council on undesirable substances in animal feed (OJ No L285 page 33, 1 November 2003).

Commission Directive 2005/86/EC of 5 December 2005 amending Annex I to Directive 2002/32/EC on undesirable substances in animal feed as regards camphechlor (OJ No L318 page 16, 6 December 2005)

Commission Directive 2005/87/EC of 5 December 2005 Annex I to Directive 2002/32/EC on undesirable substances in animal feed as regards lead, fluorine and cadmium (OJ L318 page 19, 6 December 2005)

Commission Directive 2006/13/EC of 3 February 2006 amending Annexes I and II to Directive 2002/32/EC on undesirable substances in animal feed as regards dioxins and dioxin-like PCBs (OJ L32 page 44, 4 February 2006)

Regulation (EC) No 1774/2002 of the European Parliament and of the Council laying down health rules concerning animal by-products not intended for human consumption (OJ No L273 page 1, 10 October 2002).

Directive 2002/2/EC of the European Parliament and of the Council amending Council Directive 79/373/EEC on the circulation of compound feedingstuffs and repealing Commission Directive 91/357/EEC (OJ No L63 page 23, 6 March 2002).

Regulation (EC) No 178/2002 of the European Parliament and of the Council laying down the general principles and requirements of food law, establishing the European Food Safety Authority and laying down procedures in matters of food safety (OJ No L31 page 1, 1 February 2002).

Commission Regulation (EC) No 1326/2001 laying down transitional measures to permit the changeover to the Regulation of the European Parliament and of the Council (EC) No 999/2001 laying down rules for the prevention, control and eradication of certain transmissible spongiform encephalopathies, and amending Annexes VII and XI to that Regulation (OJ No L177 page 60, 30 June 2001).

Regulation (EC) No 999/2001 of the European Parliament and of the Council laying down rules for the prevention, control and eradication of certain transmissible spongiform encephalopathies (OJ No L147 page 1, 31 May 2001).

The Transmissible Spongiform Encephalopathies (No. 2) Regulations 2006 (SI 2006 No 1228)

Council Directive 2001/102/EC amending Directive 1999/29/EC on the undesirable substances and products in animal nutrition (OJ No L6 page 45, 10 January 2002).

The Feeding Stuffs (Sampling and Analysis) Regulations 1999 (SI 1999 No 1663)

Council Directive 1999/29/EC on the undesirable substances and products in animal nutrition (OJ No L115 page 32, 4 May 1999).

Commission Directive 98/88/EC establishing guidelines for the microscopic identification and estimation of constituents of animal origin for the official control of feedingstuffs (OJ No L318 page 45, 27 November 1998).

Regulation (EC) No 258/97 of the European Parliament and of the Council concerning novel foods and novel food ingredients (OJ No L043 page 1, 14 February 1997).

Council Directive 96/51/EC amending Directive 70/524/EEC (OJ No L235 page 39, 17 September 1996).

Council Directive 96/25/EC on the circulation of feed materials, amending Directives 70/524/EEC, 74/63/EEC, 82/471/EEC and 93/74/EEC and repealing Directive 77/101/EEC (OJ No L125 page 35, 23 May 1996).

Council Directive 93/74/EEC on feedingstuffs intended for particular nutritional purposes (OJ No L237 page 23, 22 September 1993).

Commission Directive 91/357/EEC laying down the categories of ingredients which may be used for the purposes of labelling compound feedingstuffs for animals other than pet animals (OJ No L193 page 34, 17 July 1991).

Council Directive 79/373/EEC on the marketing of compound feedingstuffs

(OJ No L086 page 30, 6 April 1979).

Council Directive 70/524/EEC concerning additives in feedingstuffs (OJ No L270 page 1, 14 December 1970).

The Pollution Prevention and Control (England and Wales) (Amendment) Regulations 2002 (SI 2002 No 275)

The Waste Management (England and Wales) Regulations 2006 (SI 2006 No 937)

Directive 2000/60/EC of the European Parliament and of the Council of 23rd October 2000 establishing a framework for Community action in the field of water policy (OJ No L327 page 1, 22 December 2000)

Council Directive 91/676/EEC concerning the protection of waters against pollution caused by nitrates from agricultural sources (OJ No L375 page 1 31 December 1991)

Council Directive 98/83/EC relating to the quality of water intended for human consumption (OJ No L330 page 32 5 December 1998)

ANNEX 1

Specimen Label – Dairy Feed

AIC FEEDS Ltd, Confederation House, East of England Showground, Peterborough PE2 6XE

DAIRY Compound Nuts

This is a complementary feedingstuff for feeding with forage, to dairy cows at up to 60% of dietary dry matter. If fed with an additional source of supplemental copper a Medicated Feedingstuffs prescription may be required. Check with your veterinary surgeon.

OIL	4.50 %	VITAMIN A -retinol	8000 iu/kg
PROTEIN	18.00 %	VITAMIN D3-cholecalciferol	2000 iu/kg
FIBRE	11.00 %	VITAMIN E -alpha tocopherol	75 iu/kg
ASH	9.00 %	SODIUM SELENITE-selenium	0.85 mg/kg
MOISTURE	3.80 %	COPPER SULPHATE-copper	55 mg/kg

This product contains 56.7 g of calcined magnesite equivalent in 9.07kg ("2 in 20").
Contains the following ingredients in descending order by weight:

10-25% inclusion
WHEATFEED, MALT CULMS, MAIZE GLUTEN FEED (GM2*), SUNFLOWER EXT, WHEAT, PALM KERNEL EXP
0-10% inclusion
RAPE EXT (LOW GLUCO) MOLASSES, CALCIUM CARBONATE, BARLEY, MAIZE DISTILLERS (GM2*2), SALT, VEGETABLE OILS, MAGNESIUM OXIDE

"(GM*2) Produced from genetically modified material"
NET WEIGHT: see bag/bulk delivery order.
The stated vitamin levels will be retained until:(See Best Before)
Feeding instructions and further information available from your supplier. Store in cool dry conditions.

#SSSSSS   BEST BEFORE !D.MMM.YY   6043
VMR Est.App.No.aGBxxxxx UFAS-Compound Feeds xxxxxx

ANNEX 2

Guidance Values

Mycotoxin	Products intended for animal feed	Guidance value in mg/kg (ppm) relative to a feedingstuff with a moisture content of 12%
Deoxynivalenol	Feed materials	
	– Cereals and cereal products with the exception of maize by-products	8
	– Maize by-products	12
	Complementary and complete feedingstuffs with the exception of	5
	– complementary and complete feedingstuffs for pigs	0.9
	– complementary and complete feedingstuffs for calves (< 4 months), lambs and kids	2
Zearalenone	Feed materials	
	– Cereals and cereal products with the exception of maize by-products	2
	– Maize by-products	3
	Complementary and complete feedingstuffs	
	– Complementary and complete feedingstuffs for piglets and gilts (young sows)	0.1
	– Complementary and complete feedingstuffs for sows and fattening pigs	0.25
	– Complementary and complete feedingstuffs for calves, dairy cattle, sheep (including lamb) and goats (including kids)	0.5
Ochratoxin A	Feed materials	
	– Cereals and cereal products	0.25
	Complementary and complete feedingstuffs	
	– Complementary and complete feedingstuffs for pigs	0.05
	– Complementary and complete feedingstuffs for poultry	0.1
Fumonisin B1+B2	Feed materials	
	– maize and maize products	60
	Complementary and complete feedingstuffs for:	
	– pigs, horses (*Equidae*), rabbits and pet animals	5
	– fish	10
	– poultry, calves (< 4 months), lambs and kids	20
	– adult ruminants (> 4 months) and mink	20

ANNEX 3

The Veterinary Medicines Regulations 2005
Guidance Agreed Between AIC and the AMI

Labelling requirements

The labelling requirements for medicated premixtures, medicated feedingstuffs and feedingstuffs containing either a specified feed additive or a premixture containing a specified feed additive are laid down in Schedule 5 on medicated feedingstuffs and specified feed additives which come into operation on 1 January 2006. The guidance has been agreed with the AMI/RPSGB subject to further clarification being given once the European Commission has given an opinion on the borderline between complementary feedingstuffs and premixtures. For any queries, please contact John Millward on 02476 849260.

The wording for the labels of premixtures, feedingstuffs containing specified feed additives or veterinary medicinal products is taken from Schedule 5. Additional comments on the labelling provisions, from AIC, are given in italics after each type of feedingstuffs.

1. Additional labelling requirement for premixtures containing a veterinary medicinal product (reference paragraph 9)

    A label on a premixture containing a veterinary medicinal product must contain the information required under Article 16 of Regulation (EC) No. 1831/2003* – and in addition the following:-

    (a) the words "medicated premixture";
    (b) the proprietary name of the veterinary medicinal product and the authorisation number;
    (c) the strength;
    (d) the inclusion rate of the premixture into the feedingstuff;
    (e) the level of the active ingredient in the final feed;
    (f) warnings and contra-indications;
    (g) withdrawal period;
    (h) the expiry date;
    (i) any special storage instructions;
    (j) where a prescription is required, a statement to this effect;

    and any person who supplies such a premixture not labelled in this way is guilty of an offence.

Regulation (EC) No 1831/2003 is the Additives Regulation.

With reference to the words "medicated premixture" in (a) above, Regulation 1831/2003 requires the word "premixture" to be in capital letters; we suggest the same when declaring "MEDICATED PREMIXTURE".

The requirement to state "the strength" in (c) above refers to the level of the active ingredient in the premixture. Manufacturers could also add the level of the veterinary medicinal product incorporated into the premixture.

The requirement to state "the expiry date" in (h) above refers to the expiry date of the premixture, taking into account all ingredients, including veterinary medicinal products and specified feed additives, applying the shortest expiry date.

Please note that sub-paragraph (j) above refers to a "prescription" and not a veterinary prescription. This is because from 1 January 2006 pharmacists and Suitably Qualified Persons (SQPs) as well as veterinary surgeons can authorise the incorporation of in-feed wormers which, from that date, are being classified as POM-VPS (ie Prescription Only Medicine - Veterinarian, Pharmacist, Suitably Qualified Person).

2.   Labelling of feedingstuffs containing specified feed additives (reference paragraph 10)

Feedingstuffs containing a specified feed additive or a premixture containing a specified feed additive must be clearly and legibly labelled with the following:-

(a) the name of the specified feed additive;
(b) the name of the active substance and the level incorporated in the feedingstuff;
(c) the withdrawal period if one is specified in the authorisation;
(d) the expiry date (if there are several additives with different expiry dates, the expiry date given must be the earliest expiry date);
(e) the name and approval number of the manufacturer or the distributor;
(f) any particulars concerning the proper use of the feedingstuffs specified in the authorisation of the specified feed additive.

It is an offence to supply feedingstuffs not labelled in accordance with this paragraph.

The above declarations are in additional to the standard requirements for feedingstuffs labelling.

In keeping with feedingstuffs containing a veterinary medicinal product, detailed in 3 (b) below, we suggest the inclusion of the proprietary name of the specified feed additive and the level of inclusion in the feedingstuff.

In the provision to state "the expiry date (if there are several additives with different expiry dates the expiry date given must be the earliest expiry date)" at (d) above, the "expiry date" refers to that of the feed defined by the additive with the shortest in-feed shelf life.

Complementary Feedingstuffs

For a complementary feedingstuff (as defined by the Feeding Stuffs Regulations) into which a specified feed additive has been incorporated, and which is intended to be mixed with other feed materials the AMI has advised that such feeds fall within the definition of a premixture given in the Veterinary Medicines Regulations 2005 and, in relation to the specified feed additive, should be labelled as per article 16 of EC Regulation 1831/2003 together with the following statement in the relevant part of the label:-

"This complementary feedingstuff is a PREMIXTURE under the VM Regulations 2005 and must be mixed with other feed materials by approved manufacturers only".

We therefore advise that the "feed section" of the label is headed "Complementary feeding stuff" and details below the nutritional parameters required therein. The "medicated" section should apply the AMI statement above and the following:

Contains x kg/t of (SFA name) such that when this premixture is mixed into feed at the recommended rate of y kg/t will supply z mg/kg of (active ingredient name) in the final feed.

Other relevant statements given in sections 1f, 1h and 1i above should be applied.

3.   Labelling of feedingstuffs containing a veterinary medicinal product
     (reference paragraph 11)

A feedingstuff containing a veterinary medicinal product must be
clearly and legibly labelled with the following:-

(a) the words "Medicated Feedingstuff";
(b) the proprietary name, authorisation number and inclusion rate
     (kg/t or mg/kg) of the veterinary medicinal product incorporated
     into the feed;
(c) the name and amount of the active substance (mg/kg) in the
     feed;
(d) the species of animal for which the feed is intended;
(e) warnings and contra-indications required by the marketing
     authorisation for the veterinary medicinal product;
(f) the withdrawal period;
(g) the expiry date;
(h) any special storage instructions required by the marketing
     authorisation;
(i) a statement to the effect that the feed must only be fed in
     accordance with a prescription written by a veterinary surgeon,
     where a prescription is required *(please note that this
     requirement is new)*;
(j) the name and approval number of the manufacturer or the
     distributor.

It is an offence to supply feedingstuffs not labelled in accordance
with this paragraph.

The above declarations are in addition to the standard requirements
for feedingstuffs labelling

With reference to sub-paragraph (b) above, the requirement for
inclusion rate of the veterinary medicinal product is new, the
proprietary name and authorisation number having previously being
required.

The requirement to state "the expiry date" in (g) above refers to the
expiry date of the medicated feedingstuff taking into account all
ingredients, including veterinary medicinal products, applying the
shortest expiry date.

Complementary Feedingstuffs

For a complementary feedingstuff containing a veterinary medicinal product that is intended for direct feeding to animals without further mixing with feed materials, the labelling requirements for medicated feedingstuffs detailed in 3a to j above applies.

For a complementary feedingstuff (as defined by the Feeding Stuffs Regulations) into which a veterinary medicinal product has been incorporated, and which is intended to be mixed with other feed materials, the AMI has advised that such feeds fall within the definition of a premixture given in the Veterinary Medicines Regulations 2005 and, in relation to the veterinary medicinal product, should be labelled as per 1 above (Additional labelling requirements for premixtures containing a veterinary medicinal product) together with the following statement in the relevant part of the label:-

"This complementary feedingstuff is a MEDICATED PREMIXTURE under the VM Regulations 2005 and must be mixed with other feed materials by approved manufacturers only".

We therefore advise that the "feed section" of the label is headed "Complementary feeding stuff" and details below the nutritional parameters required therein. The "medicated" section should apply the AMI statement above and the details given as per medicated premixture given in section 1a to j.

ANNEX 4

Definition of waste: Legal Guidance Note
Use of materials resulting from the manufacture or sale of food / drink for human consumption as animal feed (with or without further processing)

1.   **Scenario 1: Materials that are always produced as an inevitable result of the process of manufacturing food and drink for human consumption (spent yeast, brewers grains, molasses, etc.)**

1.1.   **Use of these materials in the manufacture of human or animal food/ feed**

Materials: "Materials resulting from the manufacture of food or drink which are passed on directly to another undertaking for processing into food or drink (for human or animal consumption)."

Conclusion

Not waste.

Example: Brewers grains and spent yeast, where they are used to make animal feed or yeast based products; molasses and other derivatives from sugar manufacturing where they are used to make animal feed.

Rationale

Raw materials are being processed in a series of stages (albeit by different undertakings) to extract nutritional value for a number of different purposes, all of which are aimed at manufacturing food and drink from the materials. In these circumstances, the Environment Agency considers that it is appropriate to regard these food and drink by-products as not being discarded as waste but simply as another food and drink product obtained from the original raw materials. In the Agency's view, this conclusion is compatible with the aims of the Waste Framework Directive (WFD) and the need to ensure its effectiveness is not undermined.

Legal rationale (in more detail)

These substances are produced in a manufacturing/production process so the first question is whether they are products/by-products (which are *prima facie* not waste) or production residues (which are *prima facie* waste). Having regard to recent case law these substances can be classified as products/by-products. Although their nutritional value is sought at a different stage of the production process (and by different undertakings), they are nonetheless used in their entirety *for the same purposes* as the other (main product) substances sought by the operator of the initial food and drink manufacturing process – i.e. food.

In order to reach a decision as to whether something is a by-product or a production residue, it is also necessary to consider all the other relevant factors /questions (except for the questions (i) whether they can be used only in a way that involves their disappearance or (ii) whether their use must involve special measures to protect the environment, as these questions are not relevant to products/by-products). In the case of the materials identified in this scenario the answers to these questions tend to support the conclusion that it is not waste: *Is it specifically listed in Annex 1 WFD?* No. *Is it consigned to a recovery or disposal operation?* This is a rather circular question but the use of food materials in the manufacture of food/feed is not an obvious R or D operation. *Is it commonly regarded as waste?* No. *Is it a common method of recovering/disposing of waste?* No.

The final and ultimate question: *Having regard to all the circumstances and the aims of the Waste Framework Directive, would it undermine the effectiveness of the WFD not to treat this material as waste?* Answer: No. The human food and animal feed manufacturing businesses are subject to the types of controls that would ensure that any environmental risks were also addressed during the collection, transport and manufacture of this material into human food / animal feed.

1.2. Use of these materials to feed directly to animals on farm

Conclusion

In general, materials resulting from the manufacture of food and drink which are passed on to a farmer for direct use as animal feed on farm (i.e. without being manufactured into animal feed by an intermediate animal feed manufacturer) will not be regarded as waste, as long as the material is suitable for that use, there is certainty of that use and the material is only being passed on for that use. In determining whether the material is suitable for that use, compliance with the relevant animal feed legislation and recognised industry standards can be regarded as demonstrating suitability for use as animal feed. However, if the materials are unsuitable for use as animal feed and/or are being passed on in circumstances which indicate that what is really happening is waste disposal (for example a farmer is taking in excessive quantities of the material), then the Agency will treat the material as waste. Each case must be considered on its facts, having regard to all the circumstances, the aims of the Waste Framework Directive and the need to ensure the effectiveness of the Directive is not undermined.

Rationale

In this case the rationale is almost the same as above – and the conclusion indicates that they are products/by-products not production residues - but in looking at the aims of the WFD being undermined does it make a difference that the food is going directly to farms and not through a strictly controlled feed manufacturing process?

The Agency has received information from the Food Standards Agency about the obligations on animal feed manufacturers in relation to 'feedingstuffs'. From 1 January 2005 the EC Regulation 178/2002 General Food Law, amongst other things, prohibits the placing on the market, or the feeding to food-producing animals, of unsafe feed and requires feed business operators to have traceability systems in place. EC Regulation 183/2005, laying down requirements for feed hygiene, extends the approval/registration requirements to all feed businesses including food businesses selling co-products for feed use. Such businesses will have to comply with various conditions appropriate to the operations that they carry out. Annex I of the Regulation covers provisions applicable to feed businesses involved in primary production and includes hygiene standards and record keeping. The controls (178/2002 and 183/2005) apply to businesses selling and using feed materials from the human food/drink sectors and further strengthen existing controls in place for additives and undesirable substances. For example, it is illegal for the seller of feed:

*   to sell to the farmer, for use as feed, any product which contains any ingredient deleterious to the animal, or to humans through consumption of animal products; or
*   to sell feed materials that are not sound, genuine and of merchantable quality.

Further controls are to be introduced in the future, through European legislation, on matters such as transport, traceability and quality/suitability for use. It is not clear what difference if any these new controls will make to the feeding of materials from manufacturing human food/drink direct to animals.

What is clear from the information provided at the present time (including the ACAF Review of On-Farm Feeding Practices) is that:

- many 'co-products' from the manufacture of human food/drink are suitable for feeding direct to animals without being processed into animal feed; and
- there is increasing pressure for all materials, purchased by farmers for animal feeding, to come from sources and suppliers who can demonstrate compliance with recognised quality assurance standards, and for farmers themselves to use/participate in the relevant codes of practice and assurance schemes.

It is however important that any 'co products' intended to be fed directly to animals are properly identified as being suitable for use because, unlike manufactured feed, they will not have been specifically selected and processed for that purpose. In the ACAF Review they point out that:

"...primary and manufactured foods intended for direct human consumption, which are either surplus to requirements or have been rejected for quality or presentational reasons (e.g. misshapen biscuits, crisps, vegetables) may either be sold direct to farms or via intermediate processors. However, **farmers buying direct from food factories should find out why the food has been rejected and be aware of the possible hazards to livestock.**"

2. **Scenario 2: Surplus food or off-specification food from the manufacture of food and drink for human consumption (e.g. potato chips or cereals that are the wrong size or shape to go into the human food chain; leftover dough and liquid chocolate).**

2.1. **Use of these materials in the manufacture of human or animal food/feed**

Conclusion

If these materials are passed on directly to another undertaking for processing into food or drink (for human or animal consumption) then the same principles as in scenario 1.1 can be applied, with the same conclusion, i.e. they are not production residues and not waste.

Rationale

The only difference is that these are 'off-specification products' which are specifically listed in Q2 of Annex I WFD. However, an off-specification product is not necessarily waste even though it falls within Q2. Indeed, some off-specification products could also be regarded as products/by-products of a production process, in the same way as the grains, yeast etc. in scenario 1, and hence prima facie not waste. The Environment Agency also considers that in these circumstances the materials could be regarded as 'off-spec' in one sense (i.e. not of a suitable specification for use in the production of food for human consumption) but not off-spec in another sense (i.e. suitable for use in the manufacture of animal feed).

2.2. Use of these materials in animal feed to feed to animals on farm

The same principles apply as in 1.2. above and it is proposed that the same position be adopted (i.e. not usually waste if suitable for use and certain of use but may be waste if not suitable and/or passed on in circumstances that indicate it is in fact being disposed of - each case to be considered on its facts).

3.   Scenario 3: Off specification or out of date food from shops/retailers (e.g. supermarket food that's past its sell by date, bruised fruit and vegetables, stale bread).

Use of the materials in the manufacture of animal food/feed or to be fed directly to animals

The response from the FSA on this issue was:

"The vast majority of surplus or part-processed food products derive from food processors, not shops/retailers. However, some wrapped bread does come back from retailers to bakeries, as "returns". This bread is then sent to surplus food processors such as a company that is FEMAS accredited.

As far as intermediate processors are concerned, fruit and vegetables do not fit into the mix with biscuits, pasta, crisps, etc. due to their physical handling characteristics, very short shelf life, resultant perishability and general unsuitability for mono-gastric i.e. pig and poultry, outlets. Of course, ruminant livestock are very able to utilize vegetable materials e.g. carrots, which may be traded inter-farm or, presumably, bought direct from food processors. However, we would question whether shops and retailers would be able to segregate such products from less suitable materials."

We understand this to mean that it is not common practice for food to be taken from shops/retailers either for processing into animal feed or for direct use on farm. However, we are informed by the British Retail Consortium that some of their members do provide food to animal sanctuaries and urban farms (though not to commercial farms) and that the food is provided free of charge and is collected by the recipients. This food is separated out before it enters the waste stream, and it is typically fruit, vegetables and bakery products that have passed their sell-by date. (Meat products are not donated because of the restrictions in the animal by-products legislation).

In this scenario we are not dealing with a production process so there is no distinction to be made between products/by-products and production residues.

The starting point is Annex I WFD. This includes "Q2: Off-specification products" and "Q3: Products whose date for appropriate use has expired." This gives an indication that they may be waste (although as indicated above the conclusion does not necessarily follow). In this context, the terms 'off-specification' and 'appropriate use' may reasonably be interpreted to cover food from a shop/retailer that is no longer suitable for sale for human consumption. They were on sale for that purpose/use and they can no longer be sold for that purpose/put to that use.

It is then necessary to consider all the other relevant factors /questions.

- *Is it listed in Annex 1 WFD? Yes.*
- *Is it consigned to a recovery or disposal operation? The use of off-spec or out of date food from a shop/retailer as animal feed to feed directly to animals may be regarded as a R or D operation.*
- *Is it commonly regarded as waste? In some circumstances, yes.*
- *Is it a common method of recovering/disposing of waste? In some circumstances, yes.*
- *Having regard to all the circumstances and the aims of the Waste Framework Directive, would it undermine the effectiveness of the WFD not to treat this material as waste?*

Conclusions

As a general rule, we consider that it would undermine the effectiveness of the WFD not to treat this material as waste if it is unsegregated, for the following reasons:

-       The food will be of variable quantities and types.
-       The food will require some form of segregation by the user, to separate out that which is suitable for use as animal feed and that which is not (or is banned, e.g. food containing meat which has to be sent to landfill).
-       There is no certainty/continuity of use.
-       Treating some of it as waste and some as a non-waste could give rise to practical enforcement difficulties.
-       The food is less likely to be 'suitable for use' as animal feed than the food that results from a manufacturing process.
-       The materials resulting from manufacturing processes can be regarded more as a resource than a waste, whereas unsold/off-spec/out of date food from shops/retailers would normally be regarded by the shop/ retailer themselves as a waste. We understand that in most if not all circumstances the shops/retailers give this food away rather than *selling* it to farmers, which is an indication that it is being discarded.

However, where certain items of food are specifically segregated out and set aside by the retailer, for use as animal feed, before being passed on to the user, and the food is suitable for use for that purpose and there is certainty of use for that purpose, we consider that it can be regarded as non-waste without undermining the aims and effectiveness of the Waste Framework Directive. This principle would apply, for example, to the donation of pre-segregated fruit, vegetables and bakery products to animal sanctuaries and urban farms.

In addition, where surplus bread is collected from retailers, on a daily basis, and returned to the manufacturer, who then passes it on directly to an animal feed manufacturing establishment for use as a raw material, we consider that the bread can be regarded as non-waste. (The bread is effectively being passed from the original manufacturer to an animal feed manufacturer, as in scenario 2 above).

4.   **Scenario 4: Used food, e.g. used cooking oil (or partially eaten food from restaurants etc.)**

The Agency considers this material to be waste, whether it is used as animal feed (which is mostly banned under the Animal By-Products Regulation anyway; the ban on feeding used cooking oil to animals, where it has been in contact with meat, having taken effect in the UK in October 2004) or used for other purposes such as fuel.

12 October 2005

9

EUROPEAN UNION ENLARGEMENT: EFFECTS ON UK ANIMAL AGRICULTURE

ANDREW KNOWLES
BPEX, PO Box 44, Winterhill House, Snowdon Drive, Milton Keynes, MK6 1AX, UK

Introduction

Although this chapter will consider the 10 new member states of the EU, it will initially discuss the bigger picture of global livestock production and consumption trends. It will then discuss the production and consumption of animal products in the new EU member states and conclude with a consideration of the likely impact this will have on the UK Livestock Industry.

The 10 new EU member states are Latvia, Lithuania, Estonia, Poland, Czech Republic, Slovakia, Hungary, Slovenia, Malta and Cyprus (Romania and Bulgaria are due to join the EU in 2007 but will not be considered in this chapter). Figure 1 presents data on the numbers of breeding animals from which it can be seen that the new EU10 has relatively few. However it should be remembered that these data can change rapidly; there are already plans for significant increases in the sow populations in both Poland and Romania. Although incorporation of the new EU10 will increase the population of the enlarged EU by some 20%, consumption patterns of the new EU10 do not reflect that of the existing EU15. Thus figure 2 demonstrates that, whilst consumption of pig and poultry meat is similar in the 2 blocks, consumers in the new EU10 eat considerably less lamb and beef, probably a reflection of low personal income. Figure 2 also presents data for the UK where consumers eat more poultry but far less pigmeat than the mean for the EU25.

The global picture

World pigmeat trade flows are presented in figure 3. Trends are based on a number issues. The US$ is currently weak against both the € and Pound

Sterling. South America (specifically Brazil and Mexico) are increasing their exports to sustain a production boom; their targets are principally Asia and Russia although there are issues over foot and mouth disease (FMD). The EU is the second largest producer of pigmeat after China. Within the EU, Denmark dominates the export trade but is losing out to North and South America due to exchange rates, cost of legislation and relative feed prices.

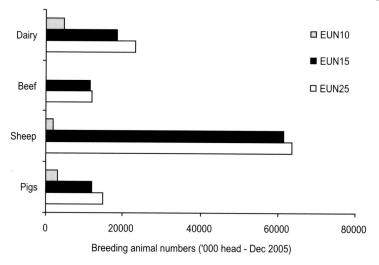

Figure 1.

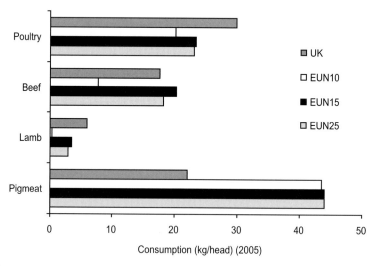

Figure 2.

Figure 4 shows data on global flows of beef. South America is the dominant global exporter but Brazil has been hit by FMD and Argentina by an economic crisis resulting in reduced exports to both the EU and Russia. Australia has been quick to replace US exports to Japan in 2005 due to Bovine Spongiform Encephalopathy (BSE). The US moved back in to the market in 2006 but Australia now has major foothold. The EU Beef import quota is unlikely to be filled due to South American restrictions.

World Pigmeat Trade Flows, 2005

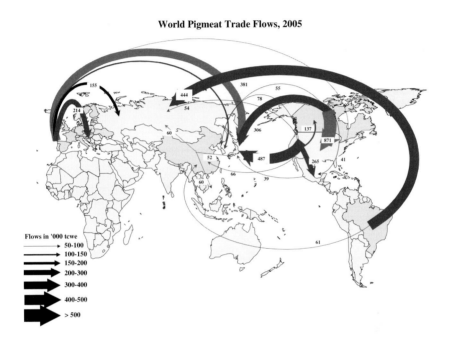

Figure 3.

Sheep meat flows are presented in figure 5. As there was a failure in the recent World Trade Association (WTO) talks, EU quotas remain. There is a move in the Australian flock from wool to meat production and Australia is targeting the US to replace drop in the domestic flock; the increase in demand in the Middle East is being supplied by Australia. The New Zealand flock is static but productivity is increasing and Asia is the new target market for the associated increased output.

World Beef Trade Flows, 2005

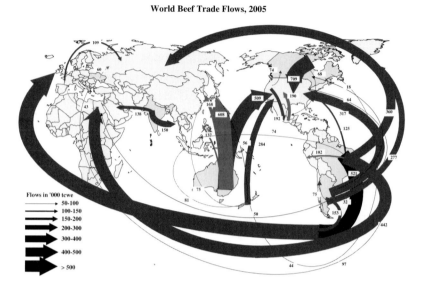

Figure 4.

World Sheepmeat Trade Flows, 2005

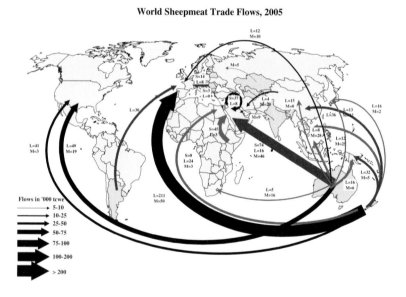

Figure 5.

Prospects for the new EU10: production and consumption

Figure 6 presents data on the beef market within the EU. It is predicted that production will be reduced by 5% by 2013 with lower customer preference

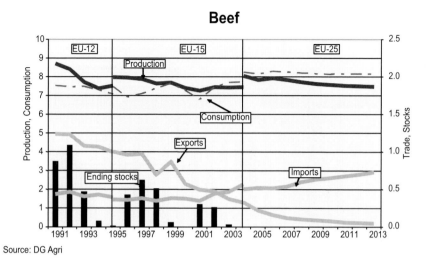

Source: DG Agri

Figure 6.

in the new EU10 offsetting increased incomes. There will probably be a steady EU supply and a tight demand, and therefore a steady increase in imports at full duty. In addition, longer term cow beef supplies will fall due to a reduction in the dairy herd. The suckler herd size is not increasing sufficiently to counter-balance the reduced cow beef supply. The milk market is detailed in figure 7. Production is expected to follow reference quantities and exceed 144 million tonnes by 2013. However, production is of course constrained by EU quotas. The 2 main features of note are increasing yields per cow but a reduction in overall size of the EU dairy herd. The cheese market will show steady growth in the medium term. It is expected that the butter balance will improve but there may be short term difficulties. The SMP market is expected to shrink from 952kt in 2005 to 876kt in 2013 which will limit availability for export.

The sheep and goat markets are presented in figure 8. Production will decline in medium term, continuing the historic trend and as a result of decoupling of the ewe premium. There will be a firming of EU prices but EU production will be substituted by imports. It should not be forgotten that consumption is slowly dropping.

Figure 9 presents data on the poultry market. The short term impact of Avian Flu is still uncertain. However there will be continued medium term growth and competitive pricing relative to other proteins, and increased use in food preparations. Import pressure from low cost world producers will focus mainly in the cooked and processed poultry meat sectors. The pig

Milk

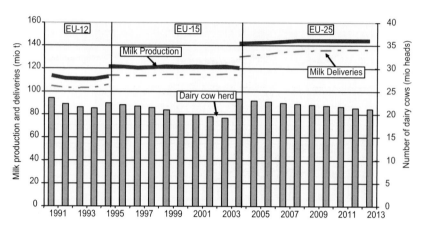

Source: DGAgri

Figure 7.

Sheep (and Goat)

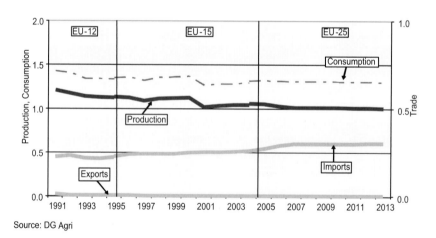

Source: DG Agri

Figure 8.

meat sector is given in figure 10. A steady increase in production is forecast as it remains the favoured meat in the EU. Per capital consumption is predicted to rise from 42.8 to 44.1 kg per capita per year by 2013. Exports have been held in check by increased competition in the Far East from North and South America. A large restructuring of the new EU10 industries, especially Poland and Hungary, is being driven by significant foreign investment.

Poultry

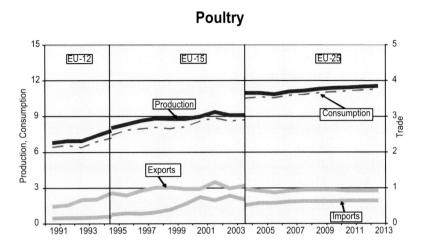

Source: DGAgri

Figure 9.

Pig meat

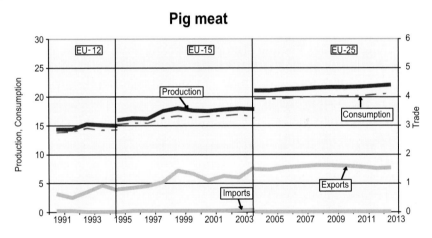

Source: DG Agri

Figure 10.

Implications for UK animal agriculture

There are many challenges facing UK Animal Agriculture. EU agricultural incomes are forecast to rise by 18% between 2006-2013. However there are significant localized effects. Thus this increase will be confined to 11% for the EU15 and much greater at 42% in the new EU10. There will be continued pressure on reducing costs in the face of internal competition but adoption of EU legislation in the medium term together with increased labour rates will narrow the gap post 2013.

There are opportunities in the context of increased availability of UK skilled labour and the quality differential which still exists. However, GDP in the new EU10 is expected to increase by 4.8% in 2007, and their consumers will 'trade up' in terms of quality expectations and price points. There will be export opportunities for the EU15 to the new EU10 up to 2013 but the speed of quality improvements will vary between sectors.

There have been significant developments in the retailer sector. Tesco, Carrefour, Alberts, Lidl, Metro have between them around 700 stores in Poland. These will be based on the same business model as the EU15, will have similar sourcing policies in terms of suppliers and will be looking to adopt regional supply policies. There will be consumer / retailer demands for provenance, food safety, quality and production standards, EUREPGAP (an equal partnership of agricultural producers and retailers that want to establish basic certification standards and procedures for Good Agricultural Practices - GAP) and labeling.

Disease factors which will have an important but hard to predict influence include the sheep sector which is still recovering from FMD and the unknown effects of blue tongue. The pig sector is suffering from Post-weaning multi-systemic wasting syndrome (PMWS) and classical swine fever (CSF). The beef sector is still vulnerable to BSE and blue tongue and the effect of avian influenza in the poultry sector.

The exchange rate factor is an additional unknown in the context of the cross-border trade (Figure 11).

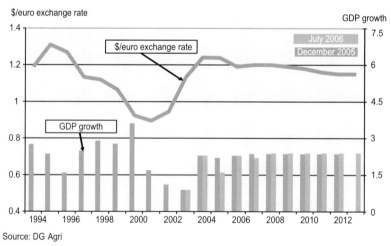

Source: DG Agri

Figure 11.

Examining one particular country, it should be noted that Poland has 1.7 million sows on 1.5 million farms. However, Smithfield Foods, which is the world's largest pig meat processor, has recently placed over 120,000 sows. Production will all be to UK assurance scheme standards including no tethers or stalls, traceability, quality and food safety. The intention is to supply Tesco Poland and, possibly, Tesco UK. Such expansion is not confined to the EU; China is planning major developments in its pig sector.

To summarise, global trade flows are increasingly volatile and the WTO is increasingly ineffective. It is probable that there will be regionalisation not globalisation in trade and commerce. Perhaps 'glocalisation' is the key which is adapting a global or regional product to local market requirements. This applies to cars, and also animal production and meat products.

All things being equal the overall impact of EU enlargement on UK animal agriculture will be positive up to 2013 in terms of exports, labour, quality and provenance issues. After 2013 the effects will be negative as new EU10 will become net importers to existing EU countries based on lower cost but similar quality. A question remains as to whether there will be similar application of EU legislation. More realistically the impact of the new EU10 will depend on retailer attitudes to sourcing policy, customer / legislative demands on assurance and labeling, disease outbreaks, exchange rate changes and global trade.

The prospects for pigs are medium to good; The EU15 is a net exporter to new EU10. There will be a tightening of supply and demand. After 2013 the UK will need to have differentiated to offset high costs of production. As regards sheep, the prospects are good given WTO breakdown. There will be little production but little demand from new EU10. The prospects for beef are medium depending on what happens to the dairy sector for which the prospects are only medium to poor.

10

BY-PRODUCTS FROM NON-FOOD AGRICULTURE: IMPLICATIONS FOR THE FEED SUPPLY INDUSTRY

TIM WILSON

ABNA, P O Box 250, Oundle Road, Peterborough PE2 9PW, UK

The current deluge of press releases heralding new investments in UK biofuels production has stimulated a debate amongst agriculturalists as to what will be the long-term effects on the UK cereals and feed markets of this major development in the use of food crops for industrial processing.

The objective of this chapter is not to provide a detailed guide to the size and shape of this new industry, nor to focus on the nutritional characteristics of the resulting co-products that may become available (others are better equipped to provide such guidance). This chapter seeks to clarify, the "drivers" of this frantic activity, the likely timescales and magnitude of any investments, and in particular, indicate how these fledgling industries may/ will impact on our activities within and the future of, the UK animal feed industry, plus provide some clear pointers as to where feed advisers and formulators should focus their strategic thinking.

The drivers

The EU has adopted a policy specifying that 5.75% of all transport fuels should come from biofuels by 2010 – the UK Government (not uniquely) chose to achieve this by putting an obligation on fuel supply companies to ensure that they meet this objective. (This is known as the Road Transport Fuel Obligation (RTFO)) There are penalties for the fuel companies if they do not achieve this objective, but equally there are significant costs to them of moving to 5% biofuels in such a short timescale.

The UK Government's objective is to let the market determine the where and how, having established the why! Other countries, noticeably Germany, have provided capital investments to underwrite such biofuels production and as a result German plants are responsible for the majority of the biofuels currently being produced in Europe (Figure 1).

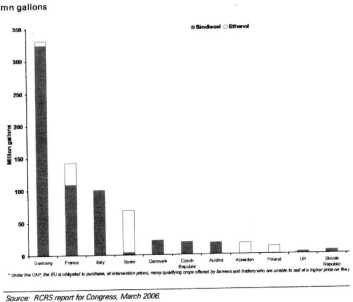

Figure 1. EU biofuel production by member state, by fuel type 2004

Throughout the EU, different countries have adopted different policy instruments but all are seeking to meet the 2010 objective.

Current thinking suggests that a 5% biofuels fuel mix is about the maximum level achievable before vehicles need modification, but with increasing worries about the security of supply and the price of mineral oil-based fuels we must conclude that 5% is the first base and 10-25% inclusion is a longer-term objective!

What are the biofuels options in the UK?

Currently the UK fuel market is comprised of approximately 21 million tonnes of petrol and 25 million tonnes of diesel. The RTFO does not specify that any one fuel should be substituted, so the 5.75% obligation could be met wholly from petrol or diesel replacing fuels.

However in reality it will be some of each, the exact scale of the investment in biodiesel or biopetrol replacers being determined by a number of factors, not least by each company's assessment of the availability and price of the raw material needed for their chosen process.

It is important to recognise that for the UK to produce this initial commitment would require either 3.5 million tonnes of wheat/cereals for biopetrol or 2.5 million tonnes of Oilseed Rape (or similar) for biodiesel. For comparison the current UK cereal output is *circa* 21-23 million tonnes and oilseed rape is 1.2-1.5 million tonnes

The risks for the biofuels investor

Once the cost of building and operating a biofuel plant is known, every investor is left with at least four key variables – energy costs, biofuel values, raw material costs and co-product values.

It is not in the author's brief (or competence) to consider the first two, but all of us are keenly interested to understand the likely impact of this industry on the last two variables, raw material cost and co-product values.

In these two areas alone the possible price variance over the initial 5-15 year life of any biofuels investment can make it unacceptably risky, which is why the current "hype" is not always matched by actions!

Let us consider these last two risks in particular:

RAW MATERIAL COST

Biopetrol

The production of bioethanol (or as announced by British Sugar/BP and DuPont – biobutanol) is as a result of the fermentation of a starch stream from cereals.

In the UK (and assuming wheat is the raw material) the process will involve an initial dry milling. The resultant meal is then put into solution and fermented to produce bioethanol and a low dry matter fermentation residue, which can be partially evaporated to produce a liquid feed stream. This stream can then be evaporated further or dried to produce a moist or dried feed.

In future new technology may allow these fuels to be produced from lignin-cellulytic material ie straw/wood, but for the next 5-10 years the cheapest and most available fermentable substrate will be starch sourced from UK cereals – almost exclusively wheat.

As indicated above, producing all the obligation as 'biopetrol' would use up all of the UK's normal exportable wheat surplus (1-5 million tonnes) and may necessitate some imports in the event of poor harvests.

We can see in Figure 2, the scale of the major UK produced cereals (wheat and barley) and the relatively small exportable surplus of each when compared with the current usage for human food and animal feed.

WHEAT		BARLEY	
UK Production	14.6	UK Production	5.5
Imports	0.9	Imports	007
Total	15.6	Total	5.6

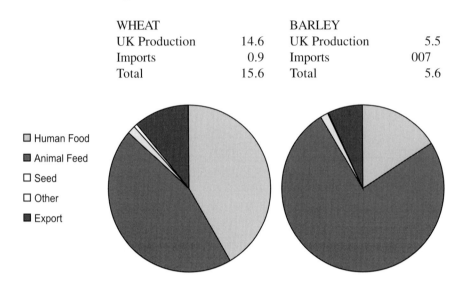

Human Food
Animal Feed
Seed
Other
Export

Figure 2. UK cereal production and usage (2005 / 2006) (million tonnes)

As a minimum this extra demand moves the UK from being a discounted market (an exporter) to being at parity with world markets – in the extreme we could become a premium market if we become a regular cereal importer. At the same time similar biofuels investments elsewhere in Europe will increase EU-wide cereal demand and may inflate both EU and world cereal markets. We must always remember that the UK's exportable surplus was/is feeding people and animals in other markets and their demand will continue to be met from other suppliers, with a commensurate impact on their overall cereal values.

The scope for growth of biofuels in the EU is significant, as on a world scale we lag far behind the US and Brazil in ethanol production (Figure 3), albeit we do have a higher percentage of diesel usage in the EU than either Brazil or the USA.

Importantly the biopetrol producer, once in production has practically no "formulation" opportunities to switch raw materials and thus will be committed to purchasing high volumes of wheat, or similar cereals, almost irrespective of price – the alternative is to shut down!

Can we predict a compensating increase in supply? We don't know at present but farmers and agronomists will need to work hard to significantly increase current yields cost effectively and bring more marginal and set-aside land back into cereal production. This may increase the available UK cereal harvest by *circa* 1 million tonnes over time.

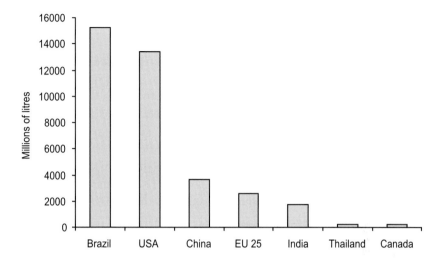

Figure 3. Main ethanol producers 2004

The feed industry, which has enjoyed relatively low cereal prices over the last 4-5 years, must now reassess other feeds in the light of higher cereal costs, and must learn a lesson from the US and Brazil where the biofuels industries' activities have resulted in price increases of between 50 and 100% in grain and sugar prices.

This new worldwide demand for cereals (or other fermentable carbohydrates) will exacerbate an already tight cereal supply and demand balance, where population growth and increasing meat consumption in the developing world is already increasing demand.

As the world enters each harvest period the current worldwide stock of cereals is only *circa* 3-4 months, and as a result any crop scares have a more than commensurate effect on prices. We have seen this in Europe over the past 2-3 years.

Potential bioethanol investors are already offering growers long term contracts to secure wheat supplies at a 20-30% premium over 2005 levels.

In the past, high EU cereal prices were partly mitigated for feed producers by the availability of low cost cereal substitutes. However, with biofuel demand using some of these raw materials, e.g. maize meals and molasses, in their home markets these alternatives may not be available to the UK feed producer in future.

Biodiesel

Biodiesel is produced from oil derived from oilseeds by extraction or expelling. The unrefined oil then is esterified with methanol, which produces biodiesel and glycerine as a by-product.

The cost structure of biodiesel will differ from cereals in two key areas – firstly – the cost of oilseed rape seed is of less consequence to the feed trade as it is not so important a raw material for feed use, and secondly the biodiesel manufacturer has the option to buy other oils from which to make biodiesel and may thus not be solely reliant on UK sourced oilseed rape.

It is generally felt that the capability of UK arable farmers to increase their oilseed rape production by 50-100% is limited (not least as it is generally used as a break crop), so demand is likely to outstrip supply and push seed prices up – in any case seed prices will need to rise to encourage producers to continue to plant rape rather than increasingly profitable cereals.

However, an excess supply of rapeseed meal may have the opposite effect and there might be scope to capture feed cost savings by better utilisation of rapemeal across a wider range of feeds.

If oils, other than rape oil, are used to manufacture biodiesel in the UK there will be very little co-product (apart from glycerine) as seed crushing will most likely take place at origin.

THE OPPORTUNITIES

Biopetrol

In these processes, approximately 30% of the raw material dry matter could be produced as a dried feed product, similar/equivalent to Dried Distillers' Dark Grains (DDGs). If conservatively 2-3 million tonnes of wheat are processed, this will put between 600,000 tonnes and 1 million tonnes of new high protein/high energy co-product into the UK market or even higher volumes if the by-product streams are marketed in their moist and / or liquid form.

This volume could be supplemented by similar materials produced by biopetrol manufacturers in Spain, France, Germany and Holland, some of which is already entering the UK market

Over the last 5 years we have seen volumes of biofuels co-products materials accessing the UK from US and Canadian producers and this may also continue – but increasingly these producers are recognising the threat to them of indigenous EU production and are working hard to develop their domestic markets in innovative ways.

The UK feed industry must learn quickly how to make better use of these new materials (or their component parts) and in return the biofuels industry will need to be cognisant of how their processes can be managed and amended to ensure that a co-product is produced with the right characteristics for new markets or increased usage.

The experience of the US and Canadian markets will be useful pointers as to how the commercial and technical requirements of producer and consumer can be better matched.

Biodiesel

With biodiesel, significant increases in feed raw materials will only occur if and when oilseed rape is crushed domestically to supply oil for biodiesel processing. As mentioned before, the scale of this activity may not match the scale of wheat processing, but a 50% increase in rapeseed meal availability may push down prices to significantly lower levels.

Again there are plant/processing modifications which can help ensure that the co-products produced have characteristics that enable the feed industry to maximise their use across a wider range of feeds, and in particular the industry will need to work hard to increase usage in monogastric feeds and in on farm feeding situations

An extra factor to consider in production of biodiesel is the large volume of glycerine that results from the esterification process. This product is described by the European Biodiesel Board as the "queen of co-products" and many believe that it will/can play a valuable role in animal nutrition.

Once human food/industrial uses are exhausted for glycerine, this valuable high energy raw material, (once the methanol content has been reduced to acceptable levels), can be accessed for use in feeds, but it may need some inventive thinking from feed formulators and mill managers to make this happen.

Alternative usage of co-product feeds

It would be a mistake to assume, however, that the biofuels industry will be wholly dependent on the feed industry for its co-product options. Increasing energy costs (which have partially driven this industry's development) have also driven a re-evaluation of the range of alternative fuels that can be combusted to produce heat or electricity.

Currently in the UK many hundreds of thousands of tonnes of palm kernel extraction meal are being burnt by UK generators to partially replace coal. This activity may switch towards biofuels co-products, particularly if they are classified as co-products from industrial crops – thereby meeting a requirement of future co-firing legislation. The decision as to whether to co-fire is driven by the value of the "green electricity" produced and a strong market for this electricity may lead to co-firers being prepared to pay better prices than the feed industry for certain feed co-products.

Nearer to home, any biofuels producer will be concerned about the future energy costs for running their plant. In this context it is feasible that it will pay to combust the co-product (rather than to dry it) and use the resulting energy for their own heat and power requirements.

These may both be costly options to adopt in terms of capital spend, but given the scale of the projected biofuels investments they may be wise investments if co-products values fall away and if their green credentials/ credits can benefit from a further reduction in their reliance on carbon fuels.

What to do?

As with any fledgling market it is hard to read what will happen and in what order, but there are several issues and actions that you should now consider when planning for the future.

TIMING

Very little biofuel will be produced in the UK before mid/late 2008 – the exceptions are biobutanol from sugar by British Sugar at Wissington and some limited increase in oilseed rape seed crushing at existing plants. However, sentiment is already inflating forward grain markets. This may be the worst of both worlds, with inflating grain values and no compensating movements in co-product prices before 2009/10.

GRAIN MARKETS

Recent experience in established biofuels markets suggests that we should model future raw material solutions with UK grain prices at least 20-30% above last year's levels.

This is of particular consequence in monogastric diets where the alternatives are/will be limited – while for ruminant feeds, there are alternatives to replace all, or part of the, cereals, hence diets will move towards a heavier reliance on co-products, albeit they will need some low protein components to balance the overall ration.

Importantly for the monogastric sector, one of our competitive advantages (discounted cereals) against other European or World producers, may be lost, which may lead to more imported (frozen) pig and poultry meat eroding our own market.

CO-PRODUCTS

We should evaluate novel raw material solutions – such as, wholly replacing molasses with distillery syrups, using glycerine instead of fat, using moist feeds into outdoor sow diets etc.

We should evaluate novel raw material/feeding solutions which can utilise the full range of co-products and co-product forms that these industries could produce. These may be dry feeds, moist feeds and/or liquids, some of which may fit a feed manufacturers needs, but others will go directly to ruminant or pig farms.

We should also consider the impact on raw material supply of biofuels development in other countries. Do these create co-products for us to use, or as in the case of molasses do they result in restricted supplies or price levels that make the raw material uncompetitive?

We must recognise that combustion or co-firing is a real option for co-products and not fall into the trap of thinking that the feed industry will be the sole beneficiary of new co-product supplies.

THE LONGER TERM

The initial target of 5.75% biofuel inclusion is going to have a significant impact on all grain and feed markets throughout Europe – longer term, a move towards a 10-20% inclusion must result in a more fundamental appraisal of land use/productivity and may prompt us to reassess how we can re-structure our livestock industries to co-exist with these new industries.

In this context, innovation and new thinking will be essential if we are to implement strategies that ensure a profitable future for the feed industry and its customers!

11

BY-PRODUCTS FROM NON-FOOD AGRICULTURE: TECHNICALITIES OF NUTRITION AND QUALITY

MATTHEW L. GIBSON AND AND KIP KARGES
Dakota Gold Marketing, Dakota Gold Research Association, Sioux Falls, South Dakota, USA

Introduction

THE ETHANOL PROCESS

Although ethanol production has been in existence for thousands of years (The Bible), it has mainly focused on production of potable product. In fact, the processes for production of modern potables is quite similar to those implemented to produce fuel ethanol.

From an overall standpoint, the process of ethanol production is quite simple (Figure 1). A grain is ground into a meal, water is added to produce a "mash" which is then cooked to gelatinize the starch. From there, enzymes are added to cleave the starch into glucose which is then fermented into ethanol by yeast. The resulting mixture is then subjected to fractional distillation to separate the ethanol from the stillage.

Although the two industries use very similar processes, the overall goals are quite different. The potable whisky distillers are interested in achieving a certain organoleptic profile with the focus being taste of the end-product. Although the production of whisky is beyond the scope of this chapter, it is noteworthy to make some observations about its production – especially in light of the fact that the stillage from whisky production is further processed into feed. In addition, although the processes may be different than fuel ethanol production, this feed product shares exactly the same AAFCO nomenclature: DDG/S. In whisky production, any number of grains may be included in the "mash bill" – essentially, the recipe which is placed into the fermenter. Furthermore, the enzyme source for potable ethanol production is from malted barley. Finally, because the potables industry is mainly concerned with taste, any number of fermentation conditions may exist.

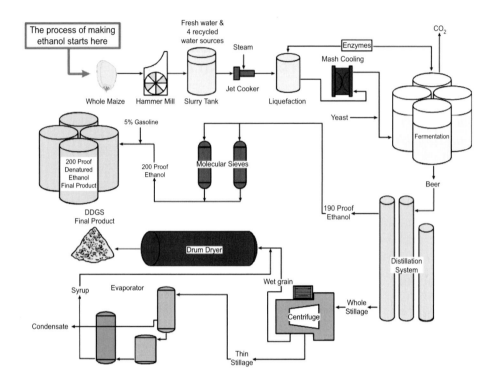

Figure 1. The ethanol production process

On the other hand, the fuel ethanol industry is focused on one objective: produce as much ethanol as possible and do it quickly and efficiently. To that end, purified fungal enzyme preparations are substituted for the barley malt and fermentation conditions are optimized to achieve very high levels of ethanol in the fermenter. Furthermore, the resulting mixture is subjected to very complete fractional distillation to achieve the azeotrope (190 proof). The azeotrope is then further processed to achieve pure ethanol (200 proof). The stillage is treated similarly to that from the potable industry – namely, centrifuged, condensed, and dried into DDG/S.

As for production volumes, one unit of maize will yield about 1/3 unit of ethanol, 1/3 unit of carbon dioxide and 1/3 unit of DDG/S.

One peculiarity of the AAFCO definitions is that the majority grain must be listed on the label. Thus, a DDG/S from a whisky distillery containing 510g maize/kg will be labelled exactly like one coming from a fuel ethanol plant using pure maize – even though we know the processes are somewhat different and the end-product may be quite different.

Some clarifications should be addressed: Although wine and beer are certainly potables produced from fermentation of glucose, for purposes of this discussion potable ethanol will indicate whisky. Additionally this chapter will focus on the "dry-grind" ethanol process which gives rise to DDG/S.

THE FUEL ETHANOL INDUSTRY

Industry resources

The uses of ethanol in the United States fuel industry have received generous press – both print and air-time – in recent weeks and months. Several resources are available with up-to-date literature on the subject. The reader is directed to the Renewable Fuels Association (RFA, www.EthanolRFA.org), the American Coalition for Ethanol (ACE, www.Ethanol.org), and the National Ethanol Vehicle Coalition (NEVC, www.E85Fuel.com). In addition, a concise review targeted to the animal nutrition industry has been published (Gibson and Karges, 2006).

Uses of ethanol

Basically, ethanol has three uses as a blending component for the fuel industry: renewable fuel, octane booster, and oxygenate molecule. Additionally, ethanol is now approved for all internal combustion uses in the USA – small engine, marine, automotive and aviation.

Although the reasons for the growth of the ethanol industry are myriad and beyond the scope of this chapter, the fact remains that it is nothing short of phenomenal. Although total production of ethanol in the USA barely reached one billion US gallons by 1995, since then it has almost quadrupled (Figure 2). Furthermore, this production is expected to double again within a few years.

Distillers grains production

Along with the dramatic growth in fuel ethanol production, DDG/S production has increased at an equally high rate (Figure 3). Obviously, a large influx of any new feed ingredient is cause for scientific investigation. However, due to the rapid evolution of the ethanol process, modern DDG/S product may be quite different from that produced by older ethanol production technology – whether it is from a potable ethanol distillery or a fuel ethanol plant.

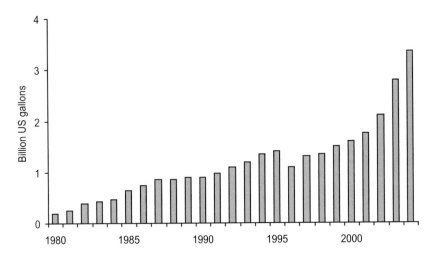

Figure 2. Growth of ethanol production

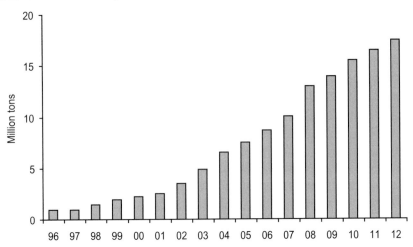

Figure 3. Growth of DDG/S production

This product is generally referred to with some colloquialism, but will usually contain the term "new" in order to differentiate it from the other products described. Therefore, we will adopt for our thesis: the DDG/S of today is not the DDG/S of even the recent past. We will investigate how it is different, how do we determine its nutritional value, and how do we determine its quality. Additinally, we will examine the extremely new products which are just recently being introduced into the marketplace.

Interest in quality of DDG/S is not new. Cromwell *et al.* (1993) noted a correlation between Hunter L* and b* scores for DDG/S and performance characteristics (weight gain and feed efficiency) in chicks. Furthermore, they noted that over-processing of DDG/S resulted in lowered lysine levels and increased acid detergent insoluble nitrogen – both of which resulted in lowered performance. They noted that the Maillard, non-enzymatic browning reaction – or lack of it – was responsible for all these effects.

This will not be an academic review of the scientific literature. First and foremost, the position of the authors is that of "industry participants." Observations on the use of the new DDG/S in the feed industry will abound. Secondly, due to the rapid evolution of the industry, very little peer-reviewed literature exists on most of the very new technology products. Appropriate references will be included; however, readers are urged to contact the authors for further discussion.

One last item: as mentioned, the USA ethanol industry is growing and evolving so fast that comments included herein should be construed in that context. That is, for future readers (probably, beyond the year 2007), these data are likely to be considered out of date.

New ethanol process – focus on feed

The new DDG/S is quite different from the old. Several nutrients are quite different than those listed in older, peer-reviewed publications and reference literature. There are probably several reasons for these phenomena. The next section will explore these reasons and observations. The effects on animal production will be reviewed later.

Most discussions of new DDG/S revolve around improvements in drying technology with the implications that over-drying results in excessive Maillard reaction products. This browning does destroy any amino acids with free amino groups. This includes the terminal amino acid residue on proteins and peptides, but most focus surrounds the epsilon amino group of in-line lysine residues. Furthermore, as lysine is the first-limiting amino acid in maize-based diets (the most common in the USA), this is of great concern for livestock production. Certainly, this over-drying is a real phenomenon and has become common knowledge.

In fact, some modern ethanol plants have begun focusing on this problem. New, modern dehydration and drying technology has become widely available to the industry. Where implemented, it may be able to reduce the rate and extent of Maillard reactions.

However, it must be noted that over-drying is but one facet of the problem. The Maillard reaction requires the presence of free reducing sugars. In the case of the ethanol process, this is in the form of glucose. Modern fuel ethanol production focuses entirely on the most complete conversion of starch to glucose to ethanol. Any glucose remaining in the fermenter is less profit for the plant. Thus, one characteristic of the new DDG/S is much less formation of Maillard reaction products – especially with reduced lysine destruction.

The real observation of this exercise is this: over-drying is not the only problem. Changes to the ethanol production process have profound effects on the resulting DDG/S.

Other nutrient differences noted between old and new DDG/S are probably related to this potential reduction in Maillard reaction products. Acid detergent insoluble nitrogen (ADIN), an indicator of unavailable protein, is the most obvious phenomenon resulting from Maillard reactions. It tends to be lower in new DDG/S. The ME value of new DDG/S is higher than old; most probably due to reduced formation of ADIN and other Maillard reaction products.

One concern when high levels of DDG/S are included in many livestock diets is in the area of mineral nutrition. In order to achieve higher levels of ethanol, greater control must be maintained over fermentation. One area which requires attention is pH of the fermenter. In order to provide pH control, both acids and bases may be added. Usually, the acids of choice are sulphuric and, possibly, phosphoric. The bases of choice are sodium hydroxide and potassium hydroxide. The resulting minerals which may be elevated in the DDG/S are sulphur, phosphorus, sodium and / or potassium.

One non-nutritive area which should receive some mention is mycotoxins. As long as maize is being processed for food use, there is little concern with mycotoxins. The processors must either screen for mycotoxins, or must remove it during the process. However, mycotoxins are not a factor in the production of fuel ethanol. Furthermore, as mycotoxins are quite robust molecules, they survive the processing, fermentation, and distillation steps. They will survive, intact, and be present in the DDG/S. Furthermore, as the maize non-fermentables are concentrated approximately three-fold in the DDG/S, the mycotoxins are similarly concentrated. Care should be taken to select suppliers who screen for mycotoxins.

NUTRIENT VARIABILITY

Given equivalent pricing, nutritionists always prefer high-quality ingredients over low-quality ingredients. However, consistency of quality is generally more important than level of quality. For most ingredients, variability tends to be quite low. In the USA, # 2 Yellow Maize tends to be fairly consistent within crop year and within region. Obviously, there may be differences between regions and there are certainly differences between crop years.

Dried distillers grains with solubles is notorious for being highly variable. As has been noted, the whisky industry uses a variety of grains in the recipe along with fermentation conditions somewhat different to those used in the fuel ethanol business. Even within the fuel ethanol business, there are still "old" plants operating. Both scenarios lend variability to the end-product.

However, even if we strictly limit the discussion to "new", fuel plants, we still see tremendous variability in DDG/S. Overall, the adoption of new technologies in fuel ethanol production has allowed for improved quality of DDG/S. However, just as with any other sector of agriculture, in order to exploit these improvements fully, there must be an integrated approach to production with an effective feedback mechanism. As most fuel ethanol producers have little affiliation with the feed industry, neither one of these events is the norm. That is, even though technology is available for producing high quality and consistent products, regular implementation is limited to a few integrated production and marketing companies.

Robinson (2004) examined several samples of DDG/S from multiple sources – all fuel ethanol plants located in the Midwest region of the USA. The product was collected randomly from either: (1) various suppliers, or (2) from a single supplier (Table 1). The product from the single supplier was of higher quality overall and, more importantly, was more consistent. Consumers are cautioned to choose their suppliers carefully.

Table 1. DDG/S Source-to-source Variability (g/kg). After Robinson (2004)

	Source	
Component	*Industry-wide*	*Dakota Gold*
Crude Protein	301 ± 26	307 ± 12
Fat	115 ± 35	119 ± 7
ADIN	289 ± 117	82 ± 23
(acid detergent insoluble nitrogen)		
Phosphorus	8.8 ± 1.4	7.0 ± 1.0

[1] Mean ± SD

NEW DDG/S FOR PIG PRODUCTION

In order to exploit the new DDG/S product to the fullest, we must define it. Furthermore, in order to define the product, we must be able to evaluate its quality. The most expensive components in North American pig diets are energy, amino acids, and phosphorus.

Metabolizable energy

The ME values for new DDG/S are quite different from those that have been observed in the past. In two trials, Spiehs *et al.* (1999) observed an ME value which averaged 3,828 kcal/kg (16.02MJ/kg) on a dry matter basis (DMB). This is significantly different than the value of 3,032kcal/kg (12.69MJ/kg) listed in the Swine NRC (1998). In a separate trial, Allee *et al.* (2005) found the ME value of new DDG/S to be 3,940 kcal/kg (16.48MJ/ kg). This result is especially compelling as they found the energy of their maize control to be 3,864 kcal/kg (16.17MJ/kg) which very closely approximates that listed in the NRC of 3,842kcal/kg (16.07MJ/kg).

As for evaluating new DDG/S for ME values, the best method is still the use of metabolism crates with full fecal and urine collections. This procedure is both costly and time-consuming. However, there is no real substitute procedure available.

Amino acid nutrition

Probably no other area of DDG/S nutrition has received more attention than amino acids. With the new processes, we have seen it is possible to conserve more lysine. The Swine NRC lists values for lysine ranging from 5.4 to 6.3g/kg for DDG/S protein levels of 240 to 280g/kg, respectively. However, the table value is listed as 6.2g/kg – at the high end of the range. After the discussion on Maillard reaction browning, it is possible that this level was optimistic, at best, for the old product, but probably accurately describes the new product.

Whitney *et al.* (1999) found lysine levels ranging from 6.8 to 8.3. Stein *et al.* (2004) found lysine levels ranging from 6.8 to 8.5g/kg. The DGRA has done extensive testing over multiple crop years and has found the lysine level in Dakota Gold® brand of DDG/S to average 9.5g/kg on an as fed basis (AFB).

The best method for evaluating protein quality for pigs is to perform ileal digestibility determination and calculate a digestibility coefficient. Several publications list the digestibility coefficients. The Swine NRC (1998) lists a single value of 0.47. However, any single value does not account for quality variation. Whitney *et al.* (2000) compared the "new" product to the "old" product and found digestibility coefficients of 0.53 and 0.00, respectively which is a broad range indeed. Stein *et al.* (2004) found a low of 0.44 and a high of 0.63 in 10 samples of varying quality – but all from "new" ethanol plants.

One problem with performing ileal digestibility trials in pigs is the intensive nature of the process. These experiments are very time-consuming which results in a long lag-time to obtain results, not to mention the very high cost.

An alternative is to use cecectomized cockerels. The benefits of this assay are: (1) a much shorter time-frame to obtain data, and (2) a much lower cost. Using such a cockerel assay, Ergul *et al.* (2003) found digestible lysine content to range from 3.8 to 6.5g/kg in product from "new" ethanol plants. In a similar experiment, Batal and Dale (2006) found the digestible lysine content to range from 1.8g/kg to 6.6g/kg.

An even quicker (and less expensive) method for determining amino acid quality has been presented by Schasteen *et al.* (2005). The IDEA™ assay uses a series of *in vitro* enzyme treatments to estimate lysine digestibility in particular. The assay can be performed on a bench-top, under non-sterile conditions, and requires only hours to complete. Using such an assay optimized for DDG/S, these researchers found a good correlation ($R^2 = 0.88$) between the IDEA™ assay and true lysine digestibility in cecectomized cockerels. Furthermore, these researchers found a good correlation ($R^2 = 0.81$) when comparing the IDEA™ estimate for lysine digestibility between pigs and poultry for soyabean meal.

Much has been made about colour of DDG/S. The Maillard reaction has been discussed previously. Evaluating colour is a natural progression for determining quality of DDG/S – especially with respect to amino acid digestibility. In the experiments of Ergul *et al.* (2003) and Batal and Dale (2006), both groups found that the products with low Hunter L* and b* scores had the lower lysine digestibilities and the products with the high Hunter L* and b* scores had the higher lysine digestibilities (Table 2). Objective determination of colour is even easier, faster, and less costly than the cockerel assay or the IDEA™ assay.

Table 2. Hunter colour score and digestible lysine

Color	Hunter L*	Hunter b*	Digestible LYS, g/kg
Dark / Brown[1]	41.8	32.9	3.8
Light / Yellow[1]	53.8	42.8	6.5
Dark / Brown[2]	50.4	7.41	1.8
Light / Yellow[2]	60.3	25.9	6.6

[1] After Ergul, *et al.* (2003)
[2] After Batal & Dale (2006)

It should be noted that there is not good agreement of the scores between trials. The scores are not absolute. However, one thing is clear – within a specific set of observations, lighter colour (Hunter L*) and more yellow colour (Hunter b*) definitely indicate higher amino acid digestibility.

Although not objective, colour of DDG/S can be estimated by merely looking at it. A good understanding of the Hunter colour scoring system is required to understand the nuances of colour determination. One may easily mistake a light product (high Hunter L* score) which has a high amount of redness (high Hunter a* score) for a darker product (low Hunter L* score). However, with a bit of practice, this is easily achievable.

Phosphorus

Phosphorus (P) digestibility for DDG/S has been estimated to range from 0.15 to 0.90 (personal observation) with the Swine NRC estimating a value of 0.77. Allee and Fent (2005) estimated P digestibility to be 0.85 using a Slope Ratio bioavailability assay with mono-sodium phosphate as the control comparison. The variables measured were piglet fibula ash and breaking strength.

Fat

Fat levels vary along with other components as discussed previously. However, many nutritionists consider the fat in DDG/S to be identical to maize oil. Analysis indicates this is not so. The fat in DDG/S has lower linoleic acid and higher omega-3, the iodine value is lower and the FFA content is higher. (Table 3).

Table 3. Fatty acid profile of maize and DDG/S (g/kg)

Item	Maize[1]	DDG/S[2]
C16:0	110	130
C18:1	240	290
C18:2	590	510
$\Omega3$	7	20
$\Omega6$	580	520
Unsat:Sat	6.5	4.6
Iodine Value	125	110
Free Fatty Acids	0 ?	100

[1] After NRC
[2] DGRA

ANIMAL PERFORMANCE

When a new ingredient is introduced to the feed market, animal nutritionists are most interested in the nutrient profile and the digestibilities of those nutrients. Following that information, the conduct of actual animal performance trials is essential.

Sow lactation

Hill *et al.* (2003) compared a control diet (with 50g beet pulp/kg) to a diet containing 150g DDG/S/kg. There was no difference (P > 0.05) in sow weight change (-6.2 kg vs -8.0 kg), day 18 litter weight (62.9 kg vs 62.3 kg), litter gain during lactation (41.7 kg vs 43.4 kg), or number of pigs weaned (10.9 vs 10.8) for control diet vs DDG/S diet, respectively.

Grow / finish

Cook *et al.* (2005) fed graded levels (0, 100, 200, and 300g/kg) of DDG/S to approximately 1,000 pigs housed with 26 head per pen and an initial weight of 42 kg with an average weight of 117 kg when finished.

Nutrient values used for formulating rations were provided by the supplier. Most importantly, an adequate number of samples were analyzed to provide accurate means and variance about those means for all necessary nutrients. Further, statistics were applied to determine formulation matrix values. Values used for ME, and digestibility of LYS and P were 3,416 kcal/kg (14.29MJ/kg), 0.70, and 0.85, respectively.

They found no overall difference in average daily gain (ADG), average daily feed intake (ADFI), or feed efficiency (FE). Mortality decreased linearly. Carcass yield decreased linearly, while lean yield and backfat were not different (Figures 4 and 5). Cook *et al.* (2005) concluded that when proper nutrient values are used, DDG/S can be used effectively at moderate levels for growing / finishing swine with few negative effects.

Gourley and Lampe (2005) fed graded levels of DDG/S to approximately 1,000 pigs housed with 26 head per pen and had an initial weight of 15 kg with an average weight of 131.5 kg when finished. This trial differed from the study of Cook *et al.* (2005) in that the DDG/S was from an even "newer" ethanol plant which incorporated the BPX™ process (described subsequently). As in the study of Cook *et al.* (2005), adequate sample nutrient analysis (with resultant statistical analysis) was provided to determine formulation matrix values. Similar digestibilities were applied for ME, LYS and P.

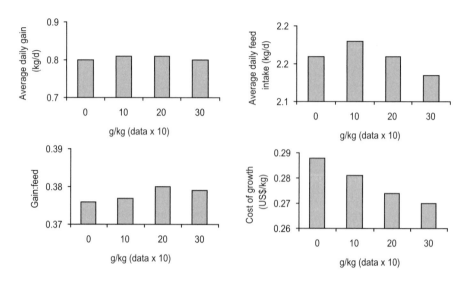

Figure 4.   Effect of feeding graded levels of DDG/S on pig performance. After Cook, *et al.* (2005)

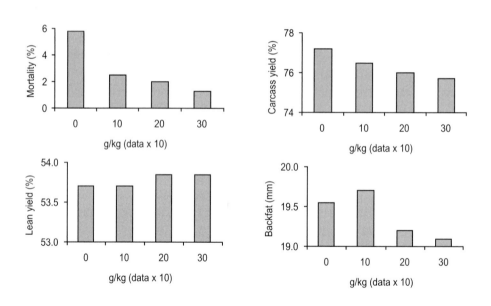

Figure 5.   Effect of feeding graded levels of DDG/S on pig performance. After Cook, *et al.* (2005)

The study of Gourley and Lampe (2005) used a different scheme for determining the DDG/S inclusion rates. In the study, a typical maize-soya diet was formulated and a calculated NDF level was determined. Then DDG/

S was included at increasing levels to raise the NDF by 150g increments. The resulting diets contained 73, 146, 219, and 293g DDG/S/kg. Due to a collection error, no data were reported for the second diet.

As in the study of Cook *et al.* (2005), Gourley and Lampe (2005) found no difference for ADG, ADFI, or pig weight sold (Figures 6 and 7). There was an improvement in FE for the higher DDG/S inclusion rates. There was no difference in carcass weight. As in the study of Cook *et al.* (2005), there was a decrease in carcass yield with increasing DDG/S, but no difference in lean yield. Interestingly, although there was no difference in lean yield, there was a non-statistical increase in both studies.

Gourley and Lampe (2005) also took fat samples from the carcasses and analyzed for Iodine Value (IV). There was a significant increase in IV at the highest DDG/S inclusion rate.

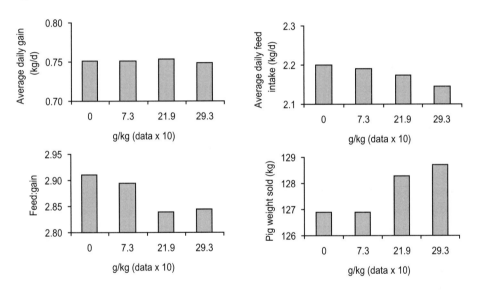

Figure 6. Effect of feeding graded levels of DDG/S on pig performance. After Gourley and Lampe (2005).

New technologies

As noted, the production of ethanol in dry-grind facilities is undergoing rapid technological evolution. In addition, as should be clearly evident at this point, any alteration of the ethanol process will result in changes to the resultant DDG/S. Some new technologies which have recently appeared in the

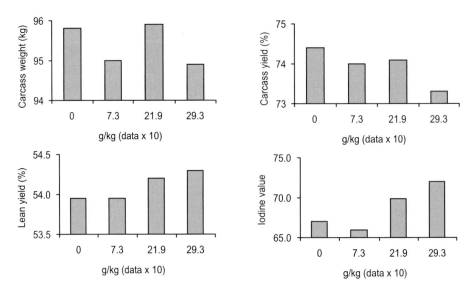

Figure 7. Effect of feeding graded levels of DDG/S on pig performance. After Gourley and Lampe (2005).

marketplace are of particular note – especially, due to their profound changes on the resulting DDG/S.

BPX™

A new technology which completely revolutionizes ethanol production has recently been introduced. The technology is named BPX™. The process is patented by the Broin Companies (B&A, 2005). Essentially, the process allows production of ethanol without "cooking" the mash to gelatinize the starch. The changes in the resultant DDG/S – although not completely understood – are profound. The BPX™ product exhibits greatly improved physical characteristics such as higher density and easier pelleting (DGRA, 2006). Most importantly, the product exhibits enhanced flowability.

BIO-REFINING

Until recently, all the product going into a dry-grind ethanol production facility has essentially become DDG/S through the process. Currently, three fully-commercialized dry-grind facilities have implemented true dry-milling operations in front of the ethanol facility. The whole maize is milled into several fractions which can then be directed into several different production streams (Figure 8).

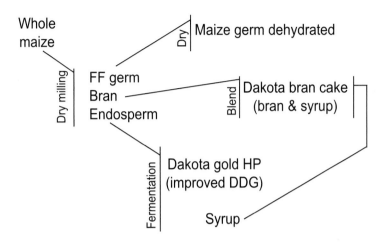

Figure 8. Process flow for dry milling biorefining process

The "endosperm" stream – actually, a "maize-starch-enriched" stream – is what ends up in the fermenter. That is, some of the bran and some of the germ – the non-fermentables – are removed from the whole kernel before fermentation. The advantages to ethanol production are fairly obvious. What is less obvious are the changes to the resultant co-product.

The co-product – marketed under the trade name Dakota Gold HP™ – is actually a true DDG. Compared with "normal" DDG/S, it has very high levels of protein (and amino acids, obviously) along with lower levels of fat and phosphorus (Table 4). The reader is cautioned that nutrient specifications for any Dakota Gold® products are not representative of the ethanol industry as a whole.

Allee *et al.* (2005) found the ME value of this product to be 4,049 kcal/kg (DMB); (16.94MJ/kg). This ME may seem high in light of the much lower fat level (compared to conventional DDG/S); it is probably due to the removal of the bran fraction which dilutes the ME in "normal" DDG/S.

As the maize is milled prior to fermentation, the "germ enriched" fraction also becomes available as a feedstuff for animal production. The product is marketed as Maize Germ Dehydrated (AAFCO, 2006). As expected this product is high in fat and phosphorus (Table 4). As the germ fraction contains the most desirable proteins in the maize kernel, the amino acid profile is quite desirable in spite of a fairly low crude protein level. As the product has not been "steeped" (as in a wet-mill), these protein fractions contain all the soluble fractions. Additionally, as this maize has not been through fermentation, the oil is in its "native" state.

Table 4. Selected components (g/kg, except metabolisable energy)[1]

Item	Dakota Gold® DDG/S	Dakota Gold HP™ DDG	Maize germ dehydrated
Crude protein	296	430	175
Crude fat	108	43	202
Met. energy, kcal/kg	1790	1842	2060
(MJ/kg)	(7.49)	(7.71)	(8.62)
Ash	46	21	62
Phosphorus	9.2	5	16.6
Lysine	10.2	14.3	8.4
Methionine	6.2	12.1	3.1
Cystine	9.3	16.0	5.4
Threonine	10.7	16.4	6
Tryptophan	3.1	5	2.4

[1] All expressed on a dry matter basis

Effects on maize supply and comparison with other feedstuffs

With the explosive growth in production of DDG/S, there will surely be effects on other feedstuffs. Maize – the major feedstock for ethanol production – is likely to be affected more than other livestock feed ingredients. Ludtke (2005) noted that during the crop year of 2004 – 2005, 36 million metric tonnes (MMT) of maize were used for production of ethanol (Table 5). This number is expected to increase significantly through 2007. However, the amount of maize available for export or used for feed will remain relatively constant. One point of interest: in the crop year 2006 – 2007, Ludtke (2005) estimated that the use of maize for ethanol will exceed that available for export – a landmark event, indeed.

Table 5. Uses of maize[1] by year

	Crop year			
Use	'04 – '05	'05 – '06	'06 – '07	'07 – '08
Feed	147	155	145	145
Export	51	43	48	48
Ethanol	36	41	53	66

[1] Million metric tonnes

Although these data may be perceived to paint a bleak picture with respect to maize availability for feed purposes, the reader is reminded that approximately 1/3 of the maize used for ethanol is returned to the feed industry in the form of DDG/S.

Another useful comparison of feedstuff usage is in the availability of different protein sources. Table 6 indicates the feed usage of the top four protein ingredients for livestock production in the USA (DGM, 2006). During the current crop year (2005 – 2006), the DDG/S will surpass both cotton seed products and canola meal in total tonnage – another landmark event.

Table 6. Protein availability – USA

	Crop year	
Ingredient	*'04 – '05*	*'05 – '06*
DDG/S	6.86	9.20
Cottonseed products	7.62	7.38
Canola meal	7.00	7.66
Soyabean meal	35.62	36.60

[1] Million metric tonnes

Summary and implications

There will be an ever-increasing supply DDG/S from the fuel ethanol industry. Most of this will be produced by ethanol plants employing newer technology than that available in the past. This new technology yields a DDG/S which may be quite suitable for feeding non-ruminant livestock. Furthermore, the growth of even newer maize milling technologies will yield a batch of even newer products. Due to the explosive growth of this industry, most of these new products are not well defined in traditionally published sources of information – namely, peer-reviewed publications, government sponsored trials on nutrient requirements, and other similar publications. Therefore, it is incumbent on both the newly-emerging ethanol industry (the supplier of these products) and on the traditional livestock producer (the consumer of these products) to work together in order to define these products. Only through a full understanding of these products may we fully exploit them for maximizing production of livestock.

References

AAFCO. 2006. Official Publication. Association of American Feed Control Officials. West Lafayette, Indiana, USA.

Allee, G.L., R.W. Fent, and S.X. Fu. 2005 Determination of the Metabolizable energy concentration of different maize byproducts of ethanol production. Univ. of Missouri – Columbia. Dakota Gold Research Assoc. Rept # 0503.

Allee, G.L. and R.W. Fent. 2005. Evaluation of the bioavailability of phosphorus in distiller's dried grains with solubles (DDGS) when fed to pigs. Univ. of Missouri – Columbia. Report to Dakota Gold Research Assoc. Rept # 0503.

B&A. 2005. Broin and Associates. Sioux Falls, South Dakota. Internal Report – Unpublished.

Batal, A.B. and N.M. Dale. 2006. True Metabolizable energy and amino acid digestibility of distillers dried grains with solubles. J App Poultry Res 15:89.

Bible. Prehistoric. Story of Noah. Genesis, chapters 5 – 9.

Cook, D.R., N.D. Paton, and M.L. Gibson. 2005. Effect of dietary level of distillers dried grains with solubles (DDGS) on growth performance, mortality, and carcass characteristics of grow-finish barrows and gilts. Midwest Amer. Soc. Anim. Sci. meeting, Des Moines, Iowa.

Cromwell, G.L., K.L. Herkelman, and T.S. Stahly. 1993. Physical, chemical, and nutritional characteristics of distillers dried grains with solubles for chicks and pigs. J. Anim. Sci. 71:679.

DGRA. 2003, 2004, 2005. Dakota Gold Research Association. Sioux Falls, South Dakota. Internal Reports – Unpublished.

DGM. 2006. Dakota Gold Marketing. Sioux Falls, South Dakota. Internal Reports – Unpublished.

Ergul, T., C. Martinez Amezcua, C. Parsons, B. Walters, J. Brannon, and S.L. Noll. 2003. Amino acid digestibility in maize distillers dried grains with solubles. Poult. Sci. Assoc. meeting, Madison, Wisconsin.

Gibson, M.L. and K. Karges. 2005. Overview of the Ethanol Industry and Production of DDG/S: A Nutritionist's Perspective. Mulit-State Poultry Feeding and Nutrition Conference. May 23 – 25, Indianapolis, Indiana.

Gourley, G., and J. Lampe. 2005. Effect of distillers dried grains and solubles formulated for % NDF on the growth and carcass performance of pigs. Swine Grafix Enterprises, Webster City, Iowa. Dakota Gold Research Assoc. Rept # 0507

Hill, G.M., J.E. Link, M.J. Rincker, K.D. Roberson, D.L. Kirkpatrick, and M.L. Gibson. 2005. Maize dried distillers grains with solubles in sow lactation diets. Midwest Amer. Soc. Anim. Sci. meeting, Des Moines, Iowa.

Ludtke, M. 2005. Demand for maize for various uses – years 1996 through 2012. Internal report to Dakota Gold Marketing. Unpublished. Commodity Marketing Company, Albert Lea, Minnesota.

NRC – Swine. 1998. Nutrient Requirements of Swine. Tenth Revised Edition. National Academy of Sciences.

Robinson, P.H. 2004. Nutritive Value of Distillers Grains. Dept. of Anim. Sci. Univ. of California – Davis. Dakota Gold Research Assoc. Rept # 0301

Schasteen, C.S., Wu, J., Yi, G., Knight, C., Parsons, C., Li, J., and D. Li. 2005. True digestibility of amino acids in raw and heat-treated soy products: comparison of values obtained with cannulated pigs, cecectomized roosters and an *in vitro* IDEA™ Assay. Midwest Amer. Soc. Anim. Sci. meeting, Des Moines, Iowa.

Spiehs, M.J., G.C. Shurson, and M.H. Whitney. 1999. Energy, nitrogen, and phosphorus digestibility of growing and finishing swine diets containing distiller's dried grains with solubles. J. Anim. Sci. 77:188 (Suppl. 1).

Stein, H.H., C. Pedersen, and M. Boersma. 2004. Amino acid and energy digestibility in ten samples of dried distillers grain with solubles by growing pigs. Report to Dakota Gold Research Assoc.

Whitney, M.H., M.J. Spiehs, G.C. Shurson, and S.K. Baidoo. 1999. Apparent ileal amino acid digestibility of maize distiller's dried grains with solubles produced from new ethanol plants in Minnesota and South Dakota. J. Anim. Sci. 77:188 (Suppl. 1)

12

EFFECTS OF MANIPULATING MUSCLE GLYCOGEN ON MEAT QUALITY IN PIGS

NIELS OKSBJERG

Danish Institute of Agricultural Sciences, Dept. of Food Science, Research Centre Foulum, DK-8830 Tjele, Denmark

Introduction

Colour and drip loss of pork are important quality traits. In the past PSE (Pale, Soft and Exudative) meat was a major problem in the meat industry. This was caused by the presence of the halothane gene due to a mutation in the ryanodine receptor. However, under Danish conditions this mutation has been eliminated. Despite of this the variation in drip loss is still considerable.

PSE is induced by a fast pH decrease together with high temperature within the first 2 hours after slaughter, but paleness and drip loss are also related to low ultimate pH (pH measured 24 hours post mortem) (Bendall and Svatland, 1988). During the conversion of muscle to meat post mortem, energy is completely released from anaerobic processes. Initially, post mortem energy is released from energy-rich compounds like ATP and CP (creatine phosphate). Subsequently, when ATP and CP are more or less depleted, energy is yielded from glycogen, which is converted to lactate and ^+H. This conversion leads to a decrease in pH. Thus, the level of muscle glycogen at slaughter is one of the factors which influence the ultimate pH and consequently colour and drip loss (Warris *et al.*, 1989). Consequently, manipulation of muscle glycogen may be used to cause changes in ultimate pH.

In the present paper a short summary of results, obtained from Danish experiments over the past 10 years, describing factors causing variation in muscle glycogen and the consequences for meat colour and drip loss (technological quality) will be given.

What is glycogen?

Glycogen is a common storage form of cabohydrates in animals. Glycogen is built up of glucose units exclusively, and the basic unit is formed by $\alpha(1\rightarrow4)$ glycosydic linkages. More than half a century ago, it was recognised that muscle glycogen from rats could be separated into "free" and "bound" moieties, depending on the degree of "binding" with proteins. Later it was recognised that these glycogen pools could be characterised on the basis of their solubility in acid (Bloom *et al.*, 1951).

The two glycogen forms are known as macroglycogen ($\sim10^4$ kDa), which is acid-soluble and has a high carbohydrate:protein ratio (99:1), and proglycogen (~400 kDa), which is acid-insoluble and has a low carbohydrate:protein ratio (10:1) (Lomako *et al.*, 1993). Proglycogen is considered a stable intermediate in glycolysis and glycogenesis of macroglycogen (Gregory, 1996). The macroglycogen fraction in humans and rats is found to increase with high muscle glycogen concentrations (Hansen *et al.*, 2000). However, the availability of the two glycogen pools for energy production during muscle contraction is dependent on the type of work. Thus, macroglycogen is mainly metabolised during aerobic exercise (Asp *et al.*, 1999), while proglycogen is predominantly metabolised during anaerobic conditions (Graham *et al.*, 2001). Until now most studies with pigs on glycogen have measured the total amount of glycogen; however I shall here present some results where glycogen has been separated in pro- and macroglycogen. In our laboratory, glycogen concentration is determined in 10-50 mg muscle samples, heated in a sealed test tube with 1-5 ml of 1 M HCL at 100°C for 2 hours. Glycogen is then analysed as glucose residues on a spectrophotometer (Passonneau, and Lowry 1973). When determining pro- and macroglycogen these are separated by TCA precipitation prior to analyses for glucose. The resting level of glycogen in Danish purebred is given in Table 1.

Relationship between muscle glycogen concentration and ultimate pH

To cause a large variation in the concentration of glycogen in *longissimus dorsi*, Henckel *et al.* (2001) treated pigs with either adrenaline (depletes glycogen) prior to slaughter or exercised pigs on a treadmill just before slaughter. Also untreated pigs were included. From these experiments the relationship between the concentration of glycogen and the ultimate pH (measured 24 hours post mortem) was calculated. They found a biphasic relationship, and below a concentration of 53 µmoles/g muscle (break point") there was a highly significant inverse linear relation (r=-0.88, P<0.001) between glycogen and ultimate pH, while beyond this glycogen level no relationship was found. Accordingly, Henckel *et al.* (1997) found a phenotypic correlation (r=0.34, P<0.001) between muscle glycogen measured at 65 kg BW (body weight) and ultimate pH measured at 100 kg slaughter weight.

Sources of variation in glycogen

STRESS AND STUNNING

In our studies on the effect of stress on muscle glycogen and pH, we used treadmill exercise prior to slaughter as a model, and to simulate muscle fatigue following long-term stress we used adrenaline injection. Thus, Henckel *et al.* (2000, 2002) studied the effect of treating slaughter pigs with 0.2 or 0.3 mg adrenaline/kg BW 15 hours prior to slaughter and exercise on a treadmill (3.8 km/h for 10 minutes) just prior to slaughter on muscle glycogen and pH. The results showed that treating animals with adrenaline decreased the muscle glycogen to 30 µmoles/g muscle compared with 70 µmoles/g muscle in controls. The ultimate pH increased to approximately 6.2 compared with pH=5.66 for control pigs. Similar results on ultimate pH were found for other muscles (*biceps femoris, semimembranosus, psoas major*). In contrast, exercise increased the rate of pH decrease during the first 3 hours post mortem resulting in a pH difference of 0.2 at 3 hours post mortem.

In another experiment Henckel (unpublished) studied the effect of stunning procedure (electrical stunning vs. stunning with CO_2) and adrenaline treatment on muscle glycogen, pH development post mortem and drip loss. Compared with CO_2 stunning, electrical stunning significantly decreased initial pH values from slaughter to 3 hours post mortem both when the pigs were treated with adrenaline or they were exercised before slaughter, and this was reflected in a higher drip loss following electrical stunning. These data clearly show that the early pH decrease post mortem plays a significant role for drip loss.

GENETIC VARIANCE WITH BREEDS

If muscle glycogen is inherited selection may be used to lower glycogen concentration in order to increased ultimate pH. Consequently we studied genetic variance in muscle glycogen in purebreds of Danish Landrace, Large White and Duroc pigs (Oksbjerg *et al.*, 2004). We sampled *M. longissimus dorsi* (300 mg) from 1643 pigs at about 85 kg BW with a biopsy device and analysed them for glycogen. We used samples from living animals, because the efficiency of selection is higher, when values are obtained on living animals instead of slaughtered relatives, and because glycogen is metabolised during transportation. The heritability (h^2) of glycogen was found to be 0.37±0.02. Several genetic correlations between glycogen and production traits and meat quality traits were found. Glycogen was positively correlated to meat percentage (r_g=0.35±0.04) and negatively correlated to the feed conversion ratio (kg feed:kg gain) (r_g=-0.25±0.06), but unrelated to daily gain. The concentration of muscle glycogen was positively correlated to L* (lightness of meat) (r_g=0.32±0.05) and a* (redness, r_g=0.12±0.03) of the loin, but inversely correlated to pH of the *longissimus dorsi* (r_g=-0.41±0.04) and of the ham (r_g=-0.27±0.04). In another study (Oksbjerg *et al.*, 2000) we examined the effect of selection by comparing the performance, muscle metabolic traits and meat quality in a genotype of Danish Landrace pigs representing the growth potential in 1976 with a genotype of Danish Landrace representing the growth potential in 1995. The pigs representing 1995 grew faster (958 vs. 670g/day) on less feed per kg gain (3.64 vs. 2.75), while the meat percentage was only slightly increased (59.9 vs. 58.1%). Although not significant, muscle glycogen was increased in Danish Landrace pigs proportionately by 1.09 compared with Danish Landrace pigs (71 vs. 65 µmoles/g wet weight). These studies suggest that it is possible to select for decreased muscle glycogen due to the heritability of glycogen and consequently improve meat pH. However, such a selection may delay the genetic improvement of some performance traits.

Effect of genotypes on muscle glycogen

We compared the glycogen concentration of *longissimus dorsi* of purebred pigs and found no differences between Danish Landrace, Danish Large White and Danish Duroc (Tabel 1, unpublished). Among these breeds the glycogen concentration was similar. However, in the Hampshire pigs the concentration of glycogen was proportionately 1.61 higher than in the other breeds. Due to the high glycogen level, Hampshire crosses produce meat with low pH and high drip loss and cooking loss. The high glycogen level is due to a dominant gene, the RN⁻ gene, named after its effect on the Napole Yield (French: Rendement Technologique Napole) (Naveau *et al.*, 1985). Initially it was reported that the low ultimate pH was developed late post mortem. However, recent studies show that the low ultimate pH develops initially between 45 minutes and 5 hours (Ylä-Ajos *et al.*, 2007).

Table 1. Muscle glycogen and colour in Danish purebred

	Duroc	*Hampshire*	*Landrace*	*Large White*	*P*
Glycogen µmoles/g wet weight	88	142	89.0	88	***
pH$_{loin}$	5.60	5.47	5.52	5.58	***
pH$_{ham}$	5.71	5.52	5.66	5.67	***
Pigment, myoglobin residues/g	1.54	1.69	1.29	1.24	***
a*	6.24	6.41	5.86	4.87	***
B*	5.94	4.84	5.84	4.71	***
L*	53.02	49.78	54.07	51.38	***
Colour	3.25	4.26	2.91	3.12	***
Gain, g/day	903	854	909	926	***

Milan *et al.* (2001) identified the gene on chromosome 15, and it was discovered that the dominant RN⁻ mutation is a substitution in the *PRKAG3* gene (Wild type=200R=rn⁺ and 200Q=RN⁻). This gene encodes for adenosine monophosphate protein kinase regulating the energy status in muscles. Later it was discovered that in *RN⁻* pigs the gene expression and the activity of UDP-glucose pyro-phosphorylase were increased (Hedegaard *et al.*, 2004).

We have studied (unpublished) the effect of the RN⁻ gene in crossbreeds of Danish Landrace x Danish Large White sows mated to Danish Hampshire males being heterozygotes for the *RN⁻* gene. Table 2 shows that the meat content in the ham is higher and the fat content lower in *RN⁻* compared with rn⁺/rn⁺ . Furthermore, it seems that the difference in meat content of the ham is exclusively due to increased fast-twitch muscles (*biceps femoris, semitendinosus, semimembranosus, gluteus*), while slow-twitch muscles (*vastus intermedius, vastus lateralis, vastus medialis*) are not different. In this study we found only small differences in meat quality traits. The temperature profile of the muscle/meat post mortem was similar between genotypes, and the pH values during the first 2 hours and 24 hours post mortem were slightly lower in RN⁻ pigs. The glycogen concentration was 2-fold higher in the RN⁻ genotype, but the decrease post mortem did not differ between genotypes. Neither did the lactate accumulation post mortem differ. On the other hand, the concentration of glucose-6-phosphate increased more and was significantly higher in RN- pigs compared with rn⁺/rn⁺ pigs 24 hours post mortem. Due to the change in pH development post mortem, the drip loss was higher and Napole yield lower in RN⁻ pigs, respectively, while the colour was unchanged.

Table 2. The composition of tissues and the weight of selected muscles in the ham of *RN⁻* and *rn⁺/rn⁺* pigs (Experiment 1).

	RN⁻	*rn⁺/rn⁺*	*SEM*	*P=*
Meat, kg	7.22	6.99	0.12	0.0546
Subcutaneous fat, kg	1.73	1.82	0.05	0.0621
Inter-muscular fat, kg	0.38	0.39	0.02	0.3020
Skeleton, kg	0.83	0.81	0.01	0.1099
	Weight of various muscles of the ham, g			
biceps femoris	1356	1301	26	0.0407
semitendinosus	491	451	14	0.0062
semimembranosus	1463	1397	29	0.0242
Gluteus	597	567	17	0.0790
vastus intermedius	292	289	5	0.4772
vastus medialis	409	409	8	0.9157
vastus lateralis	369	364	8	0.5566

Table 3. A comparison of the effect of rn⁺/rn⁺ *RN⁻* genotype on drip loss, meat colour[1], shear force and Napole Yield (Experiment 1).

	RN⁻	rn⁺/rn⁺	SEM	*P=*
Drip loss, 5	6.78	5.06	0.30	<0.0001
Meat colour				
L*	52.8	53.3	0.32	0.3414
a*	9.59	9.16	0.15	0.0456
b*	6.97	7.13	0.12	0.3392
Shear Force, N	41.6	44.2	1.9	0.3238
Napole Yield	74.9	81.1	0.53	<0.0001

Regarding the redness of meat (a*) there was an interaction between genotype and gender. The a* was larger in the RN⁻ genotype of female pigs, while no difference was apparent in castrated male pigs.

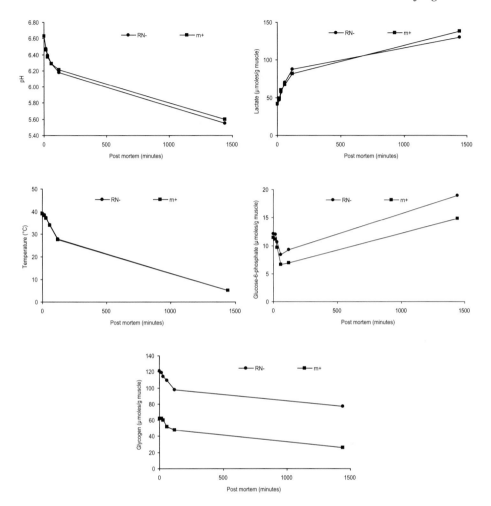

Figure 1. The influence of the RN- substitution on the development of pH and glycogen metabolism post mortem.

Together with University of Helsinki and Swedish University of Agricultural Sciences, Uppsala, we (Ylä-Ajos *et al.*, 2007) examined the effect of the RN⁻ gene in crossbreed pigs (Landrace x Large White x Hampshire) on glycogen and pH development post mortem. We found that both the rate and extent of pH (i.e., the ultimate pH) were changed. Thus, during the first three hours post mortem the rate of pH decrease was slightly faster in RN⁻ compared with the wild type (rn⁺/rn⁺), and the difference established at three hours was maintained at 24 hours. However, the difference increased further from 24 to 48 and 96 hours post mortem. In this study we measured both proglycogen and macroglycogen. In both genotypes the concentration of proglycogen was higher than the concentration of macroglycogen 30 minutes after slaughter, and the concentrations of both pro- and macroglycogen were higher in RN⁻ pigs. Again, for both genotypes, the proglycogen decreased post mortem, and in rn⁺/rn⁺ pigs the proglycogen was almost depleted at 48 hours post mortem, while in RN⁻ pigs this occurred after 96 hours. In rn⁺/rn⁺ pigs the concentration of macroglycogen did not change post mortem. However, in RN⁻ pigs a slight increase in macroglycogen was found at 96 hours post mortem. We believe this is due to accumulation of glucose-6-phosphate as discussed above. During boiling of the samples the phosphate may be separated from glucose and analysed together with the macroglycogen. Thus, glucose-6-phosphate may prevent further acidification. Thus, it seems very likely that proglycogen is responsible for the post mortem pH development.

In Denmark some production pigs are based on Hampshire crosses. Because of the higher glycogen content and lower pH leading to higher drip loss (Ylä-Ajos *et al.*, 2007 and Table 3), this gene has been eliminated from the Danish Hampshire population.

AGE

Muscle glycogen is not only important as an energy source for muscle metabolism and meat quality, but also for piglet survival. Thus, Horn *et al.* (unpublished) examined the level of muscle glycogen during various stages in gestation and at slaughter in *M. semitendinosus*. They found a dramatic increase from d 40 of gestation until d 115 (term). At d 80 of gestation the glycogen concentration was equal to the concentration measured at slaughter. However, from d 80 to term the glycogen concentration increased almost 5-fold. The large increase up to term may indicate that the piglet is equipped with a "packed lunch" consisting of glycogen, which is important for piglet survival. Oksbjerg, Henckel, Rolph and Erlandsen (1994) studied the glycogen in *M. longissimus dorsi* at various body weights (BW) from 25 kg to 90 kg BW. They found similar concentrations of glycogen at 25 and 45 kg BW. Hereafter the concentration of glycogen decreased slightly until 90 kg BW. Whether this decrease will continue beyond 90 kg BW is not known.

PHYSICAL EXERCISE, TREATMENT WITH *B*-ADRENERGIC AGONISTS; TREATMENT WITH PORCINE GROWTH HORMONE (PGH)

Nowadays there is a large variation in production systems with the extremes being the conventional system and free-range outdoor production. This suggests a large variation in physical activity of pigs among production systems. We have examined the effect of exercise training on performance, muscle metabolic traits and meat quality (Petersen *et al.*, 1997). The pigs were either individually penned (2.5 m²), individually penned and exercised-trained daily for 72 days (1 km/day at 4 km/h), or reared in large pens (36 m², containing 40 pigs). A muscle biopsy sample was taken 2 days before slaughter in the *M. longissimus dorsi* and *M. biceps femoris* and analysed for glycogen. There was no difference in the concentration of muscle glycogen in *longissimus dorsi* among treatments. On the other hand, pigs reared in large pens had a lower glycogen concentration in *biceps femoris* than control and exercise-trained pigs, which were similar. In both *longissimus dorsi* and *biceps femoris* exercise training and rearing in large pens resulted in increased pH 45 minutes after slaughter, while the ultimate pH was unaffected. The reason for this may be related to the glycolytic potential of the muscles. Thus, the activity of LDH (lactate dehydrogenase) was reduced after exercise training and when rearing pigs in large pens. In this work we did not report the drip loss. However, it is likely that increased pH 45 minutes following slaughter due to exercise training or rearing in large pens will result in a decreased drip loss.

Treatment of pigs with ß-adrenergic agonists stimulates muscle protein accretion and decreases fat accretion. Because ß-adrenergic agonists are derivates of adrenaline, it is likely that they will affect the muscle glycogen concentration. However, dietary inclusion of the ß-adrenergic agonist, Salbutamol, from 25 to 90 kg BW did not affect muscle glycogen concentration (Oksbjerg *et al.*, 1994). Similarly, treatment of pigs from 50 to 100 kg BW with daily injections of 80 µg of pGH/kg BW intramuscularly did not affect the muscle glycogen concentration compared with saline injections (Oksbjerg *et al.*, 1995). Although no effect was found on muscle glycogen, pGH treatment decreased pH during the first 4-6 hours post mortem, while the ultimate pH was similar remained unchanged We have no information from this experiment to explain this observation.

DIETARY MANIPULATION WITH THE MUSCLE GLYCOGEN

Feeding digestible carbohydrate (sugar feeding) has been investigated with the purpose to reduce or overcome the problem of inferior meat quality associated with high ultimate pH (DFD) from fatigued or long-term-stressed pigs. Thus, it has been shown that feeding sugars during overnight lairage may increase glycogen and decrease ultimate pH. In contrast, if it is possible to reduce muscle glycogen by dietary manipulation in well-rested pigs, this might be a means to increase ultimate pH and consequently reduce drip loss.

At our institute a Ph.D. study addressed this question (Rosenvold, 2002). Seven diets including the standard diet for growing pigs were formulated by varying the relative contribution of fat, protein and digestible carbohydrates. The dietary treatment commenced at 80 kg BW and lasted for three weeks. In the first week the pigs were adapted to the experimental diet by substituting the standard diet gradually with the experimental diet. The last 2 weeks the pigs were fed the experimental diets exclusively. Several of these diets prove to cause a linear reduction in glycogen with the largest effect (10-20 μ moles/ g muscle) at d 22. Two of these diets were selected for further experiments because they did not influence the performance of the pigs. One diet (INURA) was based on a high level of inulin (250g/kg) and a high level of fat (100g/ kg), and the other was based on high levels of grass meal (245g/kg) and dried sugar beet pulp (250g/kg) (GRASB). To study the temporal development in muscle glycogen, the pigs were fed the INURA diet for 4 weeks, and biopsy samples were taken repeatedly at the beginning (d 1) of the experimental period and at d 8, d 15, d 22 and d 29. When the pigs were fed the INURA diet, the glycogen decreased linearly until d 22, however, at d 29 the glycogen level returned to the same level as the control pigs. Consequently, the duration of the dietary treatment is critical. In subsequent experiments it was repeated that the INURA and GRASB diets reduced the muscle glycogen level by 15 μmole/g muscle following three weeks of dietary treatment. The INURA and GRASB diets only marginally increased the ultimate pH of *longissimus dorsi*. On the other hand, the pH 45 minutes post mortem increased, and the drip loss decreased by dietary treatment. The lightness of the meat was not influenced by dietary treatment, although Tikk *et al.* (2006) found that GRASB reduced L*.

As discussed earlier, proglycogen is responsible for the pH decrease post mortem. This was studied (Rosenvold, 2002) in relation to dietary treatment with the INURA diet for three weeks prior to slaughter. The data showed that during the experimental period, the glycogen-reducing diet reduced only macroglycogen, while the reduction in glycogen during the first 45 minutes post mortem was entirely due to a reduction in proglycogen. These results explain why dietary manipulation is not an efficient way to reduce ultimate pH. On the other hand, to change the level of macroglycogen by dietary manipulation increases pH and decreases the temperature 45 minutes post mortem, and this will lead to reduced drip loss.

Future perspectives

As mentioned above the halothane and the RN genes have been eliminated from Danish purebred pigs, and this may have reduced the initial rate of pH decrease post mortem. For Hampshire crosses the elimination of the RN gene may also increase ultimate pH. Altogether these actions may have improved colour and drip loss of the meat. However, a new substitution in the *PRKAG3* gene has been identified (Ciobanu *et al.*, 2001). This substitution termed V199I or rn* (Lindahl *et al.*, 2004) is associated with lower muscle glycogen, increased ultimate pH, lower drip loss and L*. This substitution is present in all purebred pigs varying proportionately from 0.13 in Landrace to 0.87 in Berkshire (Ciobanu *et al.*, 2001). Selection for this substitution may further improve meat quality. However, the effect of the rn* substitution on performance is not known, but should be investigated in future research.

In our opinion it is important that both pools of glycogen should be analysed in future research. This will make the understanding of the relationship between glycogen and meat quality more applicable.

Finally, to get a better understanding of the regulation of the glycogen pools we (Henckel *et al.*, unpublished) have developed a muscle cell culture where it is possible to study the effect of hormones and dietary components. In this system we can measure pro- and macroglycogen together with gene expression of enzymes important for the synthesis and degradation of muscle glycogen.

Conclusion

In conclusion, if the meat industry wish to further reduce drip loss and lightness this can be done by reducing muscle glycogen concentration in the primary production because muscle glycogen influences the rate and extent of pH. Thus, a reduction in glycogen may be obtained by selecting for lower glycogen and also by using glycogen-reducing diets. Furthermore, avoiding stress prior to slaughter is important. Biotechnological approaches may also be used. Thus under Danish conditions both the halothane and the RN⁻ substitution in the *PRKAG3* gene in Hampshire pigs have been eliminated from the populations. In the future, pigs with the rn* substitution in *PRKAG3* gene may be selected because this substitution is associated with low muscle glycogen, lower drip loss, and lower lightness of the meat. This substitution is present in all breeds.

References

Asp, S., Daugaard, J.R., Rohde, T., Adamo, K.B. and Graham, T.E. (1999) Muscle glycogen accumulation after a marathon: roles of fiber type and pro- and macroglycogen. *Journal of Applied Physiology* **86**:474-478.

Bendall, J.R. and Swatland, H.J. (1988) Rewiev of the relationship of pH with physical aspects of pork quality. *Meat Science* **24**:85-126.

Bloom, W.L., Lewis, G.T., Schumpert, M.Z. and Shen, T.M. (1951) Glycogen fractions of liver and muscle. *Journal of Biological Chemistry* **188**:631-636.

Ciobanu, D., Bastiaansen, J., Malek, M., Helm, J., Woollard, J., Plastow, G. and Rothschild, M. (2001) Evidence for new alleles in the protein kinase adenosine monophsphate-activated gamma3-subunit gene associated with low glycogen content in pig skeletal muscle and improved meat quality. *Genetics* **159**:1151-1162.

Gregory, N.G. (1996). Welfare and hygiene during preslaughter handling. *Meat Science*. **43**, no. S, S35-S46.

Hansen, B.F., Derave, W., Jensen, P. and Richter, E.A.. (2000) No limiting role for glycogenin in determining maximal attainable glycogen levels in rat skeletal muscle. *American Journal of Physiology. Endocrinology and Metabolism* **278**:E398-E404.

Henckel, P., Oksbjerg, N., Erlandsen, E., Barton-Gade, P. and Bejerholm, C. (1997) Histo- and biochemical characteristics of the longissimus dorsi muscle in pigs and their relationships to performance and meat quality. *Meat Science* **47**:311-321.

Henckel, P., Karlsson, A., Oksbjerg, N. and Petersen, J.S. (2000) Control of post mortem pH decrease in pig muscles: experimental design and testing of animal models. *Meat Sci.* **55**:131-138.

Henckel, P., Karlsson, A., Jensen, M.T., Oksbjerg, N., Petersen, J.S. 2002. Metabolic conditions in porcine longissimus muscle immediately pre-slaughter and its influence on peri- and post mortem energy metabolism. *Meat Science* **62**:145-155.

Graham, T.E., Adamo, K.B., Shearer, J., Marchand, I. and Saltin, B. (2001) Pro- and macroglycogenolysis: relationship with exercise intensity and duration. *Journal of Applied Physiology* **90**:873-879.

Lindahl, G., Enfält, A-C., von Seth, G., Josell, Å., Hedebro-Velander, I., Andersen, H.J., Braunschweig, M., Andersson, L. and Lundström, K. (2004). A second mutant allele (V199I) at the PRKAG3 (RN) locus-II. Effect on colour characteristics of pork loin. *Meat Science*. **66**:621-627.

Lomako, J., Lomako, M., Whelan, W.J., Dombro, R.S., Neary, J.T. and Norenberg, M.D. (1993) Glycogen synthesis in the astrocyte: from glycogenin to proglycogen to glycogen. *FASEB J.* **7**:1386-1393.

Oksbjerg, N., Henckel, P., Rolph, T. and Erlandsen, E. (1994) Effects of salbutamol, a $ß_2$-adrenergic agonist, on muscles of growing pigs fed different levels of dietary protein. II. Aerobic- and glycolytic capacities and glycogen metabolism of the longissimus dorsi muscle. *Acta Agriculturæ Scandinavica, Section A, Animal Science* **43**: 20-24.

Oksbjerg, N., Petersen, J.S., Sørensen, M.T., Henckel, P. and Agergaard, N. (1995) The influence of porcine growth hormone on muscle fibre characteristics, metabolic potential and meat quality. *Meat Science* **39**:375-385.

Oksbjerg, N., Petersen, J.S., Sørensen, I.L., Henckel, P., Vestergaard, M., Ertbjerg, P., Møller, A J., Bejerholm, C. and Støier, S. (2000) Long term changes in performance and meat quality of Danish Landrace pigs: a study on a current compared to an unimproved genotype. A*nimal Science* **71**:81-92.

Oksbjerg, N., Henckel, P., Andersen, S., Pedersen, B. and Nielsen, B. (2005) Genetic variation of in vivo muscle glycerol, glycogen, and pigment in Danish purebred pigs. *Acta Agriculturæ Scandinavica, Section A, Animal Science* **54**:187-192.

Passonneau, J.V. and Lowry, O.H. (1973) Enzymatic analysis – A practical guide. Totowa, New Jersey: The Humana Press.

Petersen, J.S., Henckel, P., Maribo, N. and Sørensen, M.T. (1997) Muscle metabolic traits, post mortem-pH-decline and meat quality in pigs subjected to regular physical training and spontaneous activity. *Meat Science* **46**:259-275.

Rosenvold, K. (2002) Strategic feeding - a tool in the control of technological pork quality. Doctoral thesis, Swedish University of Agricultural Sciences, Uppsala, SLU Service/repro, Uppsala.

Tikk, K., Tikk, M., Karlsson, A. and Andersen, H.J. (2006) The effect of a muscle-glycogen-reducing finishing diet on porcine meat and fat colour. *Meat Sci.* **73**:378-385.

Warris, P.D., Bevis, E.A. and Ekins, P.J. (1989) The relationship between glycogen stores and muscle ultimate pH in commercially slaughtered pigs. *British Veterinary Journal* **145**:378-383.

Ylä-Ajos, M.S.K., Lindahl, G., Young, J.F., Theil, P.K., Puolanne, E., Enfält, A.-C., Andersen, H.J. and Oksbjerg, N. (2007) Post-mortem activity of the glycogen debranching enzyme and change in the glycogen pools in porcine M. longissimus dorsi from carriers and non-carriers of the RN- gene. *Meat Science* **75**:112-119.

13

EFFECTS OF L-CARNITINE AND OTHER STRATEGIES TO INFLUENCE PRENATAL MUSCLE DEVELOPMENT AND SUBSEQUENT OFFSPRING PERFORMANCE

JASON C. WOODWORTH
Lonza Inc, 1376 1500 Ave, Enterprise, Kansas 67441, USA

Introduction

Maximizing pork output per unit of input is the ultimate goal of modern pig production and is often achieved by maximizing muscle mass in the finishing pig. Research has shown that there are a number of different methods that can be used to increase muscle expression of the finishing pig. However, the methods applied during the finishing phase can only influence the hypertrophy of the muscle fibres that are already present. A relatively new area of study centres on the idea that fetal muscle fibre number can be increased during gestation which should allow for an enhanced response from muscle development strategies used during the grow-finish phase. This should ultimately result in a carcass with more muscle mass. This chapter will briefly outline the areas of interest that have been studied to increase fetal muscle development and focus on their ability to alter the resulting offspring carcass cut out value.

Justification

The prolificacy of today's sows is increasing at an astounding rate. Genetic companies are offering sow lines that will produce over 30 pigs/sow/year with some claiming an amazing production rate of 40 pigs/sow/year. This is in relation to the 20 pigs/sow/year that was viewed as acceptable only a few years ago. However, some believe this increase in prolificacy is not without cost. In a review, Foxcroft *et al.* (2006) outlined some of the negative consequences of the introduction of hyperprolific sows into modern pig production systems. These researchers suggest that even though the sow is able to produce larger litters, the associated crowding effect that occurs within the uterus impairs fetal development. They suggest that the intrauterine growth retardation is a result of limited nutrient availability to the developing embryos which correlates to lighter birth weights and poorer survivability and postnatal growth performance. Foxcroft *et al.* (2006) also suggest that the crowding causes a negative effect on myogenesis resulting in a reduced number of muscle fibres, and consequently poorer carcass cut out of the offspring. Other research reviews have also reported that impairments to fetal development, defined as the low birth weight pigs of the litter, will exhibit the effects of reduced myogenesis with poorer subsequent muscle development and meat quality characteristics (Maltin *et al.*, 2001; Gondret *et al.*, 2006; Rehfeldt and Kuhn, 2006).

The pig industry's interest in fetal muscle development has increased considerably over the last couple of years. Research has repeatedly demonstrated the negative ramifications of poor fetal development; however, the data base of information that shows ways to improve fetal muscle development is relatively small. This appears to be due in part because of the high amount of time and money associated with this research. Over the past 30 years, three main areas have been studied to determine their effects on prenatal muscle development: exogenous hormonal control, maternal feed intake, and L-carnitine supplementation.

Influences of exogenous hormonal manipulation

Prenatal muscle development is a complex process that is influenced by a number of different factors. Some of the main regulators of fetal growth are the hormones of the somatotropic axis; of which somatotropin or growth hormone has received the most attention. Early research has shown that exogenous porcine somatotropin treatment to finishing pigs will increase muscle hypertrophy (Beermann *et al.*, 1990; Solomon *et al.*, 1990). It is known that growth hormone will influence circulating concentrations IGF-I, IGF-II, IGFBP levels as well as other growth-regulating hormones (Rehfeldt *et al.*, 2004). In addition, porcine growth hormone treatment to gestating sows has been shown to influence characteristics of the placenta (Sterle *et al.*, 2003) and has been suggested to improve amino acid delivery to the fetus resulting in the enhanced fetal muscle development (Glatford *et al.*, 2000). Therefore, the hypothesis that additional growth hormone might improve fetal growth is warranted.

Some studies have reported beneficial effects of exogenous growth hormone treatment on fetal muscle development. Rehfeldt *et al.* (2001) has shown that daily treatment with somatotropin in early gestation will affect myogenesis in the pig. These researchers injected 6 mg of porcine somatotropin daily to sows from day 10 to 27 of gestation and observed an increased number of muscle fibres and muscle fiber girth in the semitendinosus muscle as well as increased muscle protein concentration and type II to type I fibre conversion suggesting an advanced degree of differentiation. Other researchers have also found that porcine somatotropin will influence fetal muscle characteristics (Rehfeldt *et al.*, 1993; Sterle *et al.*, 1995; Gatford *et al.*, 2003). However, in many of these studies, it was observed that the positive effect of somatotropin was only observed in those pigs that had birth weights that were in the lowest 0.25 of the litter (Sterle *et al.*, 1995; Rehfeldt *et al.*, 2001). In one study, fetal development was even shown to be decreased in pigs with birth weights within the highest 0.75 of the liter (Kuhn *et al.*, 2004).

While maternal treatment with somatotropin has shown in some studies to improve fetal muscle characteristics, an observed change in carcass cut out of the offspring is hardly convincing. In one study, greater loin muscle area was observed in pigs obtained from sows treated with porcine somatotropin (Kelly *et al.*, 1995). However, other researchers have failed to find a similar response (McLaughlin *et al.*, 1996; Kuhn *et al.*, 2004). In addition, maternal treatment with growth hormone-releasing factor failed to show a beneficial response on carcass composition of the offspring (Etienne *et al.*, 1992).

Even though in some studies beneficial effects on muscle characteristics of offspring have been reported from maternal treatment with porcine growth hormone, the practical application of this hormone is for the most pat non-existent. From the logistical perspective, maternal somatotropin treatment must be accomplished through frequent (daily) injections which make it labor intensive and leads to questions regarding animal welfare. Secondly, in most countries the use of exogenous somatotropin treatment is not approved. For these reason, the application of the porcine growth hormone effects on fetal muscle development is severely limited.

Influences of maternal feed intake

Most modern pig producers limit the amount of energy that is provided to the sow during gestation. This is mainly done to prevent excess fat accumulation in the mammary glands which can impair milk production, as well as to stimulate an active appetite during lactation. However, Rehfeldt *et al.* (2004) reports that increased gestational feed intake above basal requirements might elicit changes in metabolites and reproductive hormones which will alter nutrient partitioning to the fetus ultimately resulting in enhanced fetal development. Changes in maternal nutrition will also influence the circulating concentrations of fetal growth regulating hormones (Bispham *et al.*, 2003; Thissen *et al.*, 2006). Therefore, a gestation feeding strategy that focuses on fetal development might elicit beneficial effects on fetal muscle development.

Early experiments that studied the effects of maternal nutrition on fetal development employed a model of testing a control or normal amount of feed compared to a treatment of feed restriction. Offspring growth performance and carcass composition was negatively affected when gestating sows were offered a feed restricted ration (Buitrago *et al.*, 1974; Pond *et al.*, 1985). Restriction of just the protein fraction the diet also resulted in poorer postnatal performance (Pond *et al.*, 1987; Schoknecht *et al.*, 1993). In the guinea-pig model, Dwyer *et al.* (1995) showed that maternal undernutrition will influence fetal muscle development resulting in poorer muscle fibre formation. While these studies demonstrate that fetal development can be influenced by maternal plane of nutrition, they do not offer clues as to how to improve the baseline performance.

More recent studies have focused on increased levels of maternal nutrition in an attempt to improve fetal development over a control level. Research has found that the timing of the increased nutrition will play a role in the outcome. Dwyer *et al.* (1994) found that doubling maternal feed intake from day 25 to 50 of gestation resulted in a tendency for increased number of muscle fibres whereas supplementation from day 50 to 80 or 25 to 80 had no effect. Carcass composition data were not collected and therefore it can not be determined if the increased muscle fibre number observed with the early supplementation resulted in improved carcass muscling. Post natal growth performance was also reported and shown to be improved with increased supplementation from day 25 to 80 but not with the other supplementation durations. Other researchers have also found that increased maternal nutrition from day 25 to 50 resulted in enhanced muscle fiber development (Gatford *et al.*, 2003). Penny *et al.* (2000) observed that elevated feed intake offered to sows from day 28-56 of gestation resulted in progeny with a greater lean percentage at slaughter.

Contrary to these findings, other researchers have reported minimal effects of increased maternal nutrition during gestation on offspring muscle development and postnatal performance. Nissen *et al.* (2003) did not find any effect of increased maternal nutrition from day 25 to 50 or 25 to 70 of gestation on fetal muscle fiber development, carcass composition, or meat quality. Likewise, Bee *et al.* (2004) observed that when sows were fed 40% more feed from day 0 to 50 of gestation, muscle fibre number and the resulting offspring carcass composition was not different.

Most studies have shown that maternal undernutrition will negatively affect fetal muscle development illustrating the impact of nutritional deficiencies. However, the impact of extra nutrition above the normal allocation has not consistently been shown to elicit benefits to fetal muscle development. The benefits that were shown by some studies might reflect a situation where the basal diet was deficient in a particular nutrient and therefore the extra feed allowance provided enough of that nutrient to overcome the deficiency. At this time there are not enough data to warrant increasing feed intake during gestation to improve offspring muscle development. In addition, the risk of excess fat accumulation in the mammary glands might limit the application of this technology if additional research were to show its benefits.

Influences of L-carnitine supplementation

L-carnitine is a vitamin-like compound that is essential for the transportation of long- and medium-chain fatty acids into the mitochondria for beta-oxidation and has been shown to affect several key enzymes involved in protein, carbohydrate, and lipid metabolism (Rebouche *et al.*, 1990; Owen *et al.*, 2001). Much of the early L-carnitine research focused on its effects on sow productivity, but recently there has been an emphasis on defining its role in prenatal muscle and fetal development. Reasons that supplemental L-carnitine might impact fetal development are most likely related to its ability to influence energy metabolism (Owen *et al.*, 2001), increase maternal IGF-1 concentrations (Musser *et al.*, 1999; Doberenz *et al.*, 2006), and/or influence maternal leptin concentrations (Woodworth *et al.*, 2004).

The earliest indication that L-carnitine was playing a role in fetal development was observed when piglet birth weights were measured. A number of studies have reported that when L-carnitine is included in gestation diets the piglet birth weights in the subsequent litter will be increased (Musser *et al.*, 1999; Eder *et al.*, 2001; Ramanau *et al.*, 2002; Eder *et al.*, 2003). In one study, even when the number of piglets born alive was increased, the piglet birth weight is maintained or greater when L-carnitine was included in the diet (Ramanau *et al.*, 2003). It was also shown that L-carnitine will reduce the number of non-viable piglets born (less than 800 grams) (Eder *et al.*, 2001; Ramanau *et al.*, 2002; Eder *et al.*, 2003) suggesting that L-carnitine is eliciting a beneficial effect on fetal development. More recently, Birkenfeld *et al.* (2005) showed that maternal supplementation with 50 ppm of L-carnitine during gestation will improve the postnatal growth performance of the light birth-weight piglets of the litter

Based on these findings that L-carnitine was influencing fetal development, the research focus shifted to determining its influence on fetal muscle development. Musser *et al.* (2001) reported that in two studies piglets obtained from sows fed diets containing L-carnitine during gestation had 27.8% and 6.5% more muscle fibres compared to piglets obtained from sows fed diets without L-carnitine. In a third study, Musser *et al.* (2000) confirmed that L-carnitine enhanced muscle fibre development of the offspring and observed that the benefit was maintained at slaughter as piglets from sows fed diets with L-carnitine had greater loin depth (59.4 vs 57.0 mm) and lean percent (55.1 vs 54.5%).

More recent research has been conducted to help determine why these increases in muscle fibre development might be occurring. Waylan *et al.* (2005) observed that maternal L-carnitine influenced the expression of fetal mRNA for IGF-1, IGF-2, IGFBP-3, and myogenin in isolated embryonic myoblasts, which resulted in a state of increased muscle cell proliferation and delayed differentiation. At the placental level, Brown *et al.* (2006) observed that mRNA expression of IGFBP-3, IGFBP-5, and IGF-I in the endometrium was increased when sows were supplemeated with L-carnitine. In addition Doberenz *et al.* (2006) has reported that when sows were supplemented with L-carnitine, they had heavier chorions with greater concentrations of DNA and protein which would signify an enhanced maternal/fetal interface. These researchers also observed an increased concentration of GLUT-1 transporter in the chorion which would suggest a higher potential for glucose transfer from the sow to the fetus.

Studies measuring the influence of maternal L-carnitine supplementation on fetal muscle development are relatively new. To date, the data would suggest that supplemental L-carnitine will influence the regulation of fetal development and/or nutrient flow to the fetus which will result in a state of greater fetal development, increased muscle fibre development, and offspring with improved carcass composition. In addition, at this time there does not appear to be any negative side effects resulting from L-carnitine supplementation. Additional studies are currently being conducted to further define the role that maternal L-carnitine plays in fetal development and to confirm past observations.

Conclusions

The ability to change prenatal muscle development and fetal development in general has gained a lot of interest in recent years. The idea that increasing prenatal muscle development will enhance carcass cut out of the resulting progeny is economically important for modern swine production. To date, three separate means of influencing fetal muscle development have been studied. Treatment with porcine growth hormone injections to gestating sows has been reported, but the effects on fetal muscle characteristics are inconclusive. Furthermore, the desired improvement in offspring carcass composition from maternal porcine growth hormone treatment is less than convincing. Secondly, extra maternal nutrition during certain periods of gestation was beneficial in some studies, but the overall results do not consistently yield a positive impact on fetal muscle development or carcass composition. The final area of interest is maternal supplementation with L-carnitine. Improvements in fetal muscle development and offspring carcass composition have been reported with supplemental L-carnitine, but the data set is relatively new. Additional research in all of these areas, as well as others, is sure to be conducted as industry interest in fetal muscle fiber development increases.

References

Bee, G. 2004. Effect of early gestation feeding, birth weight, and gender of progeny on muscle fiber characteristics of pigs at slaughter. *Journal of Animal Science.* 82:826-836.

Beermann, D. H, Fishell, V. K., Roneker, K., Boyd, R. D., Ambruster, G., and Souza, L. 1990. Dose-response relationships between porcine somatotropin, muscle composition, muscle fiber characteristics and pork quality. *Journal of Animal Science.* 68:2690-2697.

Birkenfeld, C., Ramanau, A., Kluge, H., and Eder, K. 2005. Effect of dietary L-carnitine supplementation on growth performance of piglets from control sows or sows treated with L-carnitine during pregnancy and lactation. *Journal of Animal Physiology and Animal Nutrition.* 89:277-283.

Bispham, J., Gopalakrishnan, G. S., Dandrea, J., Wilson, V., Budge, H., Keisler, D. H., Broughton Pipkin, F., Stephenson, T., and Symonds, M. E. 2003. Maternal endocrine adaptation throughout pregnancy to nutritional manipulation: consequences for maternal plasma leptin and cortisol and the programming of fetal adipose tissue development. *Endocrinology.* 144:3575-3585.

Brown, K. R., Goodband, R. D., Tokach, M. D., Dritz, S. S., Nelssen, J. L., Minton, J. E., Woodworth, J. C. and Johnson, B. J. 2006. Maternal supplementation of L-carnitine alters the maternal and fetal IGF axis in swine. 2006 Experimental Biology meeting abstracts [on CD-ROM]. *The FASEB Journal.* 20:266.6 (Abstr.).

Buitrago, J. A., Walker, E. G., Snyder, W. I., and Pond, W. G. 1974. Blood and tissue traits in pigs at birth and at 3 weeks from gilts fed low or high energy diets during gestation. *Journal of Animal Science.* 38-766-771.

Doberenz, J., Birkenfeld, C., Kluge, H., and Eder, K. 2006. Effects of L-carnitine supplementation in pregnant sows on plasma concentrations of insulin-like growth factors, various hormones and metabolites and chorion characteristics. *Journal of Animal Physiology and Animal Nutrition.* In press.

Dwyer, C. M., Madgwick, A. J. A., Ward, S. S., and Stickland, N. C. 1995. Effect of maternal undernutrition in early gestation on the development of fetal myofibres in the Guinea-pig. *Reproduction, Fertility, And Development.* 7:1285-1292.

Dwyer, C. M., Stickland, N. C., and Fletcher, J. M. 1994. The influence of maternal nutrition on muscle fiber number development in the porcine fetus and on subsequent postnatal growth. *Journal of Animal Science.* 72:911-917.

Eder, K., Ramanau, A., and Kluge, H. 2001. Effect of L-carnitine supplementation on performance parameters in gilts and sows. *Journal of Animal Physiology and Animal Nutrition.* 85:73-80.

Eder, K., Ramanau, A., and Kluge, H. 2003. Benefits of long term L-carnitine in sows. *International Pig Topics.* 18:25-26.

Etienne, M., Bonneay, M., Kann, G., and Deletang, F. 1992. Effects of administration of growth hormone-releasing factor (GRF) to sows during late gestation on growth hormone secretion, reproductive traits, and performance of progeny from birth to 100 kilograms live weight. *Journal of Animal Science.* 70:2212-2220.

Foxcroft, G.R., Dixon, W. T., Novak, S., Putman, C. T., Town, S. C., and Vinsky, M. D. A. 2006. The biological basis for prenatal programming of postnatal performance in pigs. *Journal of Animal Science.* 84 (E. Suppl.): E105-E112.

Gatford, K. L., Ekert, J. E., Blackmore, K., De Blasio, M. J., Boyce, J. M., Owens, J. A., Campbell, R. G., and Owens, P. C. 2003. Variable maternal nutrition and growth hormone treatment in the second quarter of pregnancy in pigs alter semitendinosus muscle in adolescent progeny. *British Journal of Nutrition.* 90:283-293.

Glatford, K. L., Owens, J. A., Campbell, R. G., Boyce, J. M., Grant, P. A., De Blasio, M. J., and Owens, P. C. 2000. Treatment of underfed pigs with

GH throughout the second quarter of pregnancy increases fetal growth. *Journal of Endocrinology.* 166: 227-234.

Gondret, F., Lefaucheur, L., Juin, H. Louveau, I., and Lebert, B. 2006. Low birth weight is associated with enlarged muscle fiber area and impaired meat tenderness of the longissimus muscle in pigs. *Journal of Animal Science.* 84: 93-103.

Kelley, R. L., Jungst, S. B., Spencer, T. E., Owsley, W. F., Rabe, C. H., and Mulvaney, D. R. 1995. Maternal treatment with somatotropin alters embryonic development and early postnatal growth of pigs. *Domestic Animal Endocrinology.* 12: 83-94.

Kuhn, G., Kanitz, E., Tuchscherer, M., Nurnberg, G., Hartung, M., Ender, K., and Rehfeldt, C., 2004. Growth and carcass quality of offspring in response to porcine somatotropin (pST) treatment of sows during early pregnancy. *Livestock Production Science.* 85:103-112.

Maltin, C. A., Delday, M. I., Sinclair, K. D., Steven, J., and Sneddon, A. A. 2001. Impact of manipulations of myogenesis *in utero* on the performance of adult skeletal muscle. *Reproduction.* 122: 359-374.

McLaughlin, C. L., Miner, C. S., Coffey, M. T., Pratt, G., and Baile, C. A. 1996. Effect of pST treatment of sows during early gestation on farrowign performance and carcass composition of offspring. *Journal of Animal Science.* 74(Suppl. 1):146.

Musser, R. E., Goodband, R. D., Tokach, M. D., Owen, K. Q., Nelssen, J. L., Blum, S. A., Dritz S. S., and Civis, C. A.. 1999. Effects of L-Carnitine Fed During Gestation and Lactation on Sow and Litter Performance. *Journal of Animal Science.* 77:3289–3295.

Musser, R. E., Dritz, S. S., Goodband, R. D., Tokach, M. D., Davis, D. L., Nelssen, J. L., Owen, K. Q., Hanni, S., Bauman, J. S., and Heintz, M. 2000. Added L-carnitine in sow gestation diets improves carcass characteristics of the offspring. *Journal of Animal Science.* 78(Suppl. 2):120(Abstr.).

Musser, R. E., Goodband, R. D., Owen, K. Q., Davis, D. L., Tokach, M. D., Dritz, S. S., and Nelssen, J. L.. 2001. Determining the effect of increasing L-carnitine additions on sow performance and muscle fiber development of the offspring. *Journal of Animal Science.* 79(Suppl. 1):65(Abstr.).

Nissen, P. M., Danielsen, V. O., Jorgensen, P. F., and Oksbjerg, N. 2003. Increased maternal nutrition of sows has no beneficial effects on muscle fiber number or postnatal growth and has no impact on the meat quality of the offspring. *Journal of Animal Science.* 81:3018-3027.

Owen, K. Q., Ji, H., Maxwell, C. V., Nelssen, J. L., Goodband, R. D., Tokach, M. D., Tremblay, G. C., and Koo, S. I. 1997. Dietary L-carnitine suppresses mitochondrial branch-chain keto acid dehydrogenase activity and enhances protein accretion and carcass characteristics of swine. *Journal of Animal Science.* 79:3104-3113.

Penny, P. C., Varley, M. A., and Tibble, S. 2000. Effect of increasing nutrient intake to sows from day 28-56 of gestation on subsequent progeny performance. *Journal of Animal Science.* 78(Suppl. 1):147(Abstr.).

Pond, W. G., Mersmann, H. J., and Yen, J. T. 1985. Severe feed restriction of pregnant swine and rats: effects on postweaning growth and body composition of progeny. *Journal of Nutrition.* 115:179-185.

Pond, W. G., Yen, J. T. and Mersmann, H. J. 1987. Effect of severe dietary protein, nonprotein calories or feed restriction during gestation on postnatal growth of progeny in swine. *Growth.* 51:355-371.

Rebouche, C. J., Panagides, D. D., and Nelson, S. E. 1990. Role of carnitine in utilization of dietary medium-chain triglycerides by term infants. *American Journal of Clinical Nutrition.* 52:820-824.

Rehfeldt, C., Fiedler, I., Weikard, R., Kanitz, E., and Ender, K. 1993. It is possible to increase skeletal muscle fibre number *in utero. Bioscience Reports.* 13: 213-220.

Rehfeldt, C. and G. Kuhn. 2006. Consequences of birth weight for postnatal growth performance and carcass quality in pigs as related to myogenesis. *Journal of Animal Science.* 84(E. Suppl.): E113-E123.

Rehfeldt, C., Kuhn, G., Nurnberg, G., Kanitz, E., Schneider, F., Beyer, M. Nurnberg, K., and Ender, K. 2001. Effects of exogenous somatotropin during early gestation on maternal performance, fetal growth and compositional traits in pigs. *Journal of Animal Science.* 79:1789-1799.

Rehfeldt, C., Nissen, P. M., Kuhn, G., Vestergaard, M., Ender, K., and Oksbjerg, N. 2004. Effects of maternal nutrition and porcine growth hormone (pGH) treatment during gestation on endocrine and metabolic factors in sows, fetuses and pigs, skeletal muscle development, and postnatal growth. *Domestic Animal Endocrinology.* 27:267-285.

Ramanau, A., Kluge, H., Spilke, J., and Eder, K. 2002. Reproductive performance of sows supplemented with dietary L-carnitine over three reproductive cycles. *Archives of Animal Nutrition.* 56:287-296.

Ramanau, A., Kluge, H., Spilke, J., and Eder, K. 2004. Supplementation of sows with L-carnitine during pregnancy and lactation improves growth of the piglets during the suckling period through increased milk production. *Journal of Nutrition.* 134:80-92.

Schoknecht, P. A., Pond, W. G., Mersmann, H. J., and Maurer, R. R. 1993. Protein restriction during pregnancy affects postnatal growth in swine progeny. *Journal of Nutrition.* 123:1818-1825.

Solomon, M. B., Campbel, R. G., and Steele, N. C. 1990. Effect of sex and exogenous porcine somatotropin on longissimus muscle fiber characteristics of growing pigs. *Journal of Animal Science.* 68:1176-1181.

Sterle, J. A., Cantley, T. C., Lamberson, W. R., Lucy, M. C., Gerrard, D. E., Matteri, R. L., and Day, B. N. 1995. Effects of recombinant porcine somatotropin on placental size, fetal growth, and IGF-I and IGF-II concentrations in pigs. *Journal of Animal Science.* 73:2980-2985.

Sterle, J. A., Cantley, T. C., Matteri, R. L., Carrol, J. A., Lucy, M. C., and Lamberson, W. R. 2003. Effect of recombinant porcine somatotropin on fetal and placental growth in gilts with reduced uterine capacity. *Journal of Animal Science.* 81:765-771.

Thissen, J. P., Ketelslegers, J., and Underwood, L. E. 1994. Nutritional regulation of the insulin-like growth factors. *Endocrine Reviews.* 15:80-101.

Woodworth, J. C., Minton, J. E., Tokach, M. D., Nelssen, J. L., Goodband, R. D., Dritz, S. S., Koo, S. I., and Owen, K. Q. 2004. Dietary L-carnitine increases plasma leptin concentrations of gestating sows fed one meal per day. *Domestic Animal Endocrinology.* 26:1-9.

Waylan, A. T., Kayser, J. P., Gnad, D. P., Higgins, J. J., Starkey, J. D., Sissom, E. K., Woodworth, J. C., and Johnson, B. J. 2005. Effects of L-carnitine on fetal growth and the IGF system in pigs. *Journal of Animal Science.* 83:1824-1831.

14

POULTRY ZOONOSES

PHILLIPPA L. CONNERTON AND IAN F. CONNERTON
Division of Food Sciences, University of Nottingham School of Biosciences, Sutton Bonington Campus, Loughborough, Leics LE12 5RD

Introduction

Zoonoses are defined by the World Health Organisation as 'diseases and infections which are transmitted naturally between vertebrate animals and man'. Zoonoses cover a broad range of diseases with different clinical and epidemiological features that require different control measures. The causative organism may be viral, bacterial, fungal, protozoal, parasitic or any other communicable agent. Zoonotic infections can be transmitted by a variety of routes, including; food, water, direct contact and through insect vectors. Despite the variety of causative agents and routes of transmission there are relatively few zoonotic infections that are transferred from poultry to humans. However the three main zoonoses of poultry are of significant economic and medical importance. The two main bacterial zoonoses arising from poultry are *Salmonella* and *Campylobacter*. Bacteria from several other genera, including *Listeria monocytogenes, Clostdrium perfringens, Yersinia enterocolitica, Staphylococcus aureus* and pathogenic *Escherichia coli* can occasionally be transmitted from poultry to man if circumstances permit but this usually involves either cross-contamination during processing and/or improper storage or inadequate cooking (reviewed by Cox *et al.* 2005). The main viral poultry zoonosis is Avian Influenza virus that has been a source of human influenza outbreaks and remains a significant threat to world health (http://www.who.int/csr/disease/avian_influenza). In addition to the bacterial and viral poultry zoonoses, the intracellular bacterium *Chlamydophila psittaci* may also affect humans causing serious illness and occasionally death. Infection with this organism is thought to be common in a number of bird species, mainly psittacines (parrots, macaws, parakeets), but it can also affect turkeys, ducks and geese (reviewed by Andersen and Vanrompay 2000; Edison

2002). Transmission to humans has occasionally been recorded in people working in pet shops (Maegawa *et al.* 2001) and poultry processing plants (Hedberg *et al.* 1987). Ectoparasites are also zoonotic agents that should be acknowledged here. Avian mite dermatitis (reviewed by Beck 1999), has been reported in poultry workers (Mazyad and Abel El-Kadi 2005) with the most common mites to be involved being *Ornithonyssus sylviarum* (Northern fowl mite) and *Dermanyssus gallinae* (red poultry mite). The clinical manifestations include itching, papules, vesicles and dermatitis. The red poultry mite *Dermanyssus gallinae* can also cause Otitis externa (infestations of the ear), which has occasionally been reported in poultry workers (Rossiter 1997).

Avian influenza virus

THE VIRUS

Avian influenza ('fowl plague' or 'bird flu') is caused by Type A influenza viruses which are members of the family Orthomyxoviridae (reviewed in Suarez *et al.* 2004). The type A viruses can infect a range of species including man, birds, pigs, horses but wild birds are the natural hosts for these viruses (http://www.cdc.gov/flu/avian/gen-info/flu-viruses.htm). The viral genome consists of eight segments of negative-sense RNA (Ghedin *et al.* 2005). An important feature of the virus is the absence of RNA proof-reading enzymes (reviewed by Webster *et al.* 1992). The RNA-dependent RNA transcriptase makes a nucleotide insertion error nearly every time a new virus is synthesised. This makes nearly every new virus particle a source of genetic variation. Added to this selective recombination of the segmented RNA strands increase the possible number of variants, and from these mutant pools virulent viruses can emerge. Influenza strains tend to be species specific due to variations in their haemagglutinins (reviewed by Webster *et al.* 1992). These are antigenic glycoproteins found on the virus surface which are responsible for binding the virus to its target cell. Mutations in the haemagglutinin gene can significantly alter the ability of viral haemagglutinin proteins to bind to receptors on the surface of host cells and potentially allow new hosts to become infected. Influenza viruses are categorised into subtypes according to the haemagglutinin (H) type and their neuraminidase (N) antigens. To date all highly pathogenic avian influenza viruses belong to either the H5 or H7 subtypes. The avian influenza viruses are closely related to human influenza viruses that cause respiratory symptoms. Transmission of avian influenza to humans in close contact with poultry or other birds occurs rarely.

However mutations in the avian viruses could change virus strains from being inefficient at attacking human cells to becoming fully virulent in humans. This may be facilitated if the virus replicates in an intermediate species such as pigs. The potential for transformation of avian influenza into a zoonotic form that causes severe disease in humans and spreads easily from person to person is a great concern for world health.

AVIAN INFLUENZA IN POULTRY

Avian influenza has been recognised as a generalised viral disease of poultry since 1901 and is a notifiable disease in the UK. Domestic fowl, ducks, geese, turkeys, guinea fowl, quail and pheasants are all susceptible to avian influenza. A particular virus isolate may be specific to a type of poultry and may, for example, cause disease in turkeys but not chickens. Wild birds, particularly water birds, are also susceptible but infections in these birds are generally subclinical (reviewed by Webster *et al.* 1992). However, aquatic birds can transmit the virus to domestic birds, which is probably the source of most outbreaks. Once established in domestic poultry, the virus is highly contagious spreading from bird to bird then from flock to flock through contact with infected birds or contaminated equipment or the apparel (footwear and overalls) of production workers. Infected birds excrete virus at high concentration in their faeces, and also via nasal and ocular discharges. Airborne transmission may occur if birds are in close proximity and with appropriate air movement. Birds become infected via instillation of virus into the conjunctival sac, nares, or the trachea. Hatching eggs from a diseased flock is considered to be a significant risk, although the possibility of direct vertical transmission remains unresolved. The incubation period following exposure is usually between 3 and 7 days, but depends on many factors, including the nature of virus, the level of exposure, the age of the bird, the species and breed of poultry.

The clinical signs of infection with avian influenza virus are quite variable. The disease usually appears suddenly in a flock leading to many deaths without previously showing any signs of illness. Some birds show signs of depression, inappetence, ruffled feathers and fever. A staggering gait is also seen in some individuals. The combs and wattles are cyanotic and oedematous, and may have petechial or ecchymotic haemorrhages at their tips. Birds frequently exhibit severe watery diarrhoea, which in turn causes dehydration. Respiratory symptoms may also be observed at this stage. Haemorrhages can be observed on exposed areas of skin. The mortality rate is variable but is generally high, ranging from 50 to 100%.

PREVENTION

Biosecurity and surveillance are the first lines of defence and the most important means of prevention (reviewed by Capua and Alexander 2006). Vaccines have been demonstrated to be effective in reducing mortality and/ or preventing disease in domestic poultry. These vaccines, however, are not without problems (reviewed by Capua and Alexander 2006). They may not prevent infection in all the individual birds of a flock, and if infected they can shed virulent virus albeit at a reduced rate compared to infected birds that were not initially vaccinated. For vaccination to be effective the antigenic type of the avian influenza virus must be known and the vaccine must represent this antigenic strain. A recombinant fowl pox virus vaccine (Qiao *et al.* 2003) containing the gene that codes for the production of the H5 antigen has recently been licensed in some countries but is not widely used at this time.

H5N1 STRAIN

The H5N1 strain causes an avian disease that is endemic in many bird populations, especially in Southeast Asia (reviewed by Webster *et al.* 2006). An H5N1 strain stemming from this Asian lineage is spreading globally and has been associated human infection. Hundreds of millions of birds have been culled as a response, in an attempt to control its spread. There is as yet no evidence of efficient human-to-human transmission or of airborne transmission of H5N1 to humans. In almost all cases, those humans that have become infected with H5N1 have been in very close contact with infected birds for prolonged periods. Of grave concern is the fact that approximately half of the individuals infected with the current Asian strain of H5N1 have died. If this strain adapted to have efficient human-to-human transmission it would have very serious global consequences. The first known strain of H5N1 killed two flocks of chickens in Scotland in 1959 but this strain was quite different from the current highly pathogenic genotype of H5N1 which, according to pre- and post surveillance data, appears to have evolved between 1999 and 2002.

H7N7

In addition to the Asian H5N1 strain another avian influenza subtype, the H7N7 strain is also of cause for concern. H7N7 can infect humans, birds, pigs, seals and horses in the wild; with the demonstration of experimental transmission to laboratory mice. Such a wide range of hosts is particularly unusual and the zoonotic potential that it represents is extremely perturbing.

An outbreak of H7N7 on several poultry farms occurred in the Netherlands in 2003, which later spread to Belgium and Germany. Some 250 farms were affected leading to the slaughter of more than 30 million poultry. In the Netherlands a total of 89 people were confirmed to have become infected with the H7N7 influenza virus as a result. Most of these had conjunctivitis, and whilst a few patients suffered respiratory symptoms in conjunction with conjunctivitis, only one death was recorded. It is not clear why this individual was so severely affected (Fouchier *et al.* 2004). The sero-prevalence of H7 antibodies in people without contact with infected poultry but with close household contact to an infected poultry worker was found to be 59%. This suggests that person to person transmission may have indeed occurred (Du Ry van Beest Holle *et al.* 2005). The final analysis of the Dutch avian influenza outbreak of H7N7 indicated much higher levels of transmission to humans had occurred than first estimated (Bosman *et al.* 2005).

The last outbreak of avian influenza in the UK was in a flock of 8000 turkeys in Norfolk in 1991. Early detection and prompt action prevented any spread to other farms. In August 2006, a low pathogenic variant of H7N7 was found during routine testing at a poultry farm in Voorthuizen in the central Netherlands. As a precautionary measure, 25,000 chickens were culled from Voorthuizen and surrounding farms.

AVIAN INFLUENZA IN HUMANS

Humans Influenza A virus symptoms include fever, cough, sore throat, muscle aches, conjunctivitis and, in severe cases, breathing problems and pneumonia that may be fatal. The symptoms of avian H5N1 flu in humans seem to be more variable. In one case, a boy with H5N1 experienced diarrhoea followed rapidly by a coma without developing respiratory or flu-like symptoms (de Jong *et al..* 2005). There have been studies of the levels of cytokines in humans infected by the H5N1 flu virus. Of particular concern is the elevated levels of tumor necrosis factor alpha, an acute phase protein that is associated with the inflammatory response to cellular damage, and leads to the production of other cytokines. Flu virus-induced increases in the levels of cytokines are associated with the typical disease symptoms that include fever, chills, vomiting and headache. Tissue damage associated with pathogenic flu virus infection can ultimately result in death. The inflammatory cascade triggered by H5N1 has been called a 'cytokine storm' by some, because of what seems to be a positive feedback process of damage to the body resulting from immune system stimulation (reviewed by Yuen and Wong 2005). H5N1 type flu virus induces higher levels of cytokines than the more common flu virus types such as H1N1.

Salmonella

THE GENUS *SALMONELLA*

Members of the genus *Salmonella* are Gram-negative rod shaped bacteria belonging to the family of Enterobacteriaceae, many of which are associated with disease in man and animals. Although the *Salmonella* bacterium was first described by Theobald Smith (1859-1934), it was named after Daniel E. Salmon who isolated a strain from pigs in 1885. There is much confusion regarding the names of individual members of this genus. In the past *Salmonellae* have been separated largely into serotypes (serovars) of which there are more than 2,400. This arose because each serotype was considered as a separate species based on antigenic differences. However as technology has progressed to enable estimates of genomic relatedness, *Salmonellae* taxonomy has undergone a radical reassessment (reviewed by Brenner *et al.* 2000). The current most commonly adopted nomenclature recognises two species, *S. enterica,* that consists of six subspecies, and *S. bongeri*. Subspecies I of *S. enterica* contains the familiar serotypes Enteritidis, Typhimurium, Typhi and Cholerasuis. These serotype names are not italicised and the first letter is capitalised. The serotypes may be further sub divided into phage types (PTs), for example, S. Enteritidis PT 4 is often associated with contaminated eggs.

Salmonellae inhabit the intestines of mammals, marsupials, birds and reptiles. Consequently they are excreted from infected animals into the environment, to contaminate soil, water, insects and plants. Here they readily survive until ingested by a new host. *Salmonellae* can be either host adapted or are generalists able to infect many hosts. For example, S. Typhi and S. Paratyphi A only infect humans and are therefore not zoonoses, whereas S. Typhimurium and S. Enteritidis are of the ubiquitous type and therefore the causative agents of zoonotic disease. The latter are sometimes referred to as non-typhoidal salmonellae

HUMAN INFECTION

Salmonellae are a well known human pathogen and is recognised to be a significant burden in terms morbidity and economic loss (Roberts and Sockett

1994; Adak et al. 2002; Roberts et al. 2003). In 2004 there were over 13,000 cases of non-typhoidal salmonelosis reported to the Heath Protection Agency in England and Wales (http://www.hpa.org.uk/infections/topics_az/ salmonella/data_human.htm). The under reporting of infectious intestinal disease is well recognised, and the true population burden is probably considerably greater than that given by national surveillance. Human *Salmonellae* infection is characterised by diarrhoea, fever, nausea, vomiting with both abdominal and muscular pains. The incubation period before onset of symptoms is usually within 48 h of exposure. The symptoms may persist for one to two weeks before recovery. Occasionally infection can result in more severe disease and even death particularly in vulnerable patients. S. Enteritidis and S. Typhimurium in particular have accounted for the majority of cases of human salmonellosis in recent years (see http://www.defra.gov.uk/ animalh/diseases/zoonoses/zoonoses_reports/zoonoses2004.pdf for a comprehensive review of the surveillance of *Salmonella* zoonoses).

POULTRY RESERVOIRS

Epidemiological investigations have often implicated poultry to be the main source of *Salmonellae* infection in the UK. This may be through consumption of eggs or inadequately cooked chicken, or where uncooked chicken has cross-contaminated other foods. In a recent survey of fresh and frozen chicken purchased in the UK (http://www.food.gov.uk/multimedia/pdfs/ campsalmsurvey.pdf) *Salmonellae* was isolated from 4.0% of fresh chicken samples and 10.4 % of frozen chicken samples. *Salmonella* Typhimurium was the most frequent of the 30 serotypes isolated, accounting for 14% of the total number of *Salmonellae* isolates. A similar survey was carried out to examine the frequency of *Salmonellae* contamination of eggs (http:// www.food.gov.uk/multimedia/pdfs/fsis5004report.pdf). The number of contaminated eggs was found to be 0.34 % in the survey carried out in 2003. This represents 9 *Salmonellae* positive eggs of the 4,753 eggs sampled and all were present only on the shell surface rather than within the egg itself.

During the mid 1980s S. Enteritidis reports associated with poultry were at relatively low levels before a dramatic increase towards the end of the 1980s (http://www.defra.gov.uk/animalh/diseases/zoonoses/zoonoses_ reports/zoonoses2004.pdf). In response to this alarming rise in numbers (nearly 2,000 incidents in 1990 from less than 500 in 1987) control measures and codes of practice for the control of *Salmonellae* were introduced in 1989. Numbers of S. Enteritidis were then observed to decline, and since the mid 1990s the reported incidents of S. Enteritidis in domestic fowl have continued to remain at low levels. The numbers of other serotypes in live poultry are still of concern, and may have only become evident due to the increased levels of monitoring.

Researchers have attempted to explain the sudden increase of S. Enteritidis in the late 1980s. It has been suggested to be connected to the reduction in two alternative serotypes, namely *S.* Gallinarum and *S.* Pullorum that rarely affect humans. These two serotypes cause an invasive rather than gastrointestinal disease of poultry that were prevalent in UK flocks before the 1970s. After this time they were virtually eradicated through culling and vaccination. It is believed that in undertaking this eradication, a niche became available that the serotype S. Enteriditis was able to exploit to become the dominant serotype in poultry until the late 1990s. However, in the following decade a variety of different serotypes were isolated, with no lasting dominance noted in the serotypes recorded.

SOURCES OF INFECTION

Salmonellea are transmitted both vertically (S. Enteritidis) where the bacteria infect the egg as it develops, and pseudovertically (any serotype) where the bacteria enter the egg after laying. In addition *Salmonella* are transmitted through contaminated feed, from contaminated equipment and the environment. Persistence of *Salmonellae* in flocks is therefore a problem and it is particularly acute in layer hens infected with S. Enteritidis as the farms are occupied continuously (reviewed by Davies 2005). Chicks usually become infected with *Salmonellae* in the first week of life with the highest prevalence being around 2 weeks of age followed by a gradual decline in numbers that may become undetectable until laying begins (Heyndrickx *et al.* 2002; Davies *et al.* 1997).

When poultry are subjected to stress such as feed withdrawal in order to induce moulting and stimulate multiple egg-laying cycles, it has been observed that they become more susceptible to S. Enteritidis infection (Holt 1993). Further more feed withdrawal may significantly affect the virulence of the infecting *Salmonellae* by increasing the expression of genes necessary for intestinal invasion (Durant *et al.* 1999).

CONTROL OF SALMONELLAE

There has been a significant decline in the incidence of isolation of *Salmonella* in poultry products since the late 1990s and cases of human infection have fallen concordantly. Most sampling of chicken flocks in Great Britain is undertaken for statutory monitoring or for surveillance purposes, so most incidents and isolations reported are not associated with clinical disease but with identification of subclinical carriage of *Salmonellae*. In 2004 there were 11 reports of S. Enteritidis incidents in chickens – 34 fewer than in 2003 (http://www.defra.gov.uk/animalh/diseases/zoonoses/zoonoses_reports/ zoonoses2004.pdf).This is partly due to improvements in the standards of egg production. In particular the implementation of the Lion Code of Practice first introduced 1998 has been of great benefit. This is an integrated programme of registration, traceability, vaccination, biosecurity, temperature controlled storage and date labelling of products. Vaccination of birds and improved biosecurity measures have also reduced the incidence of isolations of *Salmonella* on poultry reared for meat production but there is still a problem of cross-contamination occurring at the slaughter house. Competitive exclusion is another method that has been used in some countries to control *Salmonellae* (reviewed by Mead 2000). This involves the administration of usually undefined cultures of microflora to chicks that inhibits *Salmonellae* colonisation. Other methods of control include treatment of feed and drinking water, and in some countries the use of antimicrobials such as fluroquinalones although these are not permitted in the EU for non-therapeutic purposes.

Campylobacter

THE GENUS *CAMPYLOBACTER*

Members of the genus *Campylobacter* are Gram-negative, highly motile, spiral shaped bacteria. Two species, *C. jejuni* and *C. coli,* cause the majority of human disease (Friedman *et al.* 2000). Campylobacters, like Salmonellae are normally found in the intestines of animals and are excreted into the environment, although they are somewhat more fragile than *Salmonella*. In particular, campylobacters are microaerophilic requiring oxygen levels of around 5% to grow. Campylobacters are sensitive to higher atmospheric oxygen contents and are rapidly killed on exposure to the prevailing levels of oxygen in air. *Campylobacter* species appear to be particularly well adapted to colonising the intestines of birds where the partial pressures of oxygen are low and the bacteria are able to exist in large numbers without apparently causing disease in most cases (Newell and Fearnley 2003). However when infected material is consumed by humans, campylobacters cause diarrhoea and are thus an important zoonotic disease.

HUMAN INFECTION

Campylobacter infection causes diarrhoea, which may be profuse and watery, and often contains blood (reviewed by Skirrow and Blaser 2000). Infection is frequently associated with severe abdominal pain, which may mimic acute appendicitis. The symptoms usually last for one to two weeks but may persist or reoccur. Rare but serious complications such as Guillain Barré syndrome (reviewed by Hughes and Cornblath 2005) can arise. Guillain Barré is an autoimmune disorder where the peripheral nervous system is the focus of attack by antibodies thought to arise through antecedent *Campylobacter* infection (Yuki *et al.* 2004).

CURRENT SITUATION

Campylobacter is the most commonly isolated bacterial gastrointestinal pathogen in the UK. Most *Campylobacter* isolates are not routinely speciated but where this is carried out *C. jejuni* is the predominant species (90%), with the remainder largely being attributable to *C. coli* (7%) and occasional reports of *C. lari* and *C. upsaliensis* causing intestinal disease (Gillespie *et al.* 2002). Since 2001 there has been a gradual decline in the number of human cases reported each year in the UK but *Campylobacter* still represents over 40,000 reported cases, where case control studies suggest that up to eight times as many go unreported (http://www.defra.gov.uk/animalh/diseases/zoonoses/zoonoses_reports/zoonoses2004.pdf).

SOURCES OF INFECTION

Most cases of *Campylobacter* infection are sporadic and the routes of transmission remain unknown. Poultry meat may be an important vehicle of infection where surveys have shown that a significant proportion of raw poultry meat for human consumption is contaminated before cooking, where 60% (1,028/1,723) of products were recorded as *Campylobacter* positive in a survey carried out in 2004 (http://www.defra.gov.uk/animalh/diseases/zoonoses/zoonoses_reports/zoonoses2004.pdf). Evidence suggests that *Campylobacter* has a low infectious dose (Black *et al.*. 1988) and thus cross-contamination of ready to eat foods by raw meat may be an important source of infection.

CAMPYLOBACTER INFECTION LEVELS IN UK POULTRY FLOCKS AND ATTEMPTS TO AT CONTROL

The UK Food Standards Agency has set a target to work with the industry to achieve a 50% reduction in the incidence of UK produced chickens that test positive for *Campylobacter* by 2010. Reducing the numbers of campylobacters on poultry meat is a difficult problem to solve as these bacteria are well adapted to avian species such that they may be considered commensal organisms of poultry, and are certainly present in large numbers in the intestines of chickens (Newell and Fearnley 2003). When the birds are slaughtered and the intestines removed the campylobacters in the intestinal contents contaminate the surface of the poultry meat and are hard to remove (Jacobs-Reitsma 2000).

A risk assessment has estimated that a $\log_{10}$ 2.0 reduction in *Campylobacter* numbers on retail chicken carcases could reduce the frequency of human campylobacterosis by up to 30 fold (Rosenquist *et al.* 2003). To achieve this aim, intervention measures have focussed on improving farm biosecurity and/or the decontamination of poultry carcases post slaughter. Ideally decontamination techniques should not change the organoleptic or nutritional properties of the food (Corry *et al.* 1995). They should also be safe, cheap and acceptable to the public. At present no single technique fits these criteria, although a number of different approaches to reduce *Campylobacter* carcass contamination have been suggested (Newell and Wagenaar 2000).

Intervention strategies focussed at the start of the food chain (i.e. the broiler farm) are most likely to yield the greatest reductions of *Campylobacter* contaminating retail poultry meat. The upgrading of biosecurity has successfully produced *Campylobacter*-free chickens but these measures are expensive and difficult to maintain. This is largely due to the susceptibility of chickens to infection by *Campylobacter* and its ubiquity in the environment (Newell and Fearnley 2003). Moreover, unless increased biosecurity is applied globally, the benefits of reducing *Campylobacter* on some farms will be negated by cross-contamination from positive flocks at the abattoir (Herman *et al.* 2003).

A potential method for controlling campylobacters colonising poultry is through the use of Competitive Exclusion (CE). This technique has been successfully used to control *Salmonellae*, but CE trails with *Campylobacter* have produced mixed results (Newell and Wagenaar 2000). Protection has been demonstrated with a variety of layer hen leading to the conclusion that CE effect may be dependent on the genotypes of the birds to which it is to be applied (Laisney *et al.* 2004). The success of vaccination in controlling

Salmonellae in UK layer flocks has prompted studies into a similar treatment for *Campylobacter*. Although a feasible strategy, towards which some progress has been recently reported (Wyszynska *et al.* 2004), no such vaccine is currently available for commercial application (reviewed in Newell and Wagenaar 2000). Another possibility is to harness naturally occurring bacteriophage and this is discussed in the following section.

Bacteriophage

Bacteriophages are obligate pathogens of bacteria. They are naturally occurring predators of bacteria that are ubiquitous in the environment and are found in fresh and salt water, soil, manure, food and air. In fact they are found anywhere where their bacterial hosts are found. Estimates of the numbers of phage commonly found in the environment can be as high as 10^9 particle forming units (PFU) per millilitre for fresh and surface seawater (Bergh *et al.* 1989). With estimates of the total numbers of bacteriophage in the world being around 10^{31} PFU this makes them the most abundant biological entity on the planet (Rohwer and Edwards 2002).

Phage can selectively kill bacteria making them potentially useful to control pathogens and possibly combat the problem of antibiotic resistance. Their host specificity means that there is less damage to other microbial flora in contrast to other anti-microbial agents which may disturb the delicate microbial balance. Phage may be used in a number of different ways including prophylactically and/or as a remedial action such as the treatment of infection, and because they are diverse in nature they have considerable potential to overcome bacterial resistance compared to conventional antimicrobials. As stated phage are ubiquitous in the environment and their presence in poultry and poultry carcasses is no exception. Studies of the incidence of *Campylobacter* phage in UK poultry and on retail poultry products have been carried out (Atterbury *et al.* 2003 a and b; Connerton *et al.* 2004; Atterbury *et al.* 2005; El-Shibiny *et al* 2005) as a prelude to investigating their use in phage therapy aimed to reduce campylobacters in poultry, and therefore entering the human food chain from this source. As bacteriophage are already present on poultry any intervention would not constitute the addition of a new biological entity with the risk of side effects, for example allergic response. For similar reasons the use of bacteriophage for biocontrol could be considered natural and therefore consistent with "organic" or "green" production methods. All the bacteriophage isolated from these sources belong to Myoviridae family that have icosahedral heads and long contractile tails (Connerton and Connerton, 2005). The types of phage are generally lytic in nature, that is they infect, replicate and lyse the bacteria without interaction with host bacterial DNA, and as such are appropriate for use in phage therapy.

Bacteriophages have been applied as a decontamination technique to reduce campylobacters on poultry meat under experimental conditions (Atterbury *et al.* 2003b; Goode *et al.* 2003). As campylobacters are unable to multiply under refrigeration conditions, the phages may infect hosts on the surface of poultry meat but are unable to complete their replication cycle until environmental conditions are permissive for metabolic activity of their host. Whether the consumption of bacteriophage-infected campylobacters on contaminated meat would provide protection from enteric disease is unknown.

A growing number of studies have successfully used phages to treat animal diseases (reviewed in Barrow 2001; Payne and Jansen 2003). These include applications to treat *Salmonella* (Berchieri *et al.* 1991; Sklar and Joerger 2001.) and *E. coli* (Barrow *et al.* 1998; Huff *et al.* 2003; Huff *et al.* 2004) infections of young chickens. The use of phages to control *Campylobacter* in chickens diverges from these previous studies as campylobacters are considered natural commensals, not pathogens, of poultry species. Campylobacters colonise the chicken intestine to a high density, and as such are a promising target for phage therapy. Concerns have been raised that campylobacters will simply become resistant to bacteriophages rendering this strategy ineffective in the long term (Barrow 2001). Bacteria rapidly mutate to become resistant to bacteriophages *in vitro* on laboratory media (Adams 1959). However, unlike bacterial resistance to static chemotherapeutic agents such as antibiotics, bacteriophages constantly evolve to circumvent host barriers to infection. This leads to an evolutionary balance that allows both host and prey to proliferate. In our laboratory we have tested the efficacy of bacteriophage as a control agent for *Campylobacter* both *in vitro* and in vivo. Bacteriophage were administered to *Campylobacter* colonised birds at three different doses ($\log_{10}$ 5, $\log_{10}$ 7 and $\log_{10}$ 9 PFU) in antacid suspension (Loc Carrillo *et al.* 2005). The numbers of campylobacters in the caecal contents of phage treated and untreated birds were determined at 24 h intervals over 5 days. The bacteriophage treated birds showed a marked reduction in numbers of campylobacters particularly for the first 48 h after treatment. The reduction in caecal *C. jejuni* numbers varied with the phage from 2 $\log_{10}$ to 5 $\log_{10}$ (per g of caecal contents) compared to controls. The success of treatment was dependant on the bacteriophage and the colonisation strain used with some bacteriophage considerably being more virulent than others. A *Campylobacter* bacteriophage isolated **fro**m poultry meat rather than poultry excreta was found to ineffective in a similar trial despite the fact that the phage was virulent *in vitro* on laboratory media (Atterbury, 2003).

Optimization of dose and selection of appropriate phage were found to be the key elements in the use of phage therapy to reduce campylobacters in broiler chickens.

The numbers of phage resistant campylobacters present in the experimental birds following bacteriophage therapy was determined and found to be less than four per cent (Loc Carrillo *et al.* 2005). Interestingly these resistant isolates appeared to be compromised in their ability to colonise a further set of experimental birds, rapidly reverting back to the phage sensitive phenotype in the absence of phage. In contrast, when phage resistance isolates were obtained by mixing host and phage *in vitro* and culturing on laboratory media the frequency of resistance was 11% and the resistant phenotype was maintained on subculture (Loc Carrillo *et al.* 2005). This level of mutation means that phage resistant types soon can dominate phage challenged laboratory cultures but this does not happen in chickens. Other studies have noted decreased fitness when bacteria acquire phage resistance through mutation (Park *et al.* 2000; Smith *et al.* 1987). This is often because phage have evolved to target essential structures present on their outer surface as their receptors to gain entry to the cell. If bacteria alter these structures through mutation, it may prevent phage entry but can also be detrimental to their fitness such that they do not survive in competitive or environmental challenge.

Wagenaar *et al.* (2005) have reported the use of the *Campylobacter* typing phage 69 (NCTC 12669) to prevent as well as reduce *Campylobacter* colonisation of broiler chickens. The administration of phage resulted in a 3 $\log_{10}$ decline in *C. jejuni* caecal counts. Preventative phage treatment delayed the onset of *C. jejuni* colonization, and the peak titres remained two $\log_{10}$ lower than the controls. There were no adverse health effects from the phage treatments. A second phage (NCTC 12671) was added to the original, in an attempt to counter any tendency to develop phage resistance in the *Campylobacter* population. However, this strategy did not result in any significant increase in efficacy. The use of these model systems provides valuable data and indicates the potential of phage therapy to reduce campylobacters.

Conclusions

Poultry is an important part of the UK diet. The safety of food products and the biosecurity of production methods are of paramount importance to our economy and health. Zoonoses of poultry remain a significant burden on human health that require reliable surveillance data, robust biosecurity to minimise human exposure and investment in methods for their control.

References

Adak, G.K., Long, S.M, and O'Brien, S.J. (2002) Trends in indigenous foodborne disease and deaths, England and Wales: 1992 to 2000. *Gut.* **51**:832-841.

Adams, M.H. (1959). Bacteriophages. Interscience Publishers Inc, New York

Andersen, A.A. and Vanrompay, D. (2000) Avian chlamydiosis. *Rev. Sci. Tech.* **19**:396-404.

Atterbury, R.J., Connerton, P.L., Dodd, C.E.R, Rees, C.E.D. and Connerton, I.F. (2003a) Isolation and characterization of *Campylobacter* bacteriophages from retail poultry. *Appl. Environ. Microbiol.* **69**:4511-4518.

Atterbury, R.J., Connerton, P.L., Dodd, C.E.R., Rees, C.E.D. and Connerton, I.F. (2003b) Application of host-specific bacteriophages to the surface of chicken skin leads to a reduction in recovery of *Campylobacter jejuni. Appl. Environ. Microbiol.* **69**:6302-6306.

Atterbury, R.J., Dillon, E., Swift, C., Connerton, P.L., Frost, J.A., Dodd, C.E.R, Rees, C.E.D. and Connerton I.F. (2005) Correlation of *Campylobacter* bacteriophage with the reduced presence of their hosts in broiler chicken ceca. *Appl. Environ. Microbiol.* **71**:4885-4887.

Barrow, P.A. (2001). The use of bacteriophages for treatment and prevention of bacterial disease in animals and animal models of human infection *J. Chem. Technol. Biotechnol.* **76**:677-682.

Barrow, P., Lovell M. and Berchieri. A. (1998) Use of lytic bacteriophage for control of experimental *Escherichia coli* septicemia and meningitis in chickens and calves. *Clin. Diagn. Lab. Immunol.* **5**:294-298.

Beck, W. (1999) Farm animals as disease vectors of parasitic epizoonoses and zoophilic dermatophytes and their importance in dermatology. *Hautarzt.* **50**:621-628.

Berchieri, A., Lovell, M.A. and Barrow, P.A. (1991) The activity in the chicken alimentary tract of bacteriophages lytic for *Salmonella typhimurium. Res. Microbiol.* **142**:541-549.

Bergh, Ø., Børsheim, K.Y, Bratbak, G. and Heldal., M. (1989) High abundance of viruses found in aquatic environments. *Nature* **340**:467-468.

Black, R.E., Levine, M.M., Clements, M.L., Hughes, T.P. and Blaser, M.J. (1988) Experimental *Campylobacter jejuni* infection in humans. *J. Infect. Dis.* **157**:472-479.

Bosman, A., Meijer, A. and Koopmans, M. (2005) Final analysis of Netherlands avian influenza outbreaks reveals much higher levels of transmission to humans than previously thought. *Euro. Surveill.* **10**:E050106.2.

Brenner, F.W., Villar, R.G., Angulo, F.J., Tauxe, R. and Swaminathan, B. (2000) *Salmonella* nomenclature. *J. Clin. Microbiol.* **38**:2465-2467.

Capua, I. and Alexander, D.J. (2006) The challenge of avian influenza to the veterinary community. *Avian Pathol.* **35**:189-205.

Connerton, P.L., Loc Carrillo, C.M., Swift, C., Dillon, E., Scott , A., Rees, C.E.D., Dodd , C.E.R., Frost, J and. Connerton, I.F. (2004) A longitudinal study of *Campylobacter jejuni* bacteriophage and their hosts from broiler chickens. *Appl. Environ. Microbiol.* **70**:3877-3883.

Connerton, P.L. and. Connerton, I.F. (2005) Natural *Campylobacter* control with bacteriophage. *World Poultry* Salmonella & Campylobacter Special, 25-26.

Corry, J.E, James, C., James, S.J. and Hinton, M. (1995) *Salmonella, Campylobacter* and *Escherichia coli* O157:H7 decontamination techniques for the future. *Int. J. Food Microbiol.* **28**:187-196.

Cox, N.A., Richardson, L.J., Bailey, J.S., Cosby, D.E., Cason, J.A., Musgrove, M.T. and Mead, G.C. (2005). Bacterial contamination of poultry as a risk to human health. In *Food safety control in the poultry industry* pp 21-43. Ed Mead G.C., Woodhead Publishing, Cambridge.

Davies, R.H. (2005). Pathogen population on poultry farms. In *Food safety control in the poultry industry* pp101-152. Ed Mead G.C., Woodhead Publishing, Cambridge.

Davies, R.H., Nicholas, R.A., McLaren, I.M., Corkish, J.D., Lanning, D.G. and Wray, C. (1997) Bacteriological and serological investigation of persistent *Salmonella enteritidis* infection in an integrated poultry organisation. *Vet. Microbiol.* **58**:277-93.

Durant, J.A., Corrier, D.E., Byrd, J.A., Stanker, L.H. and Ricke, S.C. (1999) Feed deprivation affects crop environment and modulates *Salmonella enteritidis* colonization and invasion of leghorn hens. *Appl. Environ. Microbiol.* **65**:1919-1923.

Du Ry van Beest Holle, M., Meijer, A., Koopmans, M. and de Jager, C.M. (2005) Human-to-human transmission of avian influenza A/H7N7, The Netherlands, 2003. *Euro. Surveill.* **10**:264-268.

Eidson, M. (2002) Psittacosis/avian chlamydiosis. *J. Am. Vet. Med. Assoc.* **221**:1710-1712.

El-Shibiny, A., Connerton, P.L. and Connerton, I.F. (2005) Enumeration and diversity of campylobacters and bacteriophages isolated during the rearing cycles of free-range and organic chickens. *Appl. Environ.*

Microbiol. **71**:1259-1266.

Fouchier, R.A., Schneeberger, P.M., Rozendaal, F.W., Broekman, J.M., Kemink, S.A., Munster, V., Kuiken, T., Rimmelzwaan, G.F., Schutten, M., Van Doornum, G.J., Koch, G., Bosman, A., Koopmans, M. and Osterhaus, A.D. (2004) Avian influenza A virus (H7N7) associated with human conjunctivitis and a fatal case of acute respiratory distress syndrome. *Proc. Natl Acad Sci U S A.* **101**:1356-1361.

Friedman, C.R., Neimann, J.. Wegener, H.C. and Taux, R.V. (2000) Epidemiology of *Campylobacter jejuni* infections in the United States and other industrialized nations, p.121-138. *In* I. Nachamkin and M.J. Blaser (ed.), *Campylobacter,* 2nd ed. ASM press, Washington D.C.

Goode, D., Allen, V.M. and Barrow, P.A. (2003) Reduction of experimental *Salmonella* and *Campylobacter* contamination of chicken skin by application of lytic bacteriophages. *Appl. Environ. Microbiol.* **69**:5032-5036.

Gillespie, I.A., O'Brien, S.J., Frost, J.A., Adak, G.K., Horby, P., Swan, A.V., Painter, M.J. and. Neal. K.R. (2002) A case-case comparison of *Campylobacter coli* and *Campylobacter jejuni* infection: a tool for generating hypotheses. *Emerg. Infect. Dis.* **8**:937-942.

Hedberg, K., White, K.E., Forfang, J.C., Korlath, J.A., Friendshuh, K.A., Hedberg, C.W., MacDonald, K.L. and Osterholm, M.T. (1989). An outbreak of psittacosis in Minnesota turkey industry workers: implications for modes of transmission and control. *Am. J. Epidemiol.* **130**:569-577.

Heyndrickx, M., Vandekerchove, D., Herman, L., Rollier, I., Grijspeerdt, K. and De Zutter, L. (2002) Routes for salmonella contamination of poultry meat: epidemiological study from hatchery to slaughterhouse. *Epidemiol. Infect.* **129**:253-265.

Herman, L., Heyndrickx, M., Grijspeerdt, K., Vandekerchove, D., Rollier I. and De Zutter. L. (2003) Routes for *Campylobacter* contamination of poultry meat: epidemiological study from hatchery to slaughterhouse. *Epidemiol. Infect.* **131**: 1169-1180.

Heuer, O.E., Pedersen, K., Andersen, J.S. and Madsen, M. (2001) Prevalence and antimicrobial susceptibility of thermophilic *Campylobacter* in organic and conventional broiler flocks. *Lett. Appl. Microbiol.* **33**:269-274.

Holt, P.S. (1993) Effect of induced molting on the susceptibility of White Leghorn hens to a *Salmonella enteritidis* infection. *Avian Dis.* **37**:412-417

Huff, W.E., Huff, G.R., Rath, N.C., Balog, J.M. and Donoghue, A.M. (2003) Bacteriophage treatment of a severe *Escherichia coli* respiratory infection in broiler chickens. *Avian Dis.* **47**:1399-1405.

Huff, W.E., Huff, G.R., Rath, N.C., Balog, J.M. and Donoghue, A.M. (2004) Therapeutic efficacy of bacteriophage and Baytril (enrofloxacin) individually and in combination to treat colibacillosis in broilers. *Poult. Sci.* **47**:1944-1947.

Hughes, R.A. and Cornblath, D.R. (2005) Guillain-Barre syndrome. *Lancet.* **366**:1653-1666.

Jacobs-Reitsma, W.F. (2000) *Campylobacter* in the food supply, p. 497-509. *In* I. Nachamkin and M. J. Blaser (ed.), *Campylobacter*, 2nd ed. ASM Press, Washington, D.C.

de Jong, M.D., Simmons, C.P., Thanh, T.T., Hien, V.M., Smith, G.J., Chau, T.N., Hoang, D.M., Van Vinh Chau, N., Khanh, T.H., Dong, V.C., Qui, P.T., Van Cam, B., Ha do, Q., Guan, Y., Peiris, J.S., Chinh, N.T., Hien, T.T. and Farrar, J. (2006) Fatal outcome of human influenza A (H5N1) is associated with high viral load and hypercytokinemia. *Nat. Med.* **12**:1203-1207.

Laisney, M.J., Gillard, M.O. and Salvat, G. (2004) Influence of bird strain on competitive exclusion of *Campylobacter jejuni* in young chicks. *Br. Poult. Sci.* **45**:49-54.

Loc Carrillo, C., Atterbury, R.J., El-Shibiny, A., Connerton, P.L., Dillon, E., Scott, A. and Connerton, I.F. (2005) Bacteriophage therapy to reduce *Campylobacter jejuni* colonisation of broiler chickens. *Appl. Environ. Microbiol.* **71**:6554-6563.

Maegawa, N., Emoto, T., Mori, H., Yamaguchi, D., Fujinaga, T., Tezuka, N., Sakai, N., Ohtsuka, N. and Fukuse, T. (2001). Two cases of *Chlamydia psittaci* infection occurring in employees of the same pet shop. *Nihon Kokyuki Gakkai Zasshi.* **39**:753-757.

Mazyad, S.A. and Abel El-Kadi, M. (2005) *Ornithonyssus* (Acari: Macronyssidae) mite dermatitis in poultry field-workers in Almarg, Qalyobiya governorate. *J. Egypt. Soc. Parasitol.* **35**:213-222.

Mead, G.C. (2000) Prospects for 'competitive exclusion' treatment to control salmonellas and other foodborne pathogens in poultry. Vet J. **159**:111-23.

Newell, D.G. and Fearnley, C. (2003) Sources of *Campylobacter* colonization in broiler chickens. *Appl. Environ. Microbiol.* **69**:4343-4351.

Newell, D.G. and Wagenaar, J.A. (2000) Poultry infections and their control at farm level, p.497-510. *In* I. Nachamkin and M.J. Blaser (ed.), *Campylobacter,* 2nd ed. ASM press, Washington D.C.

Park, S.C., Shimamura, I., Fukunaga, M., Mori, K.I. and Nakai, T. (2000) Isolation of bacteriophages specific to a fish pathogen, *Pseudomonas plecoglossicida*, as a candidate for disease control. *Appl. Environ.*

Microbiol. **66**:1416-1422.

Payne, R.J. and Jansen, V.A. (2003) Pharmacokinetic principles of bacteriophage therapy. Clin. Pharmacokinet. **42**:315-325.

Qiao, C.L., Yu, K.Z., Jiang, Y.P., Jia, Y.Q., Tian, G.B., Liu, M., Deng, G.H., Wang, X.R., Meng, Q.W. and Tang, X.Y. (2003) Protection of chickens against highly lethal H5N1 and H7N1 avian influenza viruses with a recombinant fowlpox virus co-expressing H5 haemagglutinin and N1 neuraminidase genes. *Avian Pathol.*;**32**:25-32.

Ringoir, D.D. and Korolik, V. (2003) Colonisation phenotype and colonisation potential differences in *Campylobacter jejuni* strains in chickens before and after passage *in vivo*. *Vet. Microbiol.* **92**:225-235.

Roberts, J.A. and Sockett, P.N. (1994) The socio-economic impact of human *Salmonella enteritidis* infection. *Int. J. Food Microbiol.* **21**:117-129

Roberts, J.A, Cumberland, P., Sockett, P.N, Wheeler, J., Rodrigues, L.C., Sethi, D. and Roderick, P.J. (2003) The study of infectious intestinal disease in England: socio-economic impact *Epidemiol. Infect.* **130**:1-11.

Rohwer, F. and Edwards, R. (2002) The Phage Proteomic Tree: a genome-based taxonomy for phage. *J. Bacteriol* .**184**:4529-4535.

Rosenquist, H., Nielsen, N.L., Sommer, H.M., Norrung, B. and Christensen, B.B. (2003) Quantitative risk assessment of human campylobacteriosis associated with thermophilic *Campylobacter* species in chickens. *Int. J. Food. Microbiol,* **83**:87-103.

Rossiter, A. (1997) Occupational otitis externa in chicken catchers. *J. Laryngol. Otol.* **111**:366-367.

Skirrow, M.B. and Blaser, M.J. (2000) Clinical aspects of *Campylobacter* infection pp69-88. *In* I. Nachamkin and M.J. Blaser (ed.), *Campylobacter,* 2nd ed. ASM press, Washington D.C.

Sklar, I.B. and Joerger, R.D. (2001) Attempts to utilize bacteriophage to combat *Salmonella enterica* serovar Enteritidis infection in chickens. *J. Food Safety.* **21**:15-30.

Smith, H.W., Huggins, M.B. and Shaw, K.M. (1987) The control of experimental *Escherichia coli* diarrhoea in calves by means of bacteriophages. *J. Gen. Microbiol.* **133**:1111-1126.

Suarez, D.L., Senne, D.A., Banks, J., Brown, I.H., Essen, S.C., Lee, C.-W., Moreno, V., Pedersen, J.C., Panigrahy, B., Rojas, H., Spackman, E. and Alexander, D.J. (2004) Recombination resulting in virulence shift in avian influenza outbreak, Chile. *Emerg. Infect. Dis.* [serial online] 2004 Apr [27/10/06]. Available from: http://www.cdc.gov/ncidod/EID/vol10no4/03-0396.htm

Wagenaar J.A., Van Bergen, M.A.P., Mueller, M.A., Wassenaar, T.M. and Carlton, R.M. (2005) Phage therapy reduces *Campylobacter jejuni* colonization in broilers. *Vet. Microbiol.* **109**:275-283.

Webster, R.G., Bean, W.J., Gorman, O.T., Chambers, T.M. and Kawaoka, Y. (1992) Evolution and ecology of influenza A viruses. *Microbiol. Rev.* **56**:152-179.

Webster, R.G., Peiris, M., Chen, H. and Guan, Y. (2006) H5N1 outbreaks and enzootic influenza. *Emerg Infect Dis.* **12**:3-8.

Wyszynska, A., Raczko, A., Lis, M. and Jagusztyn-Krynicka, E.K. (2004) Oral immunization of chickens with avirulent *Salmonella* vaccine strain carrying *C. jejuni* 72Dz/92 *cja*A gene elicits specific humoral immune response associated with protection against challenge with wild-type *Campylobacter. Vaccine.* **22**:1379-1389.

Yuen, K.Y. and Wong, S.S. (2005) Human infection by avian influenza A H5N1. *Hong Kong Med. J.* **11**:189-99..

Yuki, N., Susuki, K., Koga, M., Nishimoto, Y., Odaka, M., Hirata, K., Taguchi, K., Miyatake, T., Furukawa, K., Kobata, T. and Yamada, M. (2004) Carbohydrate mimicry between human ganglioside GM1 and *Campylobacter jejuni* lipooligosaccharide causes Guillain-Barre syndrome. *Proc Natl Acad Sci* U S A ;**101**:11404-11409.

15

GENETICS AND NUTRITION: WHAT'S AROUND THE CORNER?

SAM HOSTE
Quantech Solutions, Orari Cottage, Howe Farm, Malton, North Yorks, YO17 6RG UK

Introduction

This chapter will start with an overview of where we are today and what is the current macro environment that we are operating in. The chapter will then focus on some of the challenges that geneticists and nutritionist share. Finally some highlights of what is around the corner will be presented.

Current market conditions are frequently described in business literature as turbulent from the effects of globalisation and agriculture generally, and animal science in particular is not immune to this situation. A visit to any UK supermarket to look at the fruit and vegetable section will show products from a vast array of countries. The decline in the numbers of farmers and the concomitant trend of increasing farm size in the Western world continues. UK farmers face global imports, downward pressure on prices from large retailer buyers (e.g. milk) uncertainty due to a new subsidy payment system (The Single Farm Payment). The UK is a market without boundaries

From all of this animal breeders predict and make selection decisions for future market needs sometimes years ahead. Although some could consider this a futile occupation, this chapter will try and develop some ideas for the future with reference to nutrition.

The nutrition and genetics of animals should be intimately linked in our thinking. Feed costs remain a major factor in the economics of animal production and therefore the optimisation of feed usage by animals is important to geneticists in making economic decisions.

Current challenges

RESEARCH

The current emphasis and funding of much Government-sponsored research is towards biotechnology and genomics (generally "-omics"). This is essential at a basic level of science; however, there is continued need for development and implementation of science. That this new science will flow linearly from scientist to users does not take into account many developments in knowledge about how innovation occurs or how knowledge is transferred (Rothwell, 2002). Generally animal science seems partly oblivious to the many social scientists and business academics with considerable expertise in innovation who work with many other types of businesses to improve their innovation stream. Research programmes also exhibit "fashions". For the last few years there has been substantial emphasis in pigs on piglet survival and in dairy cattle on fertility whereas a few years ago emphasis was elsewhere. This is to be expected in a science that responds to industry needs (so that a model of linear flow from scientist to user immediately fails) and operates within the political and social environments. Currently nutrition and genetics of farm animals does not appear "fashionable" whereas arguably they remain economically very important.

KNOWLEDGE TRANSFER

Again there is considerable scope to look outside of our own field and examine how other industries and researchers are tackling problems of knowledge transfer. From a UK animal science perspective we have dabbled and dipped our toes in the water, but we must refrain from re-inventing the wheel as there is a substantial body of work from other industries and disciplines that we can draw from (e.g. 2003 Management Science Special Issue on Managing Knowledge).

Knowledge transfer comprises a number of elements from the source, the message and the recipient. This process occurs in all sorts of contexts. One of the problems that both quantitative geneticists and nutritionists face with the new "-omics" sciences are that it is new, it is a different language and we may not be able to envisage or understand the potentials: we may not be able to ask the right questions. This is a challenge that increasingly we must address to utilise these techniques in our understanding of animals.

A gradual or multi-step approach is a possible model for learning about genomics and other molecular developments, by incrementally investing and gaining confidence. The Genesis Faraday Partnership (www.genesis-faraday.org) is an excellent example of a facilitating organisation that is actively bringing together genomics and the animal breeding and animal health companies. There are about 17 PhD studentships funded through Genesis Faraday and many other industrial sponsorships in place. I would encourage involvement and engagement as a step in learning about genomics.

That knowledge transfer or what was known as "extension" is needed is shown in a series of papers by Thirtle and Holding (http://statistics.defra.gov.uk/esg/reports/prodagri/). These papers describe the technical change in Total Factor Productivity (TFP) of UK agriculture between 1982 and 1997.

Table 1. Annual technical change and the inefficiency of the average farm.

Species	Technical change	Marginal effect of inefficiency: time
Cereals (For comparison)	0.058*	-0.008
Dairy	0.015	-0.005
Sheep	0.007	-0.0009
Poultry	0.028	-0.0016
Pigs	0.025	-0.002

* Technical change describes the production frontier through time
Paper 6 Efficiency and productivity at the farm level in England and Wales.

The second column in Table 1 shows the technical change, for example cereals the figure estimate is 0.058 which shows that the frontier is moving at nearly 6% annually, i.e. the most efficient farms – those that define the frontier – are becoming more efficient through time. The third column shows the marginal effects which indicate the strength of influence and direction the variable has on efficiency (See Wilson *et al.* (2001) for details). There are a number of variables considered in the model, however here the focus is on time which shows how the average farm changes through the period. It indicates how the average farm is keeping up with or falling behind the frontier. For cereals it indicates that the average efficiency has been declining by 0.8% per year.

Apart from sheep farms, all farms operate with high levels of efficiency and close to the frontier (not shown here, but included in the papers); however the average farm is becoming less efficient over time in all species. Thus what was previously called extension and perhaps is now called Knowledge

Transfer is increasingly important so that farmers adopt new technologies and stay close to the frontier.

Where are we now?

Animal breeding technologies are currently being applied using the latest quantitative genetics methods throughout the world. The level of technology usage in different species often reflects the industry scale. Information on actual breeding programmes is more available under publicly funded projects and less available from companies. Estimates of the improvement in livestock species since 1960 to the present are given in van der Steen *et al.* (2005), overall giving an average percentage change of over 50%.

Table 2. Improvement in livestock species from the 1960s to present

Species	Trait	1960s	Performance Present	% change
Pigs	Pigs weaned/sow/year	14	21	50
	Lean %	40	55	37
	Feed conversion ratio (FCR)	3	2.2	27
	Lean meat, kg/t of feed	85	170	100
Broliers	Days to 2kg	100	40	60
	Breast meat %	12	20	67
	FCR	3	1.7	43
Layers	Eggs/yr	230	300	30
	Eggs/t of feed	5000	9000	80
Dairy	Milk production/cow lactation, kg	6000	10000	67
Average				>50

The table provides an indication of change rather than accurate estimates

BRIEF SUMMARY INFORMATION ON EACH SECTOR

Dairy

Dairy cattle breeding shows widespread and coordinated development and processing of quantitative information using animal models. There is a relatively high concentration of companies and countries (USA, Holland, New Zealand). The use of genomic information is underway by Livestock Improvement Corporation in New Zealand. Most production of milk is from pure-breeding American Holstein (Hansen, 2006) which is in contrast to many other species where crossing is exploited to utilise heterosis. Evaluation has predominantly been selection for milk yield (where there has been tremendous genetic responses) and type traits.

Beef cattle

In beef cattle there is use of quantitative information evaluated using animal models but with relatively small herd sizes in many countries. Genetic evaluations are often undertaken at a national level rather than by individual companies in UK, USA, Australia and New Zealand. At present there is relatively little use of genomics.

Sheep

Genetic improvement of sheep is very country and breed dependent. In both Australia and New Zealand there are large flock sizes undertaking genetic improvement, whereas in the UK the relatively small individual flock size, the lack of connectedness between populations to best enable evaluation, and the stratification structure all hinder genetic improvement. In Australia, Sheep Genetics Australia was established to provide a single across flock genetic evaluation for both meat and wool sheep with over 1 million animals in the database of growth, carcase, wool, faecal eggs count and reproductive data. A complete animal model fitting the direct genetic, various maternal effects and permanent environmental effect due to the dam can be fitted (Brown, 2006). In New Zealand Landcorp with approximately 100,000 ewes utilises genetic markers to enable parentage testing so the "lambing beat" (where people assigned lambs to ewes soon after birth) is unnecessary as well as facilitating genomic evaluation.

Pigs

Pig production is increasingly concentrated in larger and fewer firms. Globally there are 2 to 3 predominant genetics companies together with a number of other smaller companies. In the USA some companies have very successfully taken the genetic supply within-house, e.g. Smithfield Premium Genetics. Genetic improvement and evaluation in contrast to ruminants is generally within company. Genetic evaluation by all these companies will be by some form of animal model. In contrast to beef and sheep, genetic evaluations are run weekly. Some companies include some form of selection for improved survival, robustness (e.g. Knap and Luiting,1999; Danavl, 2004; Koeleman, 2005) and selection using crossbred information and some utilise DNA marker information.

Chicken (layers and broilers) and turkey

Poultry breeding is concentrated in 2 to 3 companies who are responsible for over 0.9 of the global breeding stock in each sector (FABRE, 2006). Information on the state of quantitative genetics is not readily available. Some companies are currently investing in genomic technology (Avendaño, 2005).

Undesirable effects of selection for high production

There have been a number of undesirable effects of selection in farm animals which will be summarised (for an extensive review see: Rauw *et al.*, 1998). In female dairy cattle fertility, calving ease, health and survival have been ignored until recently in the USA Holstein population, whereas the Scandinavian countries have long placed considerable selection emphasis on mastitis resistance and survival (Rauw *et al.*, 1998). Inbreeding in Holsteins represents a considerable challenge with two bulls comprising 0.3 of the Holstein breed in 2005. With inbreeding increasing by about 0.15%/year heifers born in 2005 have an average inbreeding of 5.1% close to the traditional maximum recommendation of 6.25% for commercial production. The effective population size of the USA Holstein breed in 2004 calculated by the method of Falconer (1981) was only 60, despite the fact that there are 3.7 million cows in the USA.

In poultry the intense selection for growth has affected pectoral myopathy, reduced immunological competence, increased the incidence of skeletal disorders, and cardiovascular disorders such as ascites (Thorp and Luiting, 2000). Flock *et al.* (2005) describe how poultry breeding companies now focus selection on components of liveability such as feather pecking and cannibalism in layers and on leg and heart disorders in broilers to address these fitness constraints and counteract unfavourable trends.

In the pigs prior to the separation into specific sire and dam lines, selection pressure on fast growth and a reduction in backfat had a detrimental effect on sow reproduction; examples from the UK being "thin sow syndrome" and the second litter drop in performance where the second litter size was lower than in the first parity. Subsequently, selection of dam-line females for reproductive traits and the use of increased feed level for sows have largely removed this as a problem.

Traditionally there has been *ad-hoc* independent culling for feet and leg quality traits which have subsequently been incorporated into leg scores and incorporated into the selection criterion using BLUP (Knap, 2006). Knap (2006) reported a heritability estimate of around 0.25 with both favourable (+0.26) and unfavourable (-0.28) genetic correlations with production traits.

What of the future: setting the scene

In the last century (certainly in the West) there have been significant changes in the food sector. This has moved from a supply orientated production system where the goal was to increase the level of production to one of embracing a wider set of societal needs.

For animal breeding companies to be sustainable they must be profitable and therefore they must supply breeding stock that remains profitable for the whole food chain: producers, processors and retailers. At the same time they must meet ever increasing societal needs in terms of efficacy, ecological impact, welfare, health, food miles, perceived quality and safety. The agro-food sector needs to give attention not only to "prosperity", but also to "planet" and "people" (Latesteijn, 2006).

Beck (1992) in his seminal work "Risk society. Towards a new modernity" describes our society as perceiving risk in a new way that is substantially different from the risk of say cutting one's finger with a knife.

"The existence of and distribution of risks and hazards are mediated on *principle through argument* (Authors own italics)...Many of the newer risks completely escape human powers of direct observation. The focus is more and more on hazards which are neither visible nor perceptible to the victims" (Beck 1992).

There are critics of his uncritical use of some examples, however the work is a challenging thesis on modern society and he raises a number of issues regarding societal concerns that are pertinent to the livestock industry. One of his concepts is that modern society is able to question industry actions and then use a totally new vocabulary and new priority order outwith the industry – using a "different system of reference" (Beck 1992). It could be argued that, certainly in the UK, agriculture is undergoing this sort of transformation. This use of new vocabulary is important for example when we undertake surveys and ask questions based on our perceptions which may be very different from the questions that society would ask of us. An example is from meat quality assessment where the emphasis has largely been on intrinsic cues (cues that are part of the physical product, like its appearance) rather than extrinsic cues (everything else). We may be asking questions about colour, visual appearance, etc. whereas the public are concerned about food safety, GMOs and pesticide residues (Grunert, 2006).

The future therefore appears to hold a number of additional priorities and also incorporating other ways of looking at what we are doing. As usual there will be challenges and opportunities for those that embrace them.

INDUSTRY SETTING AND STRUCTURE

It is worth noting that animal breeding companies relative to other industries are not particularly large. There are small multi-national organisations (MNCs) in the dairy, poultry and to some extent in the pig sectors. The pig sector is in an intermediate position with MNCs and Small to Medium Enterprises (SME) whereas beef and sheep breeding are predominated by SMEs who record through some central recording program, often at country level.

Besides the continuing concentration across all sectors there are changes in the business model. The pig sector in the USA is characterised by vertically integrated operations combining both producer and processor. These companies have found benefit from removing market transactions and therefore costs from their organisation; however this approach involves expertise at all functions (processing and farming) and this is not always readily achievable.

The livestock sector is not especially developed in its supply chain as for example the vegetable sector in the UK (e.g. See Figure 1. The UK meat sector operates mostly in chains 1 and 2 compared with 3 and 4 as in the UK vegetable sector). Currently within the UK there are developments by the Red Meat Industry Forum to explore and utilise Lean techniques (Womack and Jones, 2003) within the supply chain, predominantly in the processing sector. More integration of the supply chain beyond a just a purely transactional basis would enable the better dissemination and exploitation and enable differentiation by the whole chain. Fundamentally producers and breeders have to convince processors and retailers that there is value to be gained from conducting business beyond a purely transactional relationship.

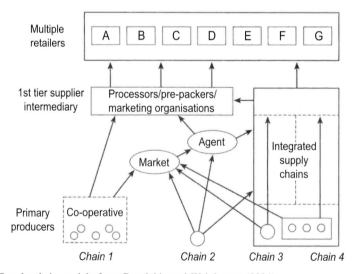

Figure 1. Supply chain models from Bourlakis and Weightman (2004)

SELECTION

Animal breeders have traditionally thought of selection objectives in terms of "production" traits. There is need for a change in emphasis towards a wider goal incorporating "planet" and "people" concomitant with "profit". The breeding goal can readily be expanded to incorporate a number of novel aspects to satisfy societal needs. A few examples of these will be suggested.

ANIMAL ROBUSTNESS

This can mean the ability of an animal to combine a high production potential with resilience to stressors (ability to regain balance after a disturbance), and resistance (allow for expression of high production potential in a wide variety of environments (Knap, 2006 ; ten Napel, 2006).

There are a number of indicator traits that can be usefully used to improve the objective traits of survival prior to weaning, survival during the growing period and survival of sows.

During the pre-weaning period such indicator traits are still birth rate, pre-weaning mortality and individual birth weight that have been described and utilised by pig breeding companies (Knol, 2001). Similarly growing pig mortality can be recorded and for sows culling age and reasons, leg and udder quality.

Many of these traits have low heritabilities, are relatively difficult to measure and are substantially affected by the production environment but also have substantial genetic variation. It would be ideal to measure these traits in the production environment but that requires individual recording of some commercial sows and piglets with semen from nucleus AI boars being used (Knap 2006), and results obtained prior to selection decisions being made at nucleus level.

An additional societal benefit from robustness is in reducing the use medicines and therefore the possible risk of residues in meat.

SENSITIVITY ACROSS ENVIRONMENTS

The sensitivity of genotypes to different environments has been an interest of geneticists for a considerable time (Lynch and Walsh, 1998). In animal breeding often this has been expressed as a genotype * environment interaction. More recently the approach using reaction norms has been described in an animal breeding context (Kolmodin *et al.*, 2002; Kolmodin

2004; Strandberg *et al.*, 2000; Knap 2005). The extension from the categorical description of the environment as 'high' versus 'low' or 'hot' versus 'cold' to a continuous scale enables a genotype to be described by two parameters. The intercept is a measure of an animal's genetic potential and the slope measures the animal's sensitivity to the environment. Once this is done, performance can be predicted across the range of environments on the horizontal axis. Knap (2006) describes the use of such a model and incorporation into the breeding goal. This approach would also seem to be interesting to evaluate against existing nutrition-genetic models where performance has to be predicted across a range of climatic environments.

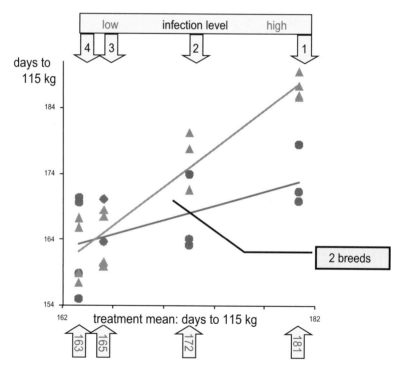

Figure 2. Growth rate of female and castrated male pigs of 2 genotypes (European and USA) in 4 health environments (1 conventional weaning and continuous flow no medication; 2 conventional weaning and continuous flow and medication; 3 segregated early weaning and no medication, and 4 all in all out housing and medication). The horizontal axis gives the mean growth rate of all sexes and genotypes in each environment. Modified from Schinckel *et al.* (1999, Fig. 1)

ENVIRONMENTAL IMPACT

A major achievement of animal breeding and one with a favourable effect on the environment has been the significant improvement in animal efficiency. There is a benefit from the improved efficiency in the animal's use of nitrogen and phosphate and therefore minimising the output of these elements into the environment (FABRE, 2006). There is also a reduction in the quantity of actual food (crops) that are needed; freeing land for other uses and reducing the transportation costs.

Further opportunities exist to improve animal efficiency: genes whose expression is regulated by nutrition and genetic variation in digestion and absorption efficiency (FABRE, 2006). Genetic improvement in crops with specific attributes for animals such as gross composition, amino acid balance, digestibility and processing properties (Warkup, 2004). Animal waste is a leading source of phosphorus pollution from agriculture (Jongbloed and Lenis, 1998). Cereal diets in pigs contain 0.33 to 0.80 of their phosphorus in the form of myo-inositol hexakis dihydrogen phosphate (phytate) complexed with minerals (Jongbloed and Kemme, 1990). Pigs do not digest this form and it is concentrated in the faeces by a factor of 3 to 4 fold (unpublished results in Phillips *et al.*, 2006). There are various nutritional methods to reduce the faecal and urinary output from pigs, and additionally plant breeders could select for more digestible cereal grains. Alternatively a pig that expresses the salivary phytase transgene, the Enviropig™ has been developed (Ward, 2000).

In dairy cattle (Garnsworthy, 2004) has modelled restoration of fertility back to 1995 levels which would reduce methane emissions by 10 to 11% and ammonia emissions by about 9%. Both genetic (Royal *et al.*, 2002) and nutritional (Garnsworthy and Webb, 1999) approaches have been suggested.

A research study in Ireland suggested that maximising dairy herd survivability would reduce the number of replacement stock needed and lower the methane emissions significantly (Berry *et al.*, 2003)

Selection for low residual feed intake (the difference between actual and expected feed intake) in feedlot cattle has demonstrated the possibility of reducing methane emissions by 28% (Nkrumah et al., 2006)

DISEASE RESISTANCE

Incorporating general or specific disease resistance into the selection goal is an area of considerable research interest at the moment and one where genomic approaches offer advantages. Minimising the use of medicines and vaccines is one direct benefit, but also tailoring medicines for specific genotypes represents another. Minimising the risk that animals will be carriers of zoonotic disease is another area where there is heightened awareness due to "Bird flu".

In New Zealand and Australian sheep population faecal egg counts are used to measure resistance to worms. There has been successful marker assisted selection (MAS) in pigs where the polymorphism in the FUT1 gene determines susceptibility of pigs to Escherichia coli F18 (Meijerink *et al.*, 2000). In sheep, MAS for the PrP allele for scrapie is compulsory in Europe and in New Zealand testing is on-going for a foot-rot marker (Hickford *et al.*, 2005; Bates and Hickford, 2005). In France collaboration between INRA, LABOGENA and 8 breeding companies are selecting for somatic cell score as an indicator for susceptibility to mastitis (Boichard *et al.*, 2002).

THE NEED FOR DATA

Satisfying the wider societal and environmental goals will need better and more sophisticated individual animal recording. The greater use of databases and animals individually identified with bar codes and electronic identification are important to obtaining accurate survival data on individuals.

Conclusion

There is an increasing number of goals that animal breeders can address through the integration of quantitative and genomic approaches to benefit society. This is an enormous opportunity to enable product differentiation between companies in their offering to the consumer. The fact the Governments may demand changes (e.g. with selection for the PrP allele) and that societal needs grow in scope should not be taken as a threat but an opportunity for animal breeders to use quantitative and genomic selection tools that can help to satisfy these needs. One of the prerequisites is that producers and breeders remain profitable. As animal feed is a major cost factor in production the research emphasis for genetics and nutrition will remain important to future profitability. There is a need for increased knowledge transfer of new "-omics" technologies both for nutritionists and quantitative geneticists.

References

Avendaño, S. (2005) 1st European Farm Animal Functional Genomics Workshop, Edinburgh.
Bates, J. and Hickford, J.G. (2005) *Final report to the Ministry of Agriculture*

and Forests - Sustainable Farming Fund. (http://www.merinoinc.co.nz/
MerinoIncReports.htm)

Beck (1992). Risk Society: Towards a New Modernity. Sage Publications Ltd.

Berry, D.P., F. Buckley, P. Dillon, R.D. Evans, M. Rath and R.F. Veerkamp.
(2003), http://www.irishgrassland.com/2003/Journal/Dairy/
Dairy%20Donagh%20Berry.PDF (Accessed 24/08/2006)

Boichard, D., Fritz, S., Rossignol, M.N., *et al.* (2002) *Proc. 7th* World Congress
on Animal Genetics Applied to Livestock Production. 7 : 22.03.

Bourlakis M and Weightman P, 2004. *Food Supply Chain Management.* Blackwell
Science.

Brown, D., (2006) Proc. 8th World Congress on Animal Genetics Applied to
Livestock Production, 7: 05-03.

Danavl. (2004) *Annual report 2004.* Landsutvalget for Svin, Copenhagen.

FABRE (2006) *Sustainable Farm Animal Breeding and Reproduction- A vision
for 2025.* FABRE Technology Platform. ISBN 90-76642-23-0. http://
www.fabretp.org/content/view/19/39/

Falconer, D.S. (1981) *Introduction to Quantitative Genetics.* Longman House,
Essex, UK.

Flock, D.K., Laughlin, K.F. and Bentley, J. (2005) *World's Poultry Sci. J.* **61** :
227-237.

Garnsworthy, P.C., (2004). *Animal Feed Science and Technology* **112**, 211-223.

Garnsworthy, P.C., Webb, R., 1999. In: Garnsworthy, P.C. Wiseman, J. (Eds.),
Recent Advances in Animal Nutrition-1999. Nottingham University Press,
Nottingham, pp. 39–57.

Grunert, K.G., (2006) *Meat Science* **74**, 149-160.

Hansen, L.B. (2006) Proc. 8th World Congress on Animal Genetics Applied to
Livestock Production, **8**: 01-01

Hickford, J.G.H., Davies, S., Zhou, H., *et al.* (2005) *Proc. N.Z. Soc. Anim. Prod.*
65 : 117-122.

Knap, P.W. and Luiting, P. (1999) *Abstr. 50th EAAP, paper GPh5.2.*

Knap, P.W. (2005) *Austr. J. Exp. Agr.* **45** : 763-773.

Knap, P. (2006) Proc. 8th World Congress on Animal Genetics Applied to
Livestock Production, **8**: 06-01.

Knol E.F., 2001. Genetic aspects of piglet survival. In. PhD Thesis. Wageningen
University.

Koeleman, E. (2005) *Pig Progress* **21** (5) : 6-7.

Kolmodin, R., Strandberg, E., Danell, B., and Jorjani, H. (2004). *Acta Agric.
Scand. Section A (Animals).* **54**: 139-151

Kolmodin, R., Strandberg, E., Madsen, P., Jensen, J., and Jorjani, H. (2002). *Acta
Agric. Scand. Section A (Animals).* **52**: 11-24

Jongbloed, A.W. and Kemme, P.A. (1990). *Neth. J. Agric. Sci.* **38**:567-575.

Jongbloed, A.W. and Lenis, N.P. (1998) *J. Anim. Sci.* **76**:2641-2648.

Latesteijn (2006). *Inventions for a sustainable development of agriculture.* Transform working paper No 1.

Lynch M, Walsh B, 1998. Genetics and Analysis. Sinauer Associates Inc.

Meijerink, E., S. Neuenschwander, R. Fries, A. Dinter, H. U., Bertschinger, G. Stranzinger, and P. Voegeli. 2000. A DNA polymorphism influencing α(1,2) fucosyltransferase activity of the pig FUT1 enzyme determines susceptibility of small intestinal epithelium to Escherichia coli F18 adhesion. *Immunogenetics*, **52**, 129-36.

Nkrumah, J.D., Okine, E.K., Mathison, G.W., Schmid, K., Li, C., Basarab, J.A., Price, M.A., Wang, Z., Moore, S.S., 2006. *J. Anim Sci.* **84**, 145-153.

Phillips, J. P., Golovan, S. P., Meidinger R.G and Forsberg C W (2006) Proc. 8th World Congress on Genetics Applied to Livestock Production. 8: 19-02

Rauw, W. M., Kanis, E., Noordhuizen-Stassen, E. N. and Grommers, F. J. (1998) *Livest. Prod.Sci.* **56**: 15-33

Rothwell, R., (2002) In *Managing Innovation and Change.*(Eds. Henry J and Mayle D.). Sage Publications Ltd. Pp 115-135.

Royal, M.D., Flint, A.P.F., Woolliams, J.A., (2002) *J. Dairy Sci.* **85**, 958–967.

Strandberg, E., Kolmodin, R., Madsen, P., Jensen, J., and Jorjani, H. (2000). *Interbull Bulletin.* **25**: 41-45

Schinckel A. P., Richert B. T., Frank J. W. and Kendall D. C. (1999) http://www.ansc.purdue.edu/swine/swineday/sday99/13.pdf

Ten Napel J. (2006) In *Inventions for a sustainable development of agriculture.* (Eds. Latesteijn, 2006). Transform working paper No 1.

Thirtle and Holding http://statistics.defra.gov.uk/esg/reports/prodagri/ (Accessed 24/08/2006)

Thorp, B.H. and Luiting, P. (2000) In *Breeding for disease resistance in farm animals* (eds. R.F.E. Axford, S.C. Bishop, F.W. Nicholas and J.B. Owen). CABI, Wallingford. Pp. 357-377.

van der Steen, H.A.M., Prall, G.F.W., Plastow, G.S. (2005) *J. Anim Sci.* **83**, E1-E8.

Ward, K. A. (2000) *Trends Biotechnol.* **18**:99-102.

Warkup, C. (2004) In *The Appliance of Pig Science* (Eds. Thompson J E, Gill B P and Varley M A) Nottingham University Press.

Wilson, P., Hadley, D., & Asby, C. 2001. The influence of management characteristics on the technical efficiency of wheat farmers in eastern England. *Agricultural Economics*, **24**, 329-338.

Womack J P and Jones D T, 2003. *Lean Thinking.* Publ. Simon and Schuster.

16

SOW AND BOAR NUTRITION: MODERN NUTRITION FOR MODERN GENOTYPES

W H CLOSE

Close Consultancy, Wokingham (Berkshire) will@closeconsultancy.com

The objective of modern pig production is to maximise the quantity and quality of pig meat produced per sow per year, or per lifetime, at minimal cost. A major component is to ensure that the sow produces an adequate number of piglets per year, or per lifetime, and nutrition is a key element in achieving this, since it has a major effect on the chief components of litter size, that is ovulation rate, fertilisation rate and embryo survival, as well as the number of litters per sow per year.

One of the major achievements in pig production over the last thirty years has been the improvement in sow productivity from about 17 to 22 piglets reared per sow per year (Table 1). However, this is well below the often quoted potential of 30 piglets per sow per year. In fact, on some farms in Denmark, 30 piglets per sow per year are reputedly consistently achieved (Jensen and Peet, 2006).

Table 1. Changes in sow performance during the last 30 years (MLC/BPEX)

	1975	1980	1985	1990	1995	2000	2005
Litters/sow/year	2.0	2.18	2.25	2.23	2.25	2.26	2.22
Piglets born alive/litter	10.4	10.3	10.4	10.7	10.8	11.0	10.9
Piglets reared/sow/year	17.5	19.8	20.9	21.1	21.6	22.4	21.5
Annual sow disposals (%)	33.9	35.9	38.1	40.0	42.6	42.0	46.2
P_2 at 100 kg (mm)	22	19	14.5	13.0	11.5	11.0	10.7

Interestingly, the improvement in sow productivity has not come about by large increases in the number of piglets born alive per litter, but more by improvements in nutritional knowledge and dietary formulation, management, husbandry, housing and stockmanship, as well as a better understanding of the healthcare needs of the animal. A contributory factor has been the reduction in weaning age. Of major benefit has been the greater understanding of the nutritional physiology of the pig, which has allowed specific strategies to be adopted and applied in the different conditions under which sows and boars are kept.

Compared with sows some 30 years ago, the modern sow has become leaner, with body fat being reduced by as much as 50%, according to the decrease in backfat thickness (Table 1). This has not only changed the metabolic needs of the sow, but has also made modern genotypes more sensitive to nutrition than their predecessors, which had ample body reserves at the start of their breeding life. These reserves helped to buffer the animal against extreme shortfalls and periods when nutrient demands outstripped nutrient supply. This situation has become further exacerbated in the modern sow, since selection for lean tissue feed efficiency may have inadvertently resulted in animals with lower voluntary feed intakes. Thus, in the design of nutritional strategies, consideration must be given to the whole cycle and lifetime performance of the animal and not just the separate phases of reproduction.

In summary, the following reflect some of the changes in the characteristics of the modern sow:

• Change in body composition: higher lean : fat ratio
• Greater mature body size
• Drive in early parities to achieve a certain lean body mass
• Higher litter size and piglet growth rates
• Higher milk yield
• Reduced appetite potential
• Greater differences in nutrient requirements
• Less flexibility in nutritional management
• Greater 'carry-over' effects from one parity to another
• Animals are more sensitive to nutrition, environment and management stressors

Targets for the modern breeding sow

Production targets for 'average' and 'good' levels of performance are suggested in Table 2.

Table 2. Production targets for the modern sow

	Average	Good
Sow replacement rate (%)	40	35
Farrowing rate (%)	85	90
Litters / sow / year	2.3	2.4
Empty days * / year	>35	<20
Piglets born alive / litter	11.3	12.5
Piglets weaned / litter	10.2	11.3
Piglets reared / sow / year	23.5	27.0
Piglet weight at weaning ** (kg)	8.0	8.0
Litter weaning weight (kg)	82	90
Sow feed consumed / piglet weaned (kg)	50	50
Litters per sow lifetime	4	5

* A 7-day weaning – mating period has been allowed
** Piglets weaned at 28 days of age

Analysis of the results of several herd recording schemes, such as that of the Meat and Livestock Commission (MLC, 1995-2002), would suggest that the major difference between the bottom- and top-producing herds is the number of piglets born and born alive, as well as the number of litters produced per sow per year (Table 3). Interestingly, the difference between the total number of piglets born and those weaned, at 2 piglets per litter, was similar across all herds, regardless of the level of productivity. This perhaps suggests that in order to improve performance, there must be an increase in either ovulation and/or fertilisation rate and a decrease in embryo losses, as well as knowledge of those factors that influence them. Similarly, in order to increase the number of litters per sow per year, there must be a reduction in the period between weaning and mating, as well as a decrease in the number of sows that return or fail to come into oestrus.

Table 3. Litter size in herds of varying productivity (MLC, 1995-2002)

	Bottom 1/3	Average	Top 1/3	Top 10 %
Piglets				
Total born	11.4	11.9	12.3	12.7
Born alive	10.5	11.0	11.4	11.8
Weaned	9.3	9.8	10.2	10.6
Sows				
Litters / sow / year	2.12	2.25	2.34	2.41
Piglets / sow / year	19.7	22.0	23.9	25.6
Non-productive days	53	37	26	13

If improvements are to be made and potential losses reduced, it is important to understand how the different components of litter size impact on reproductive performance and the major factors that influence them. These are outlined in Figure 1, demonstrating the importance not only of nutrition, but also of management.

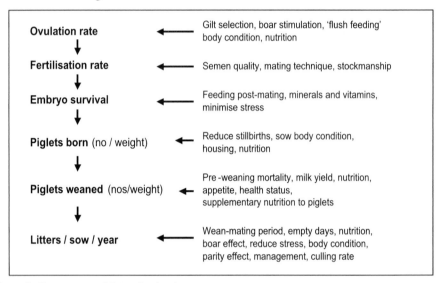

Figure 1. Components of litter size in pigs

If appropriate nutritional and management strategies are to be developed to optimise productivity, it is important to establish target values for both the body weight and body condition of the gilt and sow at the different stages of each parity and overall. Suggested values are provided in Table 4. The overall objective should be to achieve a constant body weight of 230-250 kg and a P_2 backfat thickness of about 24 mm at each mating from parity 5 onwards.

Table 4. Suggested target body weight and P2 values at mating (Close and Cole, 2000)

Parity	Body weight at mating (kg)	Net body weight change (kg)		P_2 at mating (mm)	P_2 change (mm)	
		Pregnancy	Lactation/ post-weaning		Pregnancy	Lactation / post-weaning
1	140	50	-15	20	+4	-2
2	175	40	-15	22	+3	-2
3	200	30	-10	23	+3	-2
4	220	25	-10	24	+2	-2
5	235	20	-10	24	+2	-2
6	245	15	-10	24	+2	-2

Gilt condition and management

The body condition of the gilt at first mating has a significant effect on sow lifetime performance. Animals that do not have sufficient body condition when first selected and introduced on to the farm generally fail to achieve a reasonable number of parities. The better the body condition, the better the lifetime performance of the animal (Gueblez *et al.*,1985; Gaughan *et al.*, 1995; Challinor *et al.*, 1996). The gilt must therefore be sufficiently mature, of appropriate body condition and have adequate reserves of lean and fat in her body. The latter is necessary not only to initiate the reproductive processes *per se*, but also to act as a buffer in times of nutritional inadequacy, when metabolic needs exceed nutrient intake. In addition, body reserves are also needed to protect the animal in poor environmental circumstances.

The young gilt should therefore be of sufficient age, size, maturity and achieve a certain target body condition at first mating. Suggested guidelines are:

210-230 days of age
125 - 145 kg body weight
16 - 20 mm P_2 backfat thickness
Mating at 2nd or 3rd oestrus

To achieve these, it is suggested that the young breeding gilt be selected at ~60 kg body weight and put on a special gilt rearer diet and feeding regime, as indicated in Table 5. The best practical strategy to ensure maximum ovulation rate and embryo survival in gilts is to provide a high feeding level for the oestrus cycle before mating, that is flush feeding, followed by a low feeding level for the first 21 days post-mating (Ashworth and Pickard, 1998).

Table 5. Phased feeding regime for gilts*

	Body weight (kg)	Age (days)	Backfat thickness (P_2 mm)	MJ DE per kg diet	Lysine (g) (kg/d)	Feeding strategy
Phase 1	25 - 60	60 - 100	- 7	14.0	12.0	*ad-libitum*
Phase 2	60 - 125	100 - 210	7 - 16	13.5	8.0	2.5 - 3.5
Phase 3	125 - 140	210 - 230	16 - 18	13.5	8.0	*ad-libitum*
Phase 4	early gestation	230 - 260	18	13.5	8.0	2.0

* These are suggested values. Body weight and backfat thickness may vary slightly, depending on genotype and environmental circumstances.

The gilt rearer diet should not only contain the correct level of energy and amino acids, but should also be fortified with specific minerals and vitamins that help to stimulate reproduction *per se* and ensure the strong bones and legs that are vital for a long breeding life (see Tables 12 and 14). Culling because of leg and foot problems is all too common on many farms.

Nutrition during gestation: energy and lysine requirements

During gestation, the objective should be to feed the sow for a specific body gain and increase in backfat thickness (Table 4) and to achieve a body condition score of 3.5 at parturition (Scale: 1-5).

Designing a feeding and management strategy requires knowledge of the energy and nutrient needs at all stages of the reproductive cycle. The procedures for calculating the daily energy and lysine requirements of sows during gestation are well established and are based on the maintenance requirement of the animal (dependent on its body weight and body condition), the target maternal body weight gain (that is the daily rate of protein and fat gain, which changes with parity and the maturity of the animal), conceptus tissue and mammary tissue gain (Noblet *et al.*, 1990; Close and Cole, 2000; Boyd *et al.*, 2000 and BSAS, 2003).

Table 6. provides the mean energy and lysine requirements during gestation for sows of different body weights (mid gestation) and rates of maternal gain during gestation. The mean daily requirement for conceptus tissue was taken as 0.5 MJ/day.

Table 6. The energy and lysine requirements of sows of different body weight and maternal body weight gain during gestation (BSAS, 2003)

	Maternal gain (kg)	*Energy (MJ/day)*		*Lysine (g/day)*		*Feed intake[+] (kg/day)*
		NE	*DE*	*SIDL**	*Total*	
150 kg sow	20	18.3	24.9	8.5	10.1	1.9
	40	20.9	29.4	11.7	13.9	2.2
	60	23.5	33.8	14.8	17.6	2.5
225 kg sow	15	22.9	32.1	8.0	9.5	2.4
	27.5	25.0	35.5	9.6	11.4	2.7
	37.5	26.3	37.7	11.1	13.2	2.8
	50	28.5	41.1	12.7	15.1	3.0
300 kg sow	0	23.5	34.0	7.4	8.8	2.5
	5	25.2	36.4	7.8	9.4	2.7
	15.	26.0	38.6	8.9	10.6	2.8

* Standardised ileal digestible lysine. [+] Based on diet containing 13.2 MJ DE or 9.4 MJ NE/kg

The environmental conditions under which sows are kept will influence their nutrient, and, especially, their energy requirements. In general, for every 1°C decrease in temperature below the lower critical temperature, their feed allocation needs to be increased by approximately 4%, as discussed by Close and Poornan (1993).

The values in Table 6 are mean requirements throughout gestation. However, the requirements change as gestation progresses in association with the changing body weight of the animal and hence increasing maintenance needs, as well as the change in the rate and composition of the products formed. In early gestation the main tissue deposited is fat and protein in the maternal body tissue of the sow. However, in late gestation the main tissue deposition is in the growth of the foetal and mammary tissue. There is therefore a change in both the energy and amino acid requirements of the animals within the duration of gestation, as indicated in Figure 2 for a parity-1 gilt and a phase-feeding approach is recommended.

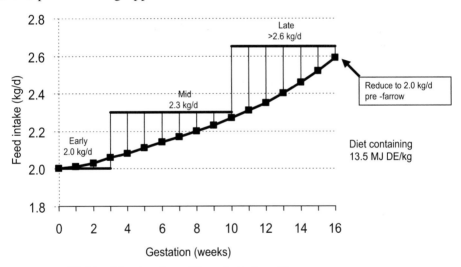

*Model predictions based on a gilt in excellent body condition

Figure 2. Feeding strategy for gilts in pregnancy

The feeding of the gilt just after mating differs from that of the mature sow, in that excessive feed intake in the gilt just after mating reduces embryo survival and hence, potential litter size. Increased embryo mortality in early pregnancy in gilts is associated with lower circulating levels of progesterone (Hughes and Pearse, 1989; Almeida *et al.*, 2000). Progesterone is required in preparing the uterus for embryo implantation and also influences the secretion of the uterine secretory hormones uteroferrin and retinol-binding protein, which enhance embryo survival (see review by van Wettere *et al.*, 2005). It is therefore recommended that gilts be fed 1.8-2.0 kg/day of a good quality gestation or gilt rearer ration for the first three weeks post mating.

On the other hand, in the mature sow, the level of feeding during early gestation does not appear to influence embryo survival. However, in sows that have lost a lot of body weight and body condition during the previous lactation, a high level of feeding may be beneficial. The amount to be fed will therefore depend on the extent of both the loss of body weight and body reserves during the previous lactation and in the post-weaning period. This is illustrated in Table 7 for a 200-kg sow at mating, but allowing for different condition scores and different levels of weight loss during the previous lactation and post weaning. Indeed, when body weight and condition loss is excessive, then it may be advisable to provide the lactation diet until the sow recovers this loss sufficiently. Once body weight and body condition have been restored, then the feed level will need to be adjusted to maintain the appropriate body condition. Feed levels will also need to be adjusted depending on both body weight and parity. A general rule is to increase feed intake by 0.2 kg/day for each parity.

Table 7. Suggested feed allowance for a 200 kg-sow in early gestation, depending on condition score and extent of body weight loss during previous lactation and post weaning

Body weight loss in lactation and post weaning (kg)	Condition score at mating (scale 1-5)	Increase in feed requirement (kg/d)	Feed intake (kg/day)
< 5 kg	3.0	0	2.4
10 – 15 kg	2.5	0.3	2.7
> 20 kg	2.0	0.5	3.0

The benefit of increased feed intake of sows in early gestation has been demonstrated by Love *et al.* (1993). They compared restricted with *ad libitum* feeding of group-housed sows under hot summer conditions. Pregnancy rates by seven weeks post-weaning were significantly higher when sows were fed *ad libitum*: 79.8, compared with 56.5% when fed restrictedly. This demonstrates the need to provide additional feed in early gestation to sows whose body condition has been compromised during lactation and post-weaning.

Maternal nutrition at key periods during gestation may influence foetal development through muscle fibre number development and consequently post-natal growth. For exampler, Dwyer *et al.* (1994) doubled sow feed intake between day 50 and 80 of gestation and found that it increased secondary muscle fibre number and form and improved subsequent growth rate and efficiency of feed utilisation in the pigs between 25 and 80 kg body weight.

However, this response was not borne out by Jagger (reported by Boyd, 2000), who fed sows 2.6 or 5.2 kg of a typical gestation ration between day 25 and 80 of gestation, but found no difference in growth rate or feed conversion efficiency of the progeny between 34 and 96 kg body weight. On the other hand, Penny *et al.* (2001) reported that higher levels of feeding between day 25 and 56 of gestation resulted in significant improvements in both growth rate (from 866 to 914 g/day) and feed conversion efficiency (from 2.18 to 2.09 g/g), compared with the progeny of control-fed sows. The response therefore is inconsistent and there may be other factors that come into play, such as the metabolic status and body condition of the sow.

Nutrition during lactation: energy and lysine requirements

During lactation, the objective should be to wean at least 10 piglets of good body weight, with minimal loss of body weight and body condition of the sow. Lactation is perhaps the most critical period in the life of the pig and the nutritional strategies implemented in this period influence both the growth and development of the piglets through to slaughter, as well as the subsequent reproductive potential of the sow and overall productivity.

Similar to gestation, the calculation of the energy and lysine requirements during lactation are based on the body weight of the sow (maintenance needs), the milk yield (dependent on the number of piglets and their growth rate) and any gain or loss of body weight - and its composition. The main energy and lysine need is for milk production, and as this increases during lactation, then the requirements for energy, lysine and feed increase (Table 8). Therefore the major objective of nutrition in lactation is to meet the requirement for milk production of the sow, which increases from about 3-4 l/day just after farrowing to 10-14 l/day in peak lactation.

The most effective feeding strategy for the sow is therefore to follow the milk yield of the sow: to feed conservatively for the first few days of lactation and then *ad libitum*, that is several times per day. Thus, the feed requirements increase with duration of lactation (Figure 3). In this respect aides, such as the Stotfold Sow Feeding Scale, are most helpful. Feeding the sow too much too soon after parturition may limit her appetite in later lactation when needs are greatest. In addition, it also helps to match feed intake more closely to the competence of the sow's digestive system; this safeguards the integrity of the gut and reduces the incidence of mastitis, metritis, agalactica (MMA).

Table 8. Energy and lysine requirements of lactating sows of different body weight and at different litter growth rates (after BSAS, 2005)

Litter growth rate (kg/d)	Energy (MJ/d)		Lysine (g/d)		Feed intake* (kg/d)
	NE	DE	SIDL[+]	Total	
Sow body weight: 150 kg					
1.5	40.7	57.5	33.1	39.4	4.10
2.0	51.5	73.6	43.2	51.4	5.25
2.5	62.3	89.7	53.3	63.5	6.40
Sow body weight: 225 kg					
2.25	61.5	89.4	49.2	58.5	6.38
2.75	72.3	105.4	59.4	70.7	7.53
3.25	83.1	121.5	69.5	82.7	8.67
Sow body weight: 300 kg					
2.50	70.9	104.5	54.3	64.6	7.46
3.20	81.7	120.6	64.4	76.6	8.61
3.50	92.5	136.7	74.5	88.7	9.76

* Based on the DE content of 14.0 MJ/kg (10.0 MJ NE/kg) [+] Standardised ileal digestible lysine

The feeding strategy during lactation aims to maximise energy and nutrient intake, that is feed intake. However, voluntary feed intake is often lower than that needed to ensure an adequate intake of energy and nutrients, and insufficient energy and nutrient intake leads to catabolism of body stores, especially body protein and fat, as well as minerals. Indeed, the higher the loss of body reserves during lactation, the lower the quality of the milk (Clowes *et al.*, 2003), the poorer the follicular development (Yang *et al.*, 2000), the greater the period between weaning and mating, the lower the ovulation rate and hence, subsequent litter size.

This is demonstrated by the work of Tritton *et al.* (1996) in relation to the lysine intake of first litter sows (Table 9). Optimum performance in terms of piglet growth rate was achieved at a lysine intake close to 60 g/day. However, at intakes below this level, both piglet growth rate and subsequent litter size was reduced. Johnson *et al.* (1993) also showed that piglet growth rate was responsive to lysine uptake up to 55 g/day in multiparous sows with a high potential for milk production.

To achieve adequate intakes in lactation, it is important to use good quality diets and soundly based feeding strategies. Some practical aids that may help in achieving good feed intakes in lactation are listed in Table 10. It may be necessary to feed several times per day, as a sow fed only twice per day may not be able to consume sufficient nutrients to meet metabolic demands, especially in late lactation. On the other hand, it is important not to over-feed in early lactation, as this may limit the animal's voluntary feed intake in later lactation when the needs are greatest; it may also predispose the sow to MMA.

Table 9. The effect of dietary lysine on the performance of sows during their first lactation and on subsequent reproductive performance (Tritton *et al.*, 1996)

Dietary lysine (g/kg)	6.2	8.4	10.6	13.1	15.1
Lysine intake (g/day)	28	37	45	60	68
Piglet growth rate (g/day)	187[a]	213[bc]	205[ab]	231[c]	210[b]
Subsequent litter size:					
Total born	10.3	9.9	10.4	11.6	11.0
Born alive	9.7	9.6	9.8	10.9	10.6

[abc] Values with different superscript are significantly different (p<0.05)

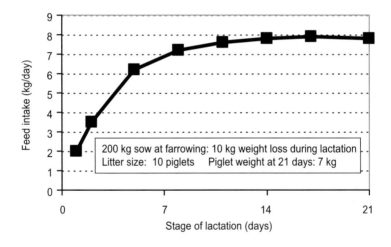

Figure 3. Feed requirement of the sow during lactation; diet containing 14.0 MJ DE (10.0 ME NE)/kg

Table 10. Practical aids to enhance appetite (Close and Cole, 2000)

- Feed a palatable, nutritious diet
- Feed a well-balanced ration of the appropriate nutrient specification
- Gradually increase daily intake over the first week, thereafter feed *ad libitum*
- Feed must be fresh, not stale or dirty
- Feed several times per day, or to appetite
- Pelleted feed is better than meal

- Ensure that fresh water is freely available at all times (consider wet-feeding)
- If nipple drinkers are provided, water flow rate must be >2 litres/minute
- Avoid exposing sow to high temperatures (>20°C) and reduce environmental stress
- Maintain good climatic control in farrowing house
- Do not overfeed in pregnancy
- Increase gut capacity by feeding high levels of soluble fibre in pregnancy diet
- Separate gestation and lactation diets are essential
- Ensure adequate feeding space
- Improve nutrient availability of diet
- Provide supplementary nutrition to piglets
- Reduce metabolic demand by cross-fostering or forward weaning
- Ensure good welfare and well-being of sow

A major limitation to achieving a good appetite during lactation is lack of water and water must always be provided in adequate quantities. If nipple drinkers are provided, then the flow rate must be at least 2 litres per minute. Large sows suckling large litters may need to consume 40 litres/day, especially under hot conditions. A lack of water restricts both the feed intake of the sow and her milk yield.

Post-weaning sows should be maintained on high intakes of the lactation ration to prompt a quick return to oestrus and to maximise subsequent litter size. Reducing the number of expensive 'empty' or non-productive days will mean more litters per sow per year.

Feeding strategy

A 3 to 5 diet feeding strategy best meets the changing nutritional and metabolic needs of the modern, hyperprolific sow and this helps to ensure optimum productivity of the sow and her offspring. During lactation, when feed intake is low, for example in first parity sows and during summer, it may be necessary to provide a diet of higher energy and nutrient specification compared with older sows and in winter, when intake is generally higher.

The following dietary specifications are therefore suggested:

Gilt rearer:	13.5	MJ DE	and	8.0 g lysine/kg
Pregnancy:	13.0	MJ DE	and	6.0 g lysine/kg
Lactation (general):	14.0	MJ DE	and	10.0 g lysine/kg
Lactation (gilts: low intake):	14.5	MJ DE	and	11.0 g lysine/kg
Lactation (sows: high intake):	13.5	MJ DE	and	9.0 g lysine/kg

As the lysine content of the diet is known, it is possible to calculate the content of other essential amino acids according to the concept of the 'ideal protein' (Table 11).

Table 11. The balance of essential amino acids for gestation and lactation in relation to lysine (=100) (Close and Cole, 2000; BSAS, 2003)

	Gestation		*Lactation*	
	Close & Cole (2000)	*BSAS (2003)*	*Close & Cole (2000)*	*BSAS (2003)*
Lysine	100	100	100	100
Threonine	70	71	59	66
Methionine	28	37	26	30
Methionine + Cystine	55	65	50	55
Valine	78	74	70	76
Isoleucine	70	70	59	60
Leucine	100	100	111	112
Phenylalanine	55	55	56	56
Phenylalanine+Tyrosine	100	100	111	114
Tryptophan	20	20	19	18
Histidine	33	33	35	40

A simple practical feeding strategy that best meets the requirements of the sow at all stages of pregnancy and lactation is illustrated in Figure 4. The feeding levels shown apply to gilts in parity 1; for older sows, feed intake in each subsequent pregnancy should therefore be increased by 0.2 kg/day, depending upon body condition.

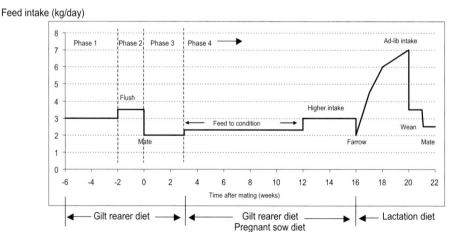

Figure 4. Overall feeding strategy (Parity 1)

Mineral requirements

Compared with energy and amino acid requirements, there is less information on the mineral needs of the modern sow. Suggested mineral allowances are provided in Table 12.

Table 12. Suggested mineral allowances for the breeding sow* (BSAS, 2003; BPEX/MLC, 2004)

	Suggested allowances (per kg diet)
Calcium (g/kg)	7.2 - 8.0
Phosphorus (digestible g/kg)	23 - 32
Sodium (g/kg)	1.7 – 2.0
Chloride (g/kg)	1.4 – 1.8
Potassium (g/kg)	2.5
Magnesium (%)	0.4
Copper (ppm)	6 – 15
Iodine (ppm)	0.2 – 2.0
Iron (ppm)	80 – 100
Manganese (ppm)	20 – 40
Zinc (ppm)	80 – 100
Selenium (ppm)	0.2 – 0.25
Cobalt (ppb)	0.2 – 0.5

* Higher values are for lactating sows

Much of the information on which current recommendations are made are based on work carried out 20-30 years ago when the productivity of sows was much lower than today. In addition, requirements are based on a per kg diet basis and do not take into account the daily metabolic needs of the sow, which changes with both body weight and level of productivity.

For example, it can be calculated that at the recommended rates of inclusion, and taking account of differences in feed intake, the mineral intake of mature sows is some 22% lower than that of first parity sows, when expressed per kg of body weight (Table 13). Mahan and Newton (1995) reported that the analysed body mineral content of sows after weaning their third litter of piglets was 15-20% lower than that of control, non-bred animals of similar age. Damgaard Poulsen (1994) has also reported a reduction in the mineral status of the sow and in suckling piglets with parity. These studies indicate that the levels of minerals recommended for the modern sow may be below those needed to optimise sow productivity. On the basis of the information presented in Table 13, the mineral content in the diet of the modern sow would need to be increased by approximately 5% with parity.

Table 13. Trace mineral intake in relation to sow body weight (BW) and parity

Mineral	Recommended[1] (mg/per kg diet)	Parity 1 (160 kg)[2] Intake		Parity 3+ (240 kg)[3] Intake		% Reduction in mineral intake (mg/kg BW)
		(mg/d)	(mg/kg BW)	(mg/d)	(mg/kg BW)	
Iron	100	300	1.87	348	1.45	22
Zinc	100	300	1.87	348	1.45	21
Copper	15	45	0.28	52	0.22	22
Manganese	40	120	0.74	139	0.58	22
Selenium	0.25	0.75	0.0047	0.87	0.0036	22

[1] MLC (2004)

[2] Animal fed 2.4 kg in gestation and 5.5 kg/day over a 26-day lactation

[3] Animal fed 2.8 kg in gestation and 6.5 kg/day over a 26-day lactation

[4] A 7-day post-weaning period has been assumed, with a feed intake of 3.5 kg/day

These results raise questions about the mineral needs of the modern sow, the actual mineral content in the diet and the availability to the animal, as well as the effect of the mineral status of the animal on overall productivity. This is especially pertinent to the sow, and Richards (1999) has shown that already in late gestation, the sow must rely on her liver iron reserves to meet foetal demands for the mineral.

Several studies have been carried out to establish if high level of dietary minerals could enhance sow productivity. For example, Cromwell *et al.* (1993) fed high levels of dietary copper to sows (250 ppm) over six parities and reported that their liver copper concentration increased by more than four-fold. There was no effect on reproductive performance, but birth weight and weaning weight of the piglets was increased. More recently, Boyd (2006) increased the mineral and vitamin content of both the gestation and lactation diets by 20-25% of sows from parity 3 onwards and reported an extra 0.6 piglet weaned per litter. This equates to 1.4 extra piglets weaned per sow per year, compared to control sows of similar parity.

Instead of increasing the mineral content of the diet with parity, an alternative would be to use more available sources of mineral, that is organic, rather than inorganic minerals. These are more bio-available and bio-active and have been reported to provide an advantage to the animal (Ammerman *et al.*, 1998).

Fehse and Close (2000) fed highly productive sows a special package of organic minerals (iron, zinc, manganese, copper, chromium and selenium) additional to the normal level of inorganic minerals over a 2-year period.

Over the peak parities (parities 3-6), 0.5 more piglets were weaned per litter from those sows fed the additional organic minerals and pre-weaning mortality was also reduced. Interestingly, it was also observed that a greater proportion of the 'supplemented' sows remained in the trial for a longer period of time compared with the 'control' sows. Similar improvements in sow productivity have been reported by Smits and Henman (2000). More recently, Lima *et al.* (2006) fed additional organic minerals to young sows from selection and reported an extra 0.7 piglets weaned during the first parity.

Mahan and Peters (2006) compared the form (inorganic or organic) and level of trace minerals (NRC (1998) or 'Industry') in the diet of sows over 6 parities. Industry levels were added, which were 50% and 200% times higher than the NRC (1998) levels for selected individual minerals. When NRC levels were fed, there was no difference in the number of live piglets born per litter. However, when industry levels were used, there was an additional piglet born per litter when organic minerals were provided compared with inorganic minerals. Performance of the sows fed the inorganic source of minerals at commercial levels was also below that of the NRC (1998) levels of inclusion, regardless of form. This suggests that when the dietary inorganic mineral inclusion may possibly be excessive, there is a reduction in the reproductive performance of sows; a response similar to that reported by Flowers *et al.* (2001). It is possible that increases in inorganic trace minerals, and especially in sulphate form, are linked to an accumulation of free radicals which may impair reproductive performance. In this respect, Mahan (2005) has suggested that organic sources of trace minerals may be more important than previously thought in preventing free radical accumulation and, as a consequence, enhancing reproductive performance.

Vitamin requirements

Although vitamins are needed for the normal functioning of the body, several play a specific role in reproduction; for example: vitamins A and B, Biotin, Folic acid and Choline. The requirements for these and the other fat- and water-soluble vitamins are presented in Table 14. Recently, Matte *et al.* (2006) have calculated in relation to B vitamins, that there is a greater need for updating information, considering the 'dietary fine-tuning' that is required for high producing pigs.

**Table 14.Suggested vitamin allowances for the breeding sow to be added per kg diet*
(BSAS, 2003; BPEX, 2004)**

Vitamin		Suggested allowances (per kg diet)
A (IU)	(Retinol)	7,500 – 12,000
D (IU)	(Calciferol)	800 – 2,000
E (IU)	(Tocopherol)	50
K (mg)	(Menadione)	1.5 – 2.0
B$_1$ (mg)	(Thiamin)	2
B$_2$ (mg)	(Riboflavin)	5
Niacin (mg)	(Nicotinic acid)	20 - 25
B$_6$ (mg)	(Pyridoxine)	3 – 4
B$_{12}$ (mg)	(Cyanocobalamin)	0.03
Pantothenic acid (mg)		15 – 20
Biotin (mg)		0.2 – 0.25
Folic acid (mg)		3
Choline (mg)		300
C	(Ascorbic acid)	-
Essential fatty acids (g)	linoleic acid	7
	arachidonic acid	5

* Higher values are for lactating sows

Nutrition of the boar

Despite the importance of the boar to herd productivity, there is only limited information available on which to base nutrient requirements.

In terms of rearing, most young boars are offered feed close to their appetite potential and at this level there is unlikely to be any effect upon sexual development or subsequent reproductive capacity.

Once they arrive on farm, boars should be managed to ensure adequate body development without becoming too large for effective service. Large boars can also have foot problems. The feeding regime should therefore aim to control body size, optimise libido and maintain a high level of fertility through good quality semen production.

ENERGY REQUIREMENT

The energy requirement of the working boar is calculated as the sum of that required for maintenance, for desired body weight gain, for semen production, as well as an extra component associated with activity at mating. As indicated in Table 15, the energy requirement increases from about 28.8 MJ DE for a 100 kg boar gaining 0.50 kg/day to 41.2 MJ DE/day for a 350 kg boar at maturity.

Table 15. Energy and feed requirements of the breeding boar (Close, 2005)

Body weight (kg)	100	150	200	250	300	350
Growth rate (kg/d)	0.50	0.40	0.30	0.20	0.10	0.0
Energy (MJ DE/d)	28.8	32.1	34.8	37.3	39.9	41.2
Feed intake (kg/d)*	2.2	2.5	2.7	2.9	3.1	3.2

* Based on a diet containing 13.0 MJ DE/kg

The major energy cost of the breeding boar is that associated with maintenance, representing between 0.6 and 0.9 of the total requirement. It is therefore important that boars are kept at or above their lower critical temperature of 20°C. If the temperature falls below this threshold, then the feed intake must be increased by 3% for every 1°C.

The energy requirement associated with semen production and mating activity is small and represents no more than 0.05 of the total requirements.

PROTEIN AND AMINO ACID REQUIREMENTS

Amino acid requirements will vary depending upon the body weight of the animal and its rate of growth. For the feed intakes provided in Table 11, a dietary requirement of approximately 7 g lysine/kg feed is proposed, with the same amino acid balance as that for the growing pig between 90 and 120 kg body weight (BSAS, 2003).

If the protein and amino acid intake of the boar is limited, then reproductive performance suffers. Louis *et al.* (1994) investigated the effects of protein alone or a combination of energy and protein intakes on semen characteristics. At similar levels of energy intakes (26.6 MJ DE/day), lowering the lysine intake of the boars from 18.1 to 7.7 g/day reduced the volume of the ejaculate and overall sperm output. Similar effects were also recorded when the energy intake was reduced from 33.6 to 26.6 MJ DE/day, at similar levels of lysine intake (18.1 g/day).

MINERAL AND VITAMIN REQUIREMENTS

Little information exists on the mineral and vitamin requirements for boars, but it is suggested that these should be the same as those used for the lactating sow. Special attention needs to be given to calcium, phosphorus and biotin, since these affect the overall soundness of the limbs. Similarly, zinc, selenium, vitamin E and vitamin C are essential for testicular and/or spermatogenic development and subsequent sperm motility. The source of the mineral may also be important and recent work by Jacyno *et al.* (2002) has shown that the addition of organic selenium + vitamin E significantly improved sperm concentration and the total number of sperm and significantly reduced the proportion of defective sperm compared with the addition of inorganic selenium + vitamin E to the diet of young boars.

FATTY ACID REQUIREMENT

Boar spermatozoa contain very high concentrations of long chain polyunsaturated fatty acids (PUFA), especially 22-carbon fatty acids: 22:6 n-3 (Docosahexaenoic acid; DHA) and 22:5 n-6 (Docosapentaenoic acid; DPA) and these are essential for sperm formation. Marine oils are good sources of long chain PUFAs and when added to the diet of boars, consistent increase in 22:6 n-3 and decrease in 22:5 n-6 concentration in sperm fatty acids have been observed (Rooke *et al.*, 2003) This has been shown to improve sperm concentration and viability and was reflected in improved sow productivity (Penny *et al.*, 2000).

Dietary implications

It is not just a question of providing a diet of correct nutrient specification to meet the needs of the modern sow and boar. Several feed ingredients generate pro-active responses and can improve sow productivity. For example, the feeding of soluble sources of fibre during gestation to enhance appetite and hence milk yield and composition in lactation (Meunier-Salaün, 2001); enhancing the anti-oxidative status through supplementation with vitamin E and selenium (Mahan, 2005); the importance of specific dietary fatty acids for both female and male reproduction (Rooke *et al.*, 2003) and ensuring the best health and immune status through nutritional manipulation.

Environmental implications

In January 2007, a new legal requirement comes into force under the IPPC and NVZ Directives to help reduce environmental pollution through the use of Best Available Practices. One way to achieve this is to reduce the total protein content of the feed, but maintain the level and balance of amino acids necessary to optimise productivity.

Studies with sows have shown that a 18% reduction in crude protein content (from 176 to 142g/kg) in the lactation diet had no effect on litter growth rate or sow weight loss at 20°C. However, at 28°C, feed intake and litter growth rate was higher, with reduced sow body weight loss when crude protein content was reduced (Renaudeau *et al.*, 2001).

A 1-2% reduction in the crude protein content of the gestation and lactation diets has been calculated to reduce N excretion by 2.05 t/year for a 750-sow herd, the herd size at which the IPPC/NVZ Directives become mandatory.

Conclusions

To achieve a high level of productivity in the modern sow, it is not sufficient to consider just the nutritional needs of the sow *per se* in terms of changes in body weight and body condition. It is equally crucial to apply nutritional and management strategies that reduce the loss of breeding potential, which is currently about 0.4 of the genetic potential of the modern hyper-prolific sow. Thus, it is important not only to supply sufficient energy and amino acids in the diet, but also minerals and vitamins in adequate quantities and in the most bio-available form. Similarly, good management practices must be applied to ensure the best health, welfare and well-being of the sow, as well as the boar, throughout their reproductive life.

References

Almeida, F.R.C.L., Kirkwood, R.N., Aherne, F.X. and Foxcroft, G.R. (2000) Consequences of different patterns of feed intake during the oestrus cycle in gilts on subsequent fertility. *Journal of Animal Science* **78**, **1556-1563.**

Ammerman, C.B., Henry, P.R. and Miles, R.D. (1998) Supplemental organically-based mineral compounds in livestock nutrition. In *Recent Advances in Animal Nutrition* pp 67-91. Edited by P.C. Garnsworthy and J. Wiseman. Nottingham University Press.

Ashworth, C.J. and Pickard, A.R. (1998) Embryo Survival and prolificacy. In *Progress in Pig Science*, pp 303-325. Edited by J. Wiseman, M.A. Varley and J.P. Chadick. Nottingham University Press, Nottingham.

Boyd, R.D. (2006) Sow mineral supplies decline with age. *Pig International, April 2006.*

Boyd, R.D., Touchette, K.J., Castro, G.C., Johnston, M.E., Lee, K.U. and Han, I.K. (2000) Recent advances in amino acid and energy nutrition of prolific sows. *Asian-Australasian Journal of Animal Science* **13**, No. 11. 1638-1652.

British Pig Executive (2006) *Pig Yearbook 2006.* BPEX, Milton Keynes.

British Pig Executive / Meat and Livestock Commission (2004) Feed formulations for Pigs. A guide and practical interpretation of the BSAS nutrient requirement standards for pigs. BPEX/MLC, Milton Keynes.

British Society of Animal Science (2003) *Nutrient Standards for Pigs.* (Authors: C.T. Whittemore, M.J. Hazzledine and W.H. Close). BSAS, Penicuik.

Challinor, C.M., Dams, G., Edwards, B. and Close, W.H. (1996) The effect of body condition of gilts at first mating on long-term sow productivity. *Animal Science,* **62,** 660 (Abstract).

Close, W.H. (2005) The role of the boar in maximising reproduction: effects of nutrition and management. In *Nutritional approaches to arresting the decline in fertility in pigs and poultry,* pp 93-115. Edited by J.A. Taylor-Pickard and L. Nollet. Nottingham University Press, Nottingham.

Close, W.H. and Cole, D.J.A. (2000) *Nutrition of Sows and Boars.* Nottingham University Press, Nottingham. 377 pages.

Close W. H. and Poornan, P.K. (1993) Outdoor pigs – their nutrient requirements, appetite and environmental responses. In *Recent Advances in Animal Nutrition 1993,* pp 175-196. Edited by P.C. Garnsworthy and D.J.A. Cole. Nottingham University Press. Nottingham.

Clowes, E.J. Aherne, F.X., Schaefer, A.L., Foxcroft, G.R. and Baracos, V.E. (2003) Parturition body size and body protein loss during lactation influences performance during lactation and ovarian function at weaning in first litter sows. *Journal of Animal Science,* **81**, 1517-1528.

Cromwell, G.L., Monegue, H.J. and Stahly, T.S. (1993) Long-term effects of feeding a high copper diet to sows during gestation and lactation. *Journal of Animal Science* **71**, 2996-3002.

Damgaard Poulsen, H. 1993. Minerals for sows. Significance of main effects and interactions on performance and biochemical traits. PhD Thesis: University of København.

Dwyer, C.M., Stickland, N.C. and Fletcher, J.M. (1994) The influence of maternal nutrition on muscle fiber number development in the porcine fetus on subsequent growth. *Journal of Animal Science* **72**, 911-917.

Fehse, R. and Close, W.H. (2000) The effect of the addition of organic trace elements on the performance of a hyperprolific sow herd. In *Biotechnology in the Feed Industry. Proceedings of the 16ᵗʰ Annual Symposium,* pp 309-325. Edited by T.P. Lyons and K.A. Jacques. Nottingham University Press, Nottingham.

Flowers, W.L., Spears, J.W. and Hill, G.M. (2001) Effect of reduced dietary Cu, Zn, Fe and Mn on reproductive performance of sows. *Journal of Animal Science,* **79** (Supplement 2): 61.

Gaughan, J.B., Cameron, R.D.A., Dryden, G.M. and Josey, M.J. (1995) Effect of selection on leanness on overall reproductive performance in Large White sows. *Animal Science* **61**: 561-564.

Gueblez, R., Gestin, J.M. and Le Henaff, G. (1985) Incidence de l'age et de l'epaisseur de lard dorsal a 100 kg sur la carriere reproductive des truies large white. *Journees de la Recherche Porcine en France,* **17**: 113-120.

Hughes, P.E. and Pearce, G.P. (1989) The endocrine basis of nutrition reproduction interactions. In *Manipulating Pig Production II,* pp 290-295. Edited by J.L. Barnett and D.P. Hennessy. Australian Pig Science Association, Werribee.

Jagger (reported by Boyd *et al.,* 2000)

Jacyno, E., Kawecka, M., Kamyczek, M., Kolodziej, A, Owsianny, J. and Delikator, B. (2002) Influence of inorganic Se + vitamin E and organic Se + vitamin E on reproductive performance of young boars. *Agricultural and Food Science in Finland* **11**, 75-184.

Jensen, H. and Peet, B. (2006) 30 Pigs per sow per year – Are we there yet? In *Advances in Pork Production. Proceedings of the 2006 Banff Pork Symposium,* pp 227-243. Eds. R.O. Ball and R.T. Zijlstra. University of Alberta, Department of Agricultrural, Food and Nutritional Sciences. Edmonton, Alberta, Canada.

Ji, F., Blantan, Jr. J.R. and Kim, S.W. (2005) Changes in weight and composition of pregnant gilts and their nutritional implications. *Journal of Animal Science* **83**: 366-375.

Ji, F., Hurley, W.L. and Kim, S.W. (2006) Characterisation of mammary gland development in pregnant gilts. *Journal of Animal Science* **84**: 579-589.

Johnston L.J., Pettigrew, J.E. and Rust, J.W. (1993) Response of Maternal-Line Sows to Dietary Protein Concentration During Lactation. *Journal of Animal Science* **71**: 2151-2156.

Kim, S.W., Hurley, W.L., Han, I.K. and Easter, R.A. (1999) Changes in tissue composition associated with mammary gland growth during lactation in sows. *Journal of Animal Science* **77**: 2510-2516.

Lima, G.J.M.M., Catunda, F., Close W.H., Ajala, L.C. and Rutz, F. (2006)

Positive effect on litter size when first parity sows were fed a mixture of organic and inorganic trace minerals. In: *Proceedings of 2006 Leman Conference.* In press.

Louis, G.F. Lewis, A.J., Weldon, W.L., Miller, P.S., Kittok, R.J. and Stroup, W.W. (1994) The effect of protein intake on boar libido, semen characteristics and plasma hormone concentrations. *Journal of Animal Science* **72**: 2038-2050.

Love R.J., Kupiec, C., Thornton, E.J. and Evans, G. (1993) Ad-libitum feeding of mated sows improves fertility during summer and autumn. In *Manipulting Pig Production IV*, p 247. Ed. E. S. Batterham, Australian Pig Science Association, Attwood.

Mahan, D. (2005) Feeding the sow and piglet to achieve maximum antioxidant and immune protection. In *Re-defining Mineral Nutrition*, pp 63-73. Edited by J.A. Taylor-Pickard and L.A. Tucker. Nottingham University Press. Nottingham.

Mahan, D. and Newton, C. A. (1995) Effect of initial breeding weight on macro- and micro-mineral composition over a three-parity period using a high-producing sow genotype. *Journal of Animal Science*, **73**: 151-158.

Mahan, D.C. and Peters, J.C. (2006) Enhancing sow reproductive performance by organic trace mineral dietary inslusions. In *Nutritional Biotechnology in the Feed and Food Industries. Proceedings of Alltech's 22nd Annual Symposium,* pp 103-108. Edited by T.P. Lyons, K.A. Jacques and J.M. Hower. Nottingham University Press, Nottingham.

Matte, J.J., Guay, F. and Girard, C.L. (2006) Folic acid and vitamin B_{12} in reproducing sows: New concepts. *Canadian Journal of Animal Science,* **86**, 197-205.

Meat and Livestock Commission (1995-2002) *Pig Yearbook.* Meat and Livestock Commission, Milton Keynes.

Meunier-Salaün, M-C. (2001) Fibre in sow diets. In *Recent Advances in Pig Nutrition 3,* pp 323-339. Edited by J. Wiseman and P.C. Garnsworthy. Nottingham University Press. Nottingham.

National Research Council (NRC) (1998) Nutrient Requirements of Swine, 10th revised Edition. *National Academy of Sciences.* Washington D.C. 183 pages.

Noblet, J., Dourmad, J.Y. and Etienne, M. (1990) Energy utilisation in pregnant and lactating sows: Modelling of energy requirements. *Journal of Animal Science,* **68**: 562-572.

Penny, P.C., Noble, R.C., Maldzian, A. and Ceroline, S. (2000) Potential role of lipids for the enhancement of boar fertility and fecundity. *Pig News and Information* **21**: 119N-126N.

Penny, P.C., Varley, M.A. and Tibble, S. (2001) Improved progeny performance by elevating nutrient intake to sows during gestation. In *Manipulting Pig Production VIII*, p 192. Ed. P.D. Cromwell, Australian Pig Science Association, Werribee.

Renaudeau, D. Quiniou, N. and Noblet, J. (2001) Effects of exposure to high ambient temperature and dietary protein level on performance of multiparous lactating sows. *Animal Science*, **79**, 1240-1249.

Richards, M.P. (1999) Zinc, copper and iron metabolism during porcine fetal development. *Biological Trace Element Research*, **69**: 27-44.

Rooke, J.A., Ferguson, E.M., Sinclair, A.G. and Speake, B.K. (2003) Fatty acids and reproduction in the pig. In *Recent Advances in Animal Nutrition, 2003*, pp 47-66. Edited by P.C. Garnsworthy and J. Wiseman. Nottingham University Press. Nottingham.

Smits, R.J. and Henman, D.H. (2000) Practical experiences with Bioplexes in intensive pig production. In *Biotechnology in the Feed Industry. Proceedings of the 16th Annual Symposium, pp 293-300*. Edited by T.P. Lyons and K.A. Jacques. Nottingham University Press, Nottingham.

Tritton, S.M., King, R.H., Campbell, R.G., Edwards, A.C. and Hughes, P.E. (1996) The effect of dietary protein and energy levels of diets offered during lactation on lactational and subsequent performance of first litter sows. *Animal Science*, **62**, 573-579.

Van Wettere, W.H.E.J., Mitchel, M., Revell, D.K. and Hughes, P.E. (2005) Management and nutritional factors affecting pubertal attainment and first litter sows in replacement gilts. In *Manipulting Pig Production X*, pp 180-187. Edited by J.E. Paterson. Australian Pig Science Association (Inc.), Werribee.

Yang, H., Foxcroft, E.R., Pettigrew, J.E., Johnston, L.J., Shurson, G.C., Costa, A.N. and Zak, L.J. (2000) Impact of dietary lysine intake during lactation on follicular development and oocyte maturation after weaning in primiparous sows. *Journal of Animal Science*, **78**, 993-1000.

17

PHYSICOCHEMICAL CHANGES TO STARCH STRUCTURE DURING PROCESSING OF RAW MATERIALS AND THEIR IMPLICATIONS FOR STARCH DIGESTIBILITY IN NEWLY-WEANED PIGLETS

FREDERIC J. DOUCET, GAVIN WHITE, JULIAN WISEMAN AND SANDRA E. HILL
School of Biosciences, University of Nottingham, Loughborough, LE12 5RD, UK

Introduction

At weaning, young piglets are faced with many challenges. Some of the most important stresses they are subjected to are their removal from the sow, their relocation to unfamiliar surroundings (often with new littermates) and a major change in their diet. These in turn may cause challenges to their digestive tract, weaning anorexia and suppressed immunity, which can all contribute to the post-weaning growth check commonly observed during this time. This growth check can greatly compromise the overall growing and finishing performance of the animal, in terms of reduced daily live-weight gain and increased days to slaughter. Marked changes in gut structure (*e.g.* villus atrophy, crypt hyperplasia) are typically observed within the first few days immediately following weaning, along with severely reduced digestive enzyme secretion and absorptive capacity of the small intestine (Miller *et al.*, 1986).

Pre-weaned piglets benefit from a digestive tract which is well adapted to the digestion of fat- and lactose-rich sow milk (Partridge & Gill, 1993). Their digestive system however becomes profoundly challenged upon weaning when a milk-based diet is suddenly replaced by a dry diet of solid food containing complex carbohydrates, primarily starch. For instance, feeding piglets with a diet based on unprocessed wheat can induce a significant reduction in starch digestibility around four days post-weaning in both the mid (0.5) and distal (0.75) regions of the small intestine (Figure 1; (White *et al.*, 2006)). Although temporary, it is apparent that starch digestion is greatly compromised, at a time when the piglet is often predisposed to malabsorption, diarrhoea and even morbidity. The recent change in European legislation, which now bans the use of in-feed antibiotics, means that the quality of the ingredients used in the weaner diet is becoming increasingly important if the post-weaning performance check is to be overcome.

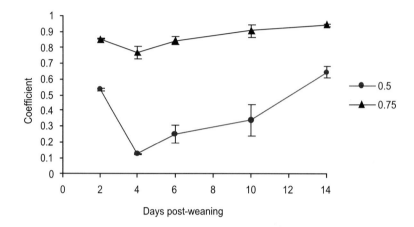

Figure 1. Coefficients of apparent starch digestibility in mid (0.5; closed circle) and distal (0.75; closed triangle) regions of the small intestine, from piglets fed an unprocessed wheat-based diet for 14 days post-weaning (White *et al.*, 2006).

Starch is generally of major importance in newly-weaned piglet diets, since by weight it constitutes the largest portion of the diet and is the major energy-yielding component. It is usually provided in the form of cereals. Starch macromolecules would be easily digestible if they readily dissolved. However, the starch molecules are laid down within the plant in a complex form. The structure of the starch granules is intricate with amylose and amylopectin organised into a pattern giving rise to a semi-crystalline structure. The crystalline bands are arranged in concentric shells within the granules. The shell and amorphous filling section are approximately 9 nm thick and there are many of these shells that make up a dense layer known as the growth ring (Jenkins & Donald, 1998). Between the growth rings there is more amorphous material. Digestion of starch granules by starch-degrading enzymes such as alpha-amylase shows that the amorphous portions between growth rings are much more readily susceptible to attack than the more crystalline regions. A decrease in the degree of crystallinity of starch can therefore result in increased susceptibility to enzyme activity (Hoover & Vasanthan, 1994) and therefore improved digestibility (Champ & Delort-Laval, 1991). An effective way of disrupting their molecular order is to subject them to thermal and/or mechanical processing (*e.g.* micronisation, extrusion, steam under pressure).

Processing of cereal starch in piglet diets

Processing of cereal starches prior to inclusion into diets for piglets is widely practised. The aim of using processed cereals is to induce severe physical changes to starch granules, and in this way increase their water-binding capacity and enzyme susceptibility (Kulp & Lorenz, 1981; van den Einde *et al.*, 2004; Anguita *et al.*, 2006). This in turn is believed to provide the animal with increased *in vivo* starch availability in a form that is more readily susceptible to amylolytic digestion, thereby providing a greater supply of energy.

Many piglet trials have been undertaken to evaluate the benefits of using various thermal or thermo-mechanical processing techniques for the improvement of *in vivo* starch digestibility. However, there is little consensus concerning the extent to which processing actually benefits animal performance. For instance, some studies have reported improved performance and digestibility in piglets following cereal processing (Skoch *et al.*, 1983; Huang *et al.*, 1997), whereas others failed to identify any significant benefits (van der Poel *et al.*, 1990; Zarkadas & Wiseman, 2001; Zarkadas & Wiseman, 2002). We believe that this discrepancy originates from a fundamental misconception about the concept of *cooking*, or more precisely *amount of cooking* (see next section). This is exemplified by the fact that precise descriptions of processing methodologies together with associated changes in physicochemical properties of cereals following processing are rarely reported in the literature (Zarkadas & Wiseman, 2002). Yet the mechanisms whereby processing techniques, such as extrusion and micronisation, damage and ultimately 'cook' starch are intrinsically different. These techniques therefore affect the physicochemical properties of starch in different ways, which in turn induce disparity in the physiological responses of animals.

Ultimately, the problem is that descriptions of processing are invariably limited to the name of the process itself with no regard whatsoever of the variables associated with each process (*e.g.* temperature, time, moisture, shear force). Descriptions of raw materials are frequently even limited to the term 'cooked' (*i.e.* no mention of the process which they were subjected to), which is completely inaccurate as a descriptor of their nutritional value.

This paper aims to argue and emphasise the importance of collecting primary information about the physicochemical properties of raw materials and the changes that they undergo on processing prior to testing experimental diets via piglet trials. The adoption of such an approach by the international animal science community will most likely help prevent further inaccurate interpretation of animal responses to changes in diets. It will also help determine the optimum processing conditions necessary for diets for post-weaned piglets. These conditions remain largely unknown in spite of several decades of intensive research on the application of processing in the manufacture of animal feeds.

Cooked starch vs amount of starch conversion

Native starch granules are insoluble, do not swell in water and can kinetically resist amylolytic digestion. Processing is therefore used to alter the structure and behaviour of starch granules in order to make starch polymers more accessible to alpha amylase (Lee *et al.*, 1985; Farhat *et al.*, 2001). However, the view whereby processing would merely supply a so-called 'cooked starch' represents a simplistic misconception. A more realistic outlook is that raw starch undergoes a continuum of complex changes during processing and reaches a different amount of cook, depending on the type of processing and the processing variables used. This continuum of changes that occur during the processing of starch has been termed 'starch conversion' (Mitchell *et al.*, 1997). The amount of starch conversion refers to the amount of starch that has been converted (sometimes erroneously called 'gelatinised') during processing, which involves destruction of the structural order of starch granules and depolymerisation of individual amylose and amylopectin molecules (Cheyne *et al.*, 2005). This process can however occur without significant changes to the overall size and shape of the starch granules. This occurs when starches are heated at high temperatures, but in limited amounts of water. During extrusion processing, on the other hand, native starch granules are subjected to high mechanical shear forces in addition to heat, with the resulting combined loss of the granule structure and the aforementioned reduction in molecular weight.

The extent of damage caused to starch granules and their components has important implications in animal nutrition and needs to be addressed. An accurate and quantitative representation of the physicochemical properties of raw materials and the changes they undergo upon processing can be achieved by means of reliable *in vitro* methodologies that are commonly used by food scientists. We show hereafter that the differences in physicochemical properties between raw and differently processed materials identified using the *in vitro* food science tests can also be perceived by weaned piglets.

In vitro characterisation of raw and processed starchy ingredients in animal feeds

Until now, little attempt has been made to quantify the effect of processing on the starch component of diets. In addition, the analysis of starchy materials (*e.g.* cereals) has generally consisted of, and is often limited to, the determination of their gross chemical composition (*i.e.* dry matter, ash, crude protein, crude fat, and starch) and of gelatinised starch as a proportion of total starch using enzymatic hydrolysis (Medel *et al.*, 1999; Medel *et al.*, 2004). However, these measurements provide no useful information on the properties of the starch component in relation to its digestibility in piglets. These limitations can now be overcome with the application of reliable quantitative laboratory tests that have been used in the field of human food development for a number of years.

The physicochemical parameters that we believe to be fundamentally associated with the quality of feed materials fall into three categories: (1) hydration properties, (2) structural properties, and (3) *in vitro* amylolytic digestion. A number of complementary tests are required to build a complete and accurate representation of starch properties.

(1) HYDRATION PROPERTIES

Hydration is considered of prime importance. It is necessary for the starch component in animal feeds to be hydrated for soluble products to be released for amylolytic degradation and for the subsequent liberation of hydrolysates of sufficient small size for absorption. Hence substantial work must concentrate on examining hydration of raw and processed starch components. Information on the hydration and interaction of the materials with water can come from different types of analysis, which are described below.

RVA measurements – The Rapid Visco Analyser (RVA) has been used extensively to study starch pasting characteristics of both raw materials (Zeng *et al.*, 1997; Jacobs *et al.*, 1999) and starch-based extruded or otherwise processed food (Whalen *et al.*, 1997; Guha *et al.*, 1998).The basic principle of this analysis involves the measurement of the resistance of starches to shearing forces under defined hydration and temperature regimes (Becker *et al.*, 2001). The RVA provides a number of pasting parameters (*e.g.* cold swelling peak, gelatinisation peak, trough, final viscosity; Figure 2), which represent a relative measure of starch gelatinisation, disintegration, swelling and gelling ability (Ruy *et al.*, 1993; Ravi et al., 1999). These parameters are particularly valuable in characterising the efficacy of processing techniques. For instance, the amount of starch conversion occurring due to extrusion processing can be related to changes in the RVA pasting profile (Whalen *et al.*, 1997). This phenomenon is best illustrated by the profiles 1, 2 and 3 in Figure 2, which show (i) a shift from a gelatinisation peak (typical of native starch) to a cold swelling peak (typical of extruded starch) following the progressive loss of starch integrity, (ii) a lowering of the trough, and (iii) a decrease in the final viscosity. An important parameter in extrusion processing,

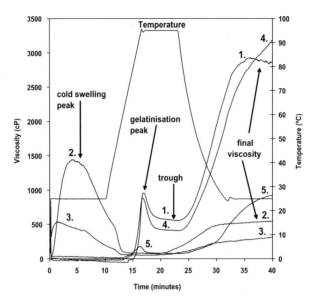

Figure 2. Typical RVA profile of raw cereal flour and processed cereal pellets (1. Raw wheat flour; 2. Wheat extruded at low SME; 3. Wheat extruded at high SME; 4. Wheat micronised at Low Cook conditions; 5. Wheat micronised at High Cook conditions).

which can affect the amount of damage caused to starch, is the specific mechanical energy (SME; defined as the net mechanical energy input divided by mass flow rate (Mercier *et al.*, 1989; Fan *et al.*, 1996)). Its effect can also be monitored using RVA, as shown in Figure 2 where differences in the cold swelling peak for high (profile 3) *vs* low (profile 2) SME indicate the influence of this extrusion parameter on the amount of particle swelling. The RVA is also able to differentiate between samples that were micronised under different moisture and temperature regimes (profiles 4 and 5 in Figure 2). The RVA is therefore a powerful and reliable technique, which is able to detect differences in starch hydration as caused by different processing methods (unprocessed *vs* extruded *vs* micronised starches), but also by different processing conditions (*e.g.* water content, thermal and mechanical input) for a specific method of processing. Finally, RVA can also assess the presence of endogenous amylase in cereals (Noda *et al.*, 2003), which is likely to affect processing and ultimately the nutritional value of cereals. For instance, it has been used successfully to demonstrate that wheat, of known variety, grown by the same breeder at the same site on two consecutive years, had very different hydration characteristics owing to differences in the amount of endogenous amylase they contained (Doucet et al., unpublished data). Semi-quantification of endogenous enzyme content in cereals can be performed using the RVA, by determining the cereals' hydration characteristics in the presence and in the absence of silver nitrate, which is a potent amylase inhibitor (Dixon & Webb, 1964; Collado & Corke, 1999). This is of prime significance since the effect of endogenous amylase on digestibility in animals and their subsequent performance is unclear. This underlines the importance of fully characterising the hydration properties of cereals and all starchy products in the laboratory before using them in animal nutrition trials. Failure to do so will certainly lead to poor interpretation of data on animal responses.

Water Absorption (WAI) and Water Solubility (WSI) Indices – WAI and WSI are two quantifiable parameters which are commonly used to assess the swelling and solubility behaviour of the starch component of cereals in excess water. They can therefore provide an indirect indication of the amount of starch conversion (Anderson *et al.*, 1969; Ollett *et al.*, 1990). WAI represents the volume occupied by the hydrated starch following swelling in excess water. It is affected by gelatinisation, granule integrity and molecular breakdown that occur during processing. For instance, an elevated WAI is generally indicative of extensively gelatinised starch with minimum molecular breakdown. On the other hand, WSI denotes the amount of soluble polysaccharides released from the granules to the aqueous phase. Typically, a high degree of molecular breakdown induces an elevated WSI. As a rule, starch that has undergone extensive conversion is expected to show high WSI and low WAI values. The wide-ranging values of WAI and WSI shown in Figure 3 for raw, extruded and micronised cereals, along with their distinct RVA pasting profiles, are a good illustration of the continuum in hydration properties that can be achieved by means of different types of processing techniques and conditions. The fact that the elevated WAI (low SME > high SME) and WSI (high SME > low SME) for extruded samples are in agreement with their corresponding RVA cold swelling peaks and final viscosities, respectively, demonstrates their usefulness in the assessment of the efficiency of the chosen processing methodologies.

(2) STRUCTURAL PROPERTIES

The structural characterisation of starch granules in raw and processed cereals is very useful in quantifying starch conversion. This can help explain the changes in hydration properties that are caused by different types of processing conditions. Two specific tests are most commonly used.

X-ray diffraction (XRD) – Native starches can be categorised into three types of semi-crystalline materials (Zobel, 1988), depending on their botanical source. These crystalline structures are characterised by different helical

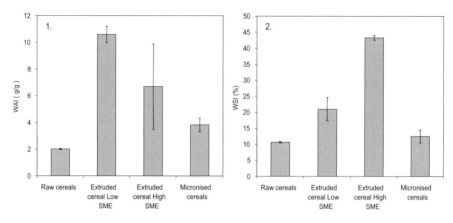

Figure 3. Typical effect of processing techniques and conditions on **1.** WAI and **2.** WSI cereals in excess water (Error bars are standard deviations; $n = 3$).

conformations which can be identified by their diffraction patterns (A-, B- or C-types; (Hizukuri, 1996)) using XRD. This instrument can also detect the loss in crystallinity (Zobel *et al.*, 1988) due to starch conversion following processing, which can be calculated from the measured degrees of crystallinity of the raw and cooked samples. This technique has already been applied to characterise micronised wheat (Zarkadas & Wiseman, 2001) and barley (Zarkadas & Wiseman, 2002) which were included in diets fed to weaned piglets. Examples of the extent of change in the degree of crystallinity of starch following micronisation and extrusion are illustrated in Figure 4. However, care must be taken in the interpretation of XRD data since a loss of crystallinity as indicated by XRD does not necessarily imply that starch granules have lost their integrity. The combined use of XRD with the above hydration measurements helps to identify possible artifacts that are inherent to specific methodologies.

Differential scanning calorimetry (DSC) – DSC has been widely used to study the thermal transitions in starches (Yu & Christie, 2001), *i.e.* the physical changes that a material undergoes when it is subjected to heating and/or cooling regimes. Of importance to animal feeds is the determination of the gelatinisation enthalpies (ΔH, expressed in J g^{-1}) of raw and processed starches, which can be used to quantify the loss of crystallinity caused by processing. Based on the principle that native starch has undergone no loss of crystallinity (0%) and that a 'theoretically fully cooked' cereal contains 100% loss of crystallinity, DSC shows that the extent to which micronisation can convert starch is highly variable whereas extrusion is a very efficient starch-converting instrument (Figure 5). Figure 5 also illustrates the wide-

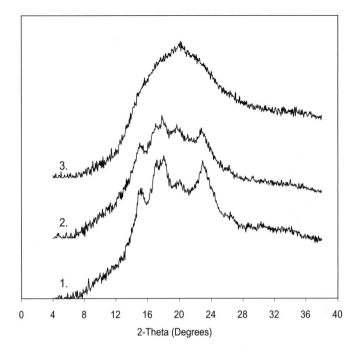

Figure 4. Wide angle X-ray diffractograms of raw and processed cereals (1. raw cereal; 2. micronised cereals; 3. extruded cereals).

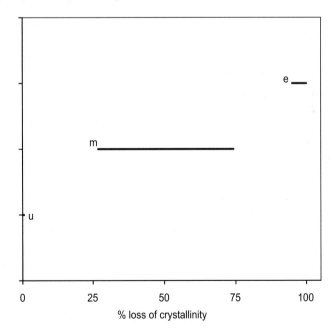

Figure 5. Typical range of loss of enthalpy, denoting loss of starch crystallinity, for **u.** unprocessed, **m.** micronised and **e.** extruded cereals, as determined by DSC.

ranging amounts of native starch still left after micronisation. This suggests that the micronisation cooking processing regimes used were very mild and much of the starch had not undergone even the first stages of loss of order. Several samples could be considered uncooked.

(3) *IN VITRO* AMYLOLYTIC DIGESTION

The botanical source of the starch and how it is processed influences the intrinsic hydration and structural characteristics of raw and processed starches and this in turn affects the rate and extent of starch hydrolysis by alpha-amylase (Gallant *et al.*, 1992; Slaughter *et al.*, 2001). This process of amylolytic digestion can be monitored using an *in vitro* digestibility test (Englyst & Cummings, 1987). Figure 6 illustrates the usefulness of this test in distinguishing between different processing techniques (unprocessed *vs* micronisation *vs* extrusion) and between different processing conditions for a same cooking technique (profiles 2 and 3). In the main, the kinetic of the action of alpha-amylase on starches altered structurally by processing can vary drastically and is generally more rapid in the following order: extruded > micronised > unprocessed starch (Figure 6). In addition, changes in the temperature and water content during *e.g.* micronisation also induce significant differences in the rate of amylolytic degradation. The elucidation of the effect of SME during extrusion on the *in vitro* digestibility test is however more challenging, presumably due to the high amount of converted starch caused by this effective form of thermo-mechanical processing, which becomes completely susceptible to *in vitro* amylolytic digestion. This is exemplified by the rapid (< 5 min) completion of the enzymatic reaction (see profile 4 in Figure 6).

Influence of processing variables on *in vivo* starch digestibility

The lack of consensus on the effectiveness of processing on *in vivo* starch digestibility in newly-weaned piglets originates from the limited information reported on the processing methodologies used in comparison studies. Very often only the named process is given, whilst processing variables (*e.g.* moisture, temperature, mechanical input) are seldom mentioned. Variations in processing techniques and variables are known to affect the physicochemical properties of starch differently, as illustrated by the above *in vitro* tests. The Nottingham contribution to the NUTWEAN project has demonstrated that the effects of these variations are also apparent in the biological responses of piglets.

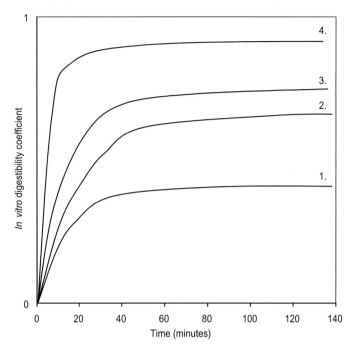

Figure 6. *In vitro* digestibility of raw and processed cereals (**1.** raw cereal; **2.** micronised cereal at low cook conditions; **3.** micronised cereal at high cook conditions; **4.** extruded cereal).

The choice of the processing technique is a fundamental consideration as it can have a marked effect on *in vivo* starch digestibility (Figure 7). Regardless of the processing variables used, the overall trend indicates that extrusion processing promotes high starch digestibility (coefficient of > 0.8 at mid region and > 0.87 at distal region) within the small intestine of young piglets, whereas data on micronisation are much lower and very similar to those obtained on raw materials and therefore less conclusive. A comparison between the effects of different extrusion variables (low *vs* high SME) on the digestibility of soft endosperm texture wheat indicates the importance of carefully selecting processing parameters. For instance, within the 0.5 region, there was a positive correlation between SME and starch digestibility (Figure 8). This difference however became insignificant in the 0.75 region. The higher digestibility coefficient found within the 0.5 region for the high SME diet suggests enhanced digestion and a more rapid release of starch. However, it is unclear whether a diet containing rapidly, in contrast to slowly, digestible starch is more beneficial for the piglet, although there is some evidence that the latter may lead to better overall performance in broiler chickens (Weurding *et al.*, 2003). This is an important area of interest in relation to the rate of

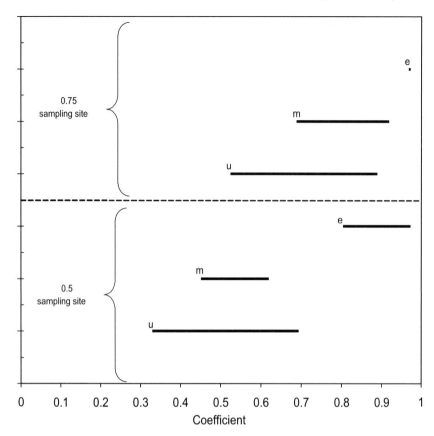

Figure 7. Typical range of digestibility coefficients of starch found in the 0.5 and 0.75 sites of the small intestine for piglets fed unprocessed and processed starchy materials (u: unprocessed; m: micronised; e: extruded).

starch breakdown in the weaned piglet, which may have implications in alleviating the post-weaning growth check. For instance, we have recently found that specific processing techniques and variables can significantly overcome the reduction in starch digestibility commonly observed around four days post-weaning in piglets (White et al., unpublished data; Figure 9).

Figures 7 and 8 illustrate the influence of processing techniques and variables on the amount of starch that escapes digestion in the small intestine in piglets. It is interesting to note that errors are higher for animals fed raw wheat-based diets; thus processing, in addition to improving digestibility, may also reduce animal variability. There is considerable interest in this resistant starch fraction, which generally becomes fermented within the large intestine. For instance, digestibility of raw and micronised hull-less barley at the ileum in piglets was found to be different to that measured over the total

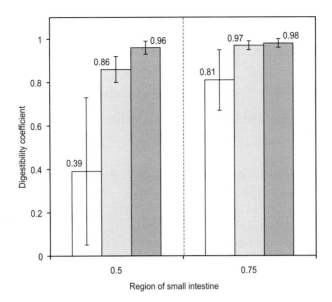

Figure 8. Effect of extruding conditions (low *vs* high SME) on apparent starch digestibility at the 0.5 and 0.75 sites of the small intestine for weaned piglets fed soft endosperm wheat diets. Initial bar is for raw wheat.

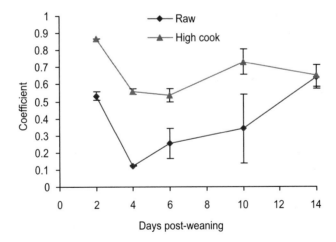

Figure 9. Effect of processing on overcoming partially the decline in wheat starch digestibility post-weaning in the 0.5 region of the small intestine. Raw (◆) vs Extruded at high SEM (▲).

tract, which was indicative of the considerable digestion of raw cereals that can occur within the large intestine (Huang *et al.*, 1998). Opinion is divided as to whether this starch fermentation in the hind gut is beneficial (creating a more acidic environment via volatile fatty acid production and their subsequent absorption by colonocytes, together with possible reduction in pathogen colonisation) or detrimental (encouraging proliferation of pathogenic microbes through supplying a readily fermentable substrate which may lead to diarrhoea and dehydration)).

Linking *in vitro* tests to the nutritional value of raw and processed starch in piglets

The above discussion demonstrates that careful consideration must be taken when selecting processing techniques and variables for the inclusion of 'cooked' cereals in newly-weaned piglet diets. It first showed that *in vitro* food science tests can detect differences in the physicochemical properties of processed cereals, which are strongly correlated with the types and conditions of processing. It then followed with an examination of the positive correlation between *in vivo* starch digestibility in piglets and processing variables, which illustrates that animals are also good indicators of the effectiveness of processing. However, this can only be fully appreciated if a thorough characterisation of the physicochemical properties of raw and processed cereals is carried out prior to animal trials. For instance, a comparative examination of the *in vitro* (RVA, WAI, WSI, XRD, DSC and amylolytic digestion) and *in vivo* starch digestibility data presented above revealed that the combination of the appearance of a cold swelling peak and a lowering of the final viscosity in the RVA, an increase in WSI, a high degree of starch conversion (as indicated by XRD and DSC) and a more rapid *in vitro* amylolytic degradation appeared to correlate fairly well with an enhanced *in vivo* starch digestibility. This review therefore provides the first strong direct confirmation that precise descriptions of processing methodologies (*e.g.* processing name, moisture content, temperature, SME, screw speed, drying conditions) together with associated changes in physicochemical properties of cereals following processing must be reported in animal trials, which is in agreement with previously published claims (Zarkadas & Wiseman, 2001, 2002). The adoption of this approach will provide more accurate interpretation of animal responses to changes in diets.

Conclusions

There are serious challenges facing the pig industry following the withdrawal of in-feed antibiotic growth promoters. Because of the susceptibility of the newly-weaned piglet to the disorders described above, efforts have concentrated on developing sustainable nutritional strategies which seek to overcome these problems that are, invariably, linked to the weaning process itself and the transition from a liquid to solid diet. Whilst many approaches have been considered, the current paper has focussed on starch as it is the major component of dry diets. Processing of cereals (that contain starch) is commonly practised but, up until now, not in a controlled fashion. Variables associated with processing will have a quantifiable influence on starch structure and in vitro assessment of its physico-chemical composition which relate to starch digestibility in vivo and hence nutritional value of diets in which cereals are contained. Ultimately, designing diets for the newly-weaned piglet can be based more on the increased precision of processing so that these diets are better able to allow animals to overcome the post-weaning growth check.

Acknowledgements

Some of the data in this paper were from research financially supported by UK sponsors: ABNA Ltd, Frank Wright Ltd, Home-Grown Cereals Authority, Meat and Livestock Commission/British Pig Executive, Primary Diets Ltd and Provimi Ltd with match funding from Defra, through the Sustainable Livestock Production LINK programme.

References

Anderson RA, Conway HF, Pfeifer VF & Griffin EL (1969) Roll and extrusion cooking of grain sorghum grits. *Cereal Science Today* **14**, 4-11.

Anguita M, Gasa J, Martin-Orue SM & Perez JF (2006) Study of the effect of technological processes on starch hydrolysis, non-starch polysaccharides solubilisation and physicochemical properties of different ingredients using a two-step *in vitro* system. *Animal Feed Science and Technology* **129**, 99-115.

Becker A, Hill SE & Mitchell JR (2001) Milling - A further parameter affecting the Rapid Visco Analyser (RVA) profile. *Cereal Chemistry* **78**, 166-172.

Champ M & Delort-Laval J (1991) Effects of processing on chemical characteristics and nutritive value of cereals. *Animal Production* **52**, 564-565.

Cheyne A, Barnes J, Gedney S & Wilson DI (2005) Extrusion behaviour of cohesive potato starch pastes. II. Microstructure-process interactions.

Journal of Food Engineering **66**, 13-24.

Collado LS & Corke H (1999) Accurate estimation of sweetpotato amylase activity by four viscosity analysis. *Journal of Agriculture and Food Chemistry* **47**, 832-835.

Dixon M & Webb (1964) Enzyme inhibitors. In *Enzymes*, pp. 344-347. London: Longmans, Green and Co.

Englyst HN & Cummings JH (1987) Digestion of polysaccharides of potato in the small intestine of man. *American Journal of Clinical Nutrition* **153**, 423-431.

Fan J, Mitchell JR & Blanshard JMV (1996) The effects of sugars on the extrusion of maize grits. I. The role of the glass transition in determining product density and shape. *International Journal of Food Science and Technology* **31**, 55-65.

Farhat IA, Protzmann J, Becker A, Valles-Pamies B, Neale R & Hill SE (2001) Effect of the extent of conversion and retrogradation on the digestibility of potato starch. *Starch/Starke* **53**, 431-436.

Gallant DJ, Bouchet B, Buleon A & Perez S (1992) Physical characteristics of starch granules and susceptibility to enzymatic degradation. *European Journal of Clinical Nutrition* **46**, S3-S16.

Guha M, Ali SZ & Bhattacharrya S (1998) Effect of barrel temperature and screw speed on rapid viscoanalyser pasting behaviour of rice extrudate. *International Journal of Food Science and Technology* **33**, 259-266.

Hizukuri S (1996) Starch: Analytical aspects. In *Carbohydrates in Food*, pp. 403 [AC Eliasson, editor]. New York: Marcel Dekker.

Hoover R & Vasanthan T (1994) Effect of heat-moisture treatment on the structure and physicochemical properties of cereal, legume and tuber starches. *Carbohydrate Research* **252**, 33-53.

Huang SX, Sauer WC, Pickard M, Li S & Hardin RT (1998) Effect of micronization on energy, starch and amino acid digestibility in hulless barley for young pigs. *Canadian Journal of Animal Science* **78**, 81-87.

Jacobs H, Eerlingen RC, Clauwaert W & Delcour JA (1999) Influence of annealing on the pasting properties of starches from varying botanical sources. *Cereal Chemistry* **72**, 480-487.

Jenkins PJ & Donald AM (1998) Gelatinisation of starch: a combined SAXS/WAXS/DSC and SANS study. *Carbohydrate Research* **308**, 133-147.

Kulp K & Lorenz K (1981) Heat-moisture treatment of starches. 1. Physicochemical properties. *Cereal Chemistry* **58**, 46-48.

Lee PC, Brooks SP, Kim O, Heitlinger LA & Lebenthal E (1985) Digestibility of native and modified starches - *in vitro* studies with human and rabbit pancreatic amylases and *in vivo* in rabbits. *Journal of Nutrition* **153**, 93-103.

Medel P, Latorre MA, de Blas JC, Lazaro R & Mateos GG (2004) Heat processing of cereals in mash or pellet diets for young pigs. *Animal Feed Science and Technology* **113**, 127-140.

Medel P, Salado S, de Blas JC & Mateos GG (1999) Processed cereals in diets for early-weaned piglets. *Animal Feed Science and Technology* **82**, 145-156.

Mercier C, Linko P & Harper JM (1989) *Extrusion cooking*. St Paul, MN, USA: American Association of Cereal Chemists, inc.

Miller BG, James PS, Smith MW & Bourne FJ (1986) Effects of weaning on the capacity of pig intestinal villi to digest and absorb nutrients. *Journal of Agricultural Science - Cambridge* **107**, 579-589.

Mitchell JR, Hill SE, Paterson L, Valles B, Barclay F & Blashard JM (1997) The role of molecular weight in the conversion of starch. In *Starch structure and functionality* [PJ Frazier, AM Donald and P Richmond, editors]. Cambridge, UK: Royal Society of Chemistry.

Noda T, Ichinose Y, Takigawa S, Matsuura-Endo C, Abe H, Saito K, Hashimoto N & Yamauchi H (2003) The pasting properties of flour and starch in wheat grain damaged by alpha-amylase. *Food Science and Technology Research* **9**, 387-391.

Ollett AL, Parker R, Smith AC, Miles MJ & Morris VJ (1990) Microstructural changes during the twin-screw extrusion cooking of maize grits. *Carbohydrate Polymers* **13**, 69-84.

Partridge GG & Gill BP (1993) New approaches with pig weaner diets. In *Recent Advances in Animal Nutrition*, pp. 221-248 [PC Garnsworthy and DG Cole, editors]. Nottingham, UK: Nottingham University Press.

Ravi R, Sai Manohar R & Haridas Rao P (1999) Use of Rapid Visco Analyser (RVA) for measuring the pasting characteristics of wheat flour as influenced by additives. *Journal of the Science of Food and Agriculture* **79**, 1571-1576.

Ruy GH, Neumann PE & Walker CE (1993) Pasting of wheat flour extrudates containing conventional baking ingredients. *Journal of Food Science* **58**, 567-573.

Skoch ER, Binder SF, Deyoe CW, Allee GL & Behnke KC (1983) Effects of steam pelleting conditions and extrusion cooking on a swine diet containing wheat middlings. *Journal of Animal Science* **57**, 929-935.

Slaughter SL, Ellis PR & Butterworth PJ (2001) An investigation of the action of porcine pancreatic alpha-amylase on native and gelatinised starches. *Biochimica et Biophysica Acta* **1525**, 29-36.

van den Einde RM, Akkermans C, van der Goot AJ & Boom RM (2004) Molecular breakdown of corn starch by thermal and mechanical effects. *Carbohydrate Polymers* **56**, 415-422.

van der Poel AFB, Den Hartog LA, Van Stiphout WAA, Bremmers R & Huisman J (1990) Effects of extrusion of maize on ileal and faecal digestibility of nutrients and performance of young piglets. *Animal Feed Science and Technology* **29**, 309-320.

Weurding RE, Enting H & Verstegen MWA (2003) The effect of site of starch digestion on performance of broiler chickens. *Animal Feed Science and Technology* **110**, 175-184.

Whalen PJ, Bason ML, Booth RI, Walker CE & Williams PJ (1997) Measurement of extrusion effects by viscosity profile using the rapid viscoanalyser. *Cereal Foods World* **42**, 469-475.

White G, Doucet FJ, Hill SE & Wiseman J (2006) The effect of wheat endosperm texture on nutritional value for weaned piglets. *Proceedings of the British Society of Animal Science*, p. 29.

Yu L & Christie G (2001) Measurement of starch thermal transitions using differential scanning calorimetry. *Carbohydrate Polymers* **46**, 179-184.

Zarkadas LN & Wiseman J (2001) Influence of processing variables during micronization of wheat on starch structure and subsequent performance and digestibility in weaned piglets fed wheat-based diets. *Animal Feed Science and Technology* **93**, 93-107.

Zarkadas LN & Wiseman J (2002) Influence of micronization temperature and pre-conditioning on performance and digestiblity in piglets fed barley-based diets. *Animal Feed Science and Technology* **95**, 73-82.

Zeng M, Morris CF, Batey IL & Wrigley CW (1997) Sources of variation for starch gelatinisation, pasting and gelation properties in wheat. *Cereal Chemistry* **71**, 63-71.

Zobel HF (1988) Starch crystal transformations and their industrial importance. *Starch/Starke* **40**, 1-7.

Zobel HF, Young SN & Rocca LA (1988) Starch gelatinization: An X-ray diffraction study. *Cereal Chemistry* **65**, 443-446.

18

NUTRITIONAL VALUE OF LEGUMES (PEA AND FABA BEAN) AND ECONOMICS OF THEIR USE

KATELL CRÉPON
Union Nationale Interprofessionnelle des Plantes riches en Protéines 12, avenue George V - PARIS

Introduction

Despite successive agricultural policies, the EU is in deficit of protein sources for livestock. European livestock depends to a very large extent on the importation of soyabean meal which represents more than 0.4 of the protein supply of European feed. Pulses represent about 0.03 of the total protein supply of animals, and this proportion tends to be decreasing mainly because of the inadequate supplies of pulses on the European market. Analysis of pulse areas in the EU shows that, after strong growth corresponding to favourable agricultural policies, increase stopped in 1998 when the EU established maximum guaranteed areas. Since 1998, the decrease in the area may be attributed to technical problems (crop diseases with peas) or economic problems (unattractive prices) (Crépon, 2004).

In 2005, the EU produced 3.9 million tonnes of pulses, most of which were peas (2.4 million tonnes) and faba beans (1.4 million tonnes). This paper will consider these two crops. The two main producers are France (1.7 million tonnes) and the United-Kingdom (0.9 million tonnes) but France produced mainly peas (0.76 of pulse production), the UK produced mainly faba beans (0.76 of pulse production) (PROLEA, 2006).

All the peas grown in the EU for animal nutrition belong to the same botanical species (*Pisum sativum* L.), but two major types of peas can be distinguished according to the presence or absence of tannins in the pericarp (Bastianelli *et al.*, 1998). In the same way, for EU faba beans (*Vicia faba* L.) four types can be distinguished according to the presence or absence of tannins in the pericarp and to the vicine and convicine content (low or high content) in the cotyledons (Duc *et al.*, 1999).

Chemical composition of peas and faba beans (Table 1)

Table 1. Chemical composition of peas and faba beans *(standard deviation in italic)*

	Bastianelli *et al.* (1998)	Sauvant *et al.* (2004)
Feed pea (white-flowered pea)		
Crude protein g/kg DM)	251 *(14.8)*	239 *(12.7)*
Starch (g/kg DM)	485 *(20.4)*	516 *(23.1)*
Crude fibre (g/kg DM)	68.3 *(8.2)*	60.2 *(6.9)*
Sugars (g/kg DM)	54.9 *(6.6)*	45.1 *(4.6)*
Fat (g/kg DM)	19.1 *(1.2)*	11.6 *(2.3)*
TIA (UTI/mg DM)	4.2 *(3.8)*	
Condensed tannins (mg/g DM)	0.07 *(0.02)*	
Coloured-flowered pea		
Crude protein (g/kg DM)	276 *(22.4)*	
Starch (g/kg DM)	430 *(32.3)*	
Crude fibre (g/kg DM)	85.4 *(12.0)*	
Sugars (g/kg DM)	50.8 *(5.6)*	
Fat (g/kg DM)	17.6 *(1.9)*	
TIA (UTI/mg DM)	2.5 (9.7)	
Condensed tannins (mg/g DM)	5.49 *(1.92)*	

	Duc *et al.* (1999)	Sauvant *et al.* (2004)
Coloured faba bean		
Crude protein (g/kg DM)	305 *(25)*	294 *(25.4)*
Starch (g/kg DM)	426	443 *(31.2)*
Crude fibre (g/kg DM)	87	91.3 *(12.7)*
Sugars (g/kg DM)	39.6	34.7 *(9.2)*
Fat (g/kg DM)	21	15 *(3.5)*
TIA (UTI/mg DM)	2.9	
Condensed tannins (mg/g DM)	6.6	
Vicine+convicine (g/kg DM)	8.3	
White faba bean		
Crude protein g/kg DM)	319	311 *(25.5)*
Starch (g/kg DM)	427	433 *(26.7)*
Crude fibre (g/kg DM)	88	87.1 *(10.4)*
Sugars (g/kg DM)	43.5	42.9 *(8.1)*
Fat (g/kg DM)	20	12.8 *(2.3)*
TIA (UTI/mg DM)	2.9	
Condensed tannins (mg/g DM)	0.1	
Vicine+convicine (g/kg DM)	7.6	

(sd)

PROTEIN AND AMINO ACID CONTENTS

White-coloured peas (feed peas) have an average crude protein content of 239 g/kg DM (Sauvant, 2004), which is lower than the crude protein content quoted by Gatel and Grosjean (1990) or Bastianelli *et al.* (1998) who mentioned an average crude protein content of 250 g/kg DM, but totally in accordance with the value quoted by Métayer *et al.* (1992). However, this crude protein content is variable and depends both on cultivar and on growing conditions (Biarnès, 2005, Biarnès and Dubois, 2005). The crude protein content of coloured-flowered pea is slightly higher than that of feed pea (Bastianelli *et al.*, 1998) but this is not always significant (Gatel and Grosjean, 1990).

Whatever the category of pea, the amino acid profile can be determined using the regressions proposed by Huet *et al.* (1987). These regressions have been updated recently using new cultivars grown in different places in France (UNIP, ITCF, Ajinomoto, 2001, unpublished) but the relationship between crude protein and amino acid contents was not significantly different from that published in 1987. Neither cultivar nor growing conditions have an effect on the amino acid profile of peas. Pea protein is rich in lysine (17.3 g/kg DM), but poor in sulphur amino acids (methionine + cystine: 5.5 g/kg DM) and tryptophan (2 g/kg DM).

Faba beans, with an average crude protein content of 300 g/kg DM, are significantly richer in protein than peas, and there is no significant relationship between crude protein and vicine–convicine content or between crude protein and tannin content if gene zt1 is involved in tannin reduction. On the other hand, if gene zt2 is involved in tannin reduction, isogenic comparison shows that tannin-free cultivars are significantly richer in protein (Duc *et al*, 1999). However, white-flowered cultivars seem to have a higher crude protein content (311 g/kg DM) than coloured-flowered cultivars (294 g/kg DM) (Sauvant *et al.*, 2004).

A linear relationship between the contents of amino acids and nitrogen has also been shown for faba beans (Mossé, 1990) and this relationship does not depend on the genotype of faba bean (Duc *et al.*, 1999).

CARBOHYDRATE CONTENT

Starch is quantitatively the most important component of peas. The average starch content of peas is 516.2 g/kg DM (Sauvant *et al.*, 2004), and there is no significant difference between the starch content of feed peas and coloured-flowered peas (Bastianelli *et al.*, 1998). The variation in starch content may be explained partially by the variation in protein content, since starch content is negatively correlated with protein content, in both feed peas and coloured-flowered peas. The mean crude fibre content is 60.2 g/kg DM (Sauvant *et al.*, 2004) but coloured peas may have a higher crude fibre content (Bastianelli *et al*, 1998) due to their smaller seed size and lower thousand-seed weight (TSW). Indeed, crude fibre content is negatively correlated with TSW, while TSW is positively correlated with starch content.

The sugar content of peas is low, and contents ranging from 66 to 83 g/kg DM have been reported by Canibe (1997) in accordance with Bastianelli *et al.* (1998) and Sauvant *et al.* (2004).

The starch content of faba beans is lower than that of peas, ranging from 413 to 439 g/kg DM according to Duc *et al.* (1999). Starch content may vary according to growing conditions but does not depend on the presence of tannins or vicine–convicine (Duc *et al.*, 1999). As already mentioned for peas, a negative correlation between crude protein and starch content also exists for faba beans. Faba beans are richer than peas in crude fibre, with an average content of 91.3 g/kg DM (Sauvant *et al.*, 2004). Reducing vicine–convicine content has no impact on crude fibre content, but reducing the tannin content may have a positive impact on crude fibre content if the gene zt2 is involved in the reduction of tannin content.

LIPID CONTENT

Lipid content is low both for peas (11.6 g/kg DM) and faba beans (15 g/kg DM) (Sauvant *et al.*, 2004). Linoleic acid represents about half the oil content of peas and faba beans.

MAJOR ANTI-NUTRITIONAL FACTORS

Trypsin inhibitor activity (TIA) in peas is generally low, but some cultivars can reach 10 to 15 UTI/mg DM. Among 905 samples, representing 195 cultivars tested, Muel *et al.* (1998) found values ranging from 1.0 to 17.7 UTI/mg DM. These values are in accordance with previous references (Valdebouze, 1980; Leterme, 1992, Gdala *et al*, 1991). The main cause of the variation in TIA is genetic and, among the environmental causes of variability, the influence of the date of sowing is not clear but its impact remains low (Grosjean *et al.*, 1993). The highest values of TIA observed in winter types are related to their genetic history: most of them are derived from the cultivar Champagne known to have high TIA. Currently, most of the cultivars grown in France present low TIA (less than 5 UTI/mg DM).

In faba beans TIA is less well documented but seems to be low. Valdebouze *et al.* (1980) reported a range from 3.3 to 6.2 UTI/mg DM among 26 cultivars, while Duc *et al.* (1999) reported a range from 0.3 to 5.3 UTI/mg DM.

Tannins are polyphenols that are able to form complexes with proteins and lead to a decrease in protein digestibility. Tannins are concentrated in the seed coat, and the presence of tannins is related to the colour of the flower. Tannins can be removed by genetic improvement. In feed peas, the average condensed tannins level is very low: 0.07 mg/g DM ranging from 0.04 to 0.14 mg/g. Coloured-flowered peas have an average condensed tannin content of 5.49 mg/g DM, and range from 0.55 to 7.45 mg/g DM (Bastianelli *et al.*, 1998).

Conventional faba bean genotypes have a mean condensed tannin content of 5 to 10 mg/g DM (Duc *et al* 1999). Alleles at two distinct genetic loci (zt1 and zt2) have been discovered in *Vicia faba* genetic resources (Picard *et al.*, 1976), either of which eliminates tannins from the seed. Tannin-free cultivars have a mean condensed tannin content of 0.1 mg/g DM (Duc *et al*, 1998, Bond and Duc, 1993). In Europe, most of the cultivars grown are still coloured-flowered faba beans.

Vicine and convicine are glucopyranosides present in mature faba bean seeds (Griffiths and Ramsay, 1993). It is known that vicine–convicine may have a strong effect on the metabolism of laying hens, through their derivatives aglycones. It has been suggested that vicine may produce pro-oxydants that cause lipid peroxidation, erythrocyte haemolysis and interfere with normal lipid metabolism in the (Muduuli *et al.*, 1981). In conventional cultivars, vicine–convicine contents range from 6 to 14 mg/g DM (Duc *et al*, 1999). Vicine and convicine are thermostable seed constituents, located principally in the cotyledons and not easily removed by technological processes. In *V. faba* genetic resources a gene vc- has been discovered that reduces the content of both vicine and convicine by 90% to 95% (Duc *et al.*, 1989, Duc *et al.* 1998). In France, five varieties with low vicine–convicine content are registered and they represent 0.15 of the market share. Moreover, one variety with both low tannin and low vicine–convicine contents is registered but not often grown because of its low yield.

Nutritive value for pigs

DIGESTIBILITY AND ENERGY CONTENT (TABLES 2 AND 3)

The mean digestible energy content of feed peas is 16.2 MJ/kg DM, and may vary from 15.2 to 17.3 MJ/kg DM. These values, measured in different

Table 2. Nutritive value of feed peas and coloured peas in pig

Feed peas	Coefficient of apparent digestibility		Digestible energy content (MJ/kg DM)	Coefficient of Ileal apparent digestibility		References
Cultivar	Crude protein	Energy		Crude protein	Lysine	References
NR	0.887	0.935	17.2			Bourdon *et al.*, 1977
Frimas	0.826	0.868	16.5			
Amino	0.864	0.868	15.9			Bourdon *et al.*, 1982
Finale	0.887	0.925	17.1			
Finale	0.913	0.906				Sève *et al.*, 1985
Finale	0.848	0.842	15.6			Grosjean *et al.*, 1989
Frisson	0.869	0.860	15.7			
Solara	0.849	0.850	15.8	0.852	0.830	Grosjean *et al.*, 1991
Frijaune	0.778	0.879	16.4	0.620	0.659	Joindreville *et al.*, 1992
Laser	0.903	0.903	16.9	0.609	0.665	
Solara	0.840	0.889	16.9	0.802	0.828	
NR	0.899	0.921	17.1	0.696	0.763	
Frisson	0.883	0.871	15.9			Grosjean *et al.*, 1992
Finale	0.876	0.890	16.5			
Victor	0.837	0.838	15.5			Grosjean *et al.*, 1994
Mistral	0.779	0.848	15.7			
Solara	0.838	0.857	16.1			
19 cultivars	0.840	0.880	16.3			Grosjean *et al.*, 1998
	(0.760 to 0.910)	(0.849 to 0.936)	(15.4 to 17.3)			
Solara		0.861	16.1			Van Cauwenberghe *et al.*, 1997
Commercial			15.6			Van Cauwenberghe *et al.*, 1997
Commercial	0.770	0.808	15.2			Noblet *et al.*, 1997
Messire	0.818	0.857	16.3	0.827	0.858	Grosjean *et al.*, 1998
Baccara	0.810	0.850	15.6	0.812	0.839	
Baccara	0.835	0.885	16.4	0.821	0.855	
Baccara	0.844	0.859	15.9			
Baccara	0.838	0.856	15.8	0.822	0.869	
Baccara	0.880	0.891	16.5			
Baccara	0.843	0.873	16.1			
Baccara	0.876	0.903	16.7			
Baccara	0.872	0.892	16.5			
Baccara	0.868	0.887	16.4	0.807	0.843	
Baccara	0.793	0.862	15.8	0.776	0.831	
Messire	0.845	0.894	16.7	0.854	0.886	
Baccara	0.813	0.831	15.4	0.837	0.861	
Messire	0.869	0.905	17.1	0.837	0.867	
Messire	0.867	0.873	16.4	0.805	0.838	
Baccara	0.793	0.826	15.3	0.819	0.848	
Baccara	0.843	0.876	16.3	0.813	0.839	
Baccara	0.854	0.862	15.9	0.813	0.832	
Messire	0.879	0.866	16.2	0.811	0.846	
Baccara	0.843	0.872	16.2	0.793	0.826	

Table 2. Contd.

Feed peas	Coefficient of apparent digestibility		Digestible energy content (MJ/kg DM)	Coefficient of Ileal apparent digestibility		
Cultivar	Crude protein	Energy		Crude protein	Lysine	References
Baccara	0.886	0.895	16.6	0.821	0.870	
Baccara	0.846	0.901	16.7	0.753	0.858	
Baccara	0.817	0.876	16.1	0.830	0.876	
Messire	0.818	0.857	16.3	0.844	0.864	
Solara				0.786	0.856	Hess *et al.*, 1998
Amino				0.734	0.808	
Solara				0.754	0.820	
Madria				0.670	0.766	
Eiffel				0.748	0.815	
Névé				0.783	0.829	Grosjean *et al.*, 2000
Baroness				0.771	0.792	
Radley				0.771	0.821	
Rafale				0.762	0.809	
Aravis				0.767	0.817	
Cheyenne				0.782	0.814	
Blizard				0.787	0.842	
Victor				0.823	0.854	
Brévent				0.807	0.855	
Victor				0.816	0.839	
Baccara				0.828	0.854	
Baccara				0.822	0.869	
Froidure				0.769	0.804	
Athos	0.873	0.869	16.0		0.891	Skiba *et al.*, 2003
NR				0.823	0.877	Vilarino *et al.*, 2006
NR				0.796	0.866	
NR				0.782	0.862	
Mean	0.832	0.876	16.2	0.788	0.833	
Min	0.770	0.808	15.2	0.609	0.659	
Max	0.913	0.936	17.3	0.854	0.891	
Mean INRA-AFZ	0.840	0.880	16.1	0.800	0.830	Sauvant *et al.*, 2004

NR : not registered

Coloured peas	Coefficient of apparent digestibility		Digestible energy content (MJ/kg DM)	Coefficient of Ileal apparent digestibility		
Cultivar	Crude protein	Energy		Crude protein	Lysine	References
Norda	0.840	0.877	16.18			Bourdon *et al.*, 1977
Commercial	0.670	0.794	14.76			Grosjean *et al.*, 1991
Commercial	0.756	0.798	14.84			
Gali	0.745	0.795	14.80	0.813	0.776	
6 cultivars	0.760 (0.676 to 0.809)	0.812 (0.787 to 0.840)	15.06 (14.50 to 15.6)			
						Grosjean *et al.*, 1998

Table 2. Contd.

Coloured peas	Coefficient of apparent digestibility		Digestible energy content (MJ/kg DM)	Coefficient of Ileal apparent digestibility		
Cultivar	Crude protein	Energy		Crude protein	Lysine	References
Mean	0.757	0.814	15.09			
Min	0.670	0.787	14.50			
Max	0.840	0.877	16.18			
Io-7	0.767	0.811	15.08			Association Française de Zootechnie

Table 3. Nutritive value of coloured and white faba beans in pigs

Coloured faba beans	Coefficient of apparent digestibility		Digestible energy content (MJ/kg DM)	Coefficient of Ileal apparent digestibility		
Cultivar	Crude protein	Energy		Crude protein	Lysine	References
High VC content						
Talo	0.719	0.785	14.5			Bourdon *et al.*, 1984
Alfred				0.818	0.867	Maillard *et al.*, 1990
Alfred		0.805	15.1	0.827	0.798	Grosjean *et al.*, 1995
Castel		0.805	15.0	0.842	0.885	
NR	0.829	0.767	14.4			Grosjean *et al.*, 2001
cv Fabiola	0.789	0.785	14.5			
NR	0.792	0.779	14.7			
cv Robin	0.793	0.796	14.8			
Maya	0.820	0.820	15.2	0.825	0.907	Vilariño *et al.*, 2004
Méli				0.767	0.853	
Olan				0.776	0.874	
Low VC content						
NR	0.795	0.810	15.2			Grosjean *et al.*, 2001
Divine	0.803	0.793	14.9	0.823	0.883	Vilariño *et al.*, 2004
Mean	0.793	0.795	14.8	0.811	0.867	
Min	0.719	0.767	14.4	0.767	0.798	
Max	0.829	0.820	15.2	0.842	0.907	
INRA AFZ	0.810	0.830	15.6	0.800	0.850	Sauvant *et al.*, 2004

NR : not registered

White faba beans	Coefficient of apparent digestibility		Digestible energy content (MJ/kg DM)	Coefficient of Ileal apparent digestibility		
Cultivar	Crude protein	Energy		Crude protein	Lysine	References
High VC content						
NR	0.802	0.803	14.8			Bourdon *et al.*, 1984
NR	0.758	0.809	15.1			
Blandine				0.846	0.882	Maillard *et al.*, 1990

Table 3. Contd.

White faba beans	Coefficient of apparent digestibility		Digestible energy content (MJ/kg DM)	Coefficient of Ileal apparent digestibility		References
Cultivar	Crude protein	Energy		Crude protein	Lysine	
Albatross		0.903	17.1			Grosjean *et al.*, 1995
NR	0.907	0.943	17.5			Grosjean *et al.*, 2001
Fabiola	0.852	0.863	15.8			
NR	0.867	0.898	16.7			
Gloria	0.739	0.833	15.4	0.788	0.883	Vilariño *et al.*, 2004
Low VC content						
NR				0.779	0.851	Hess *et al.*, 2000
NR				0.784	0.840	
NR				0.758	0.858	
NR	0.891	0.882	16.4			Grosjean *et al.*, 2001
NR	0.902	0.916	17.1			
NR				0.832	0.892	Vilariño *et al.*, 2004
Mean	0.840	0.872	16.2	0.798	0.868	
Min	0.739	0.803	14.8	0.758	0.840	
Max	0.907	0.943	17.5	0.846	0.892	
INRA AFZ	0.830	0.860	16.1	0.840	0.880	Sauvant *et al.*, 2004

NR : not registered

cultivars of feed pea agree well with the value quoted by Sauvant *et al.* (2004). The gross energy of feed peas is highly digestible, with coefficients on average 0.876, but varying from 0.808 to 0.936. The gross energy digestibility of feed pea is very similar to that of cereals. Apparent faecal crude protein digestibility is lower than that of soyabean meal (0.84 vs. 0.87, Sauvant *et al.*, 2004) and may vary from 0.770 to 0.913 according to the different measurements made on different pea cultivars. The main causes of variability in digestibility for both energy and protein are not very clear but could be the crude fibre, starch and fat content but also TIA (Grosjean *et al.*, 1998b). It has been shown that standardised ileal digestibility of protein and amino acids of peas decreased with increasing TIA (expressed per unit of protein) but was not affected by fibre content (Grosjean *et al.*, 2000).

Coloured-flowered peas have lower apparent digestibility for crude protein and energy, and consequently a lower digestible energy content (15.1 vs. 16.2 MJ/kg DM). This is obviously due to the presence of tannins in the seed coat that decrease the digestibility of protein and starch (Jansman, 1993).

The impact of vicine and convicine on digestibility is very low (Grosjean *et al.*, 2001) but not very well documented. Tannin content has a negative impact on apparent crude protein digestibility (0.793 vs 0.840). This result has been observed in numerous research papers (Bourdon, 1984, Grosjean *et al.*, 1995, Grosjean *et al.*, 2001), but is not confirmed in the most recent trial (Vilariño *et al.*, 2004). These contradictory results could be due to an interaction with crude fibre content. Tannins also have a negative impact on the apparent gross energy digestibility (0.795 vs. 0.870), but this effect is debated since some researchers do not notice a significant effect of tannin content on gross energy digestibility (Bourdon *et al.*, 1984, Vilariño *et al.*, 2004).

IMPACT OF TECHNOLOGICAL TREATMENTS ON THE NUTRITIVE VALUE

The extrusion of peas increases their gross energy and nitrogen digestibility. This could be explained by the modification of starch structure but also by the decrease in TIA (Bengala Freire *et al.*, 1991, Mariscal-Landin *et al*, 2002). Pelleting does not have a significant effect on gross energy or nitrogen digestibility (Grosjean *et al.*, 1989). Since the gross energy digestibility of peas is high and their TIA low, a technological treatment is not necessary before using peas in pig diets.

NUTRITIVE VALUE FOR POULTRY

IMPACT OF TECHNOLOGICAL TREATMENTS ON THE NUTRITIVE VALUE

Pelleting has a very positive and significant effect on the apparent metabolisable energy value (AMEn) of peas fed to adult cockerels (Carré *et al.*, 1987), broiler chickens, laying hens or turkeys (Barrier-Guillot *et al.*, 1995). The improvement is most marked when peas are coarsely ground (Conan *et al.*, 1992), birds are young (Barrier-Guillot *et al.*, 1995) or peas contain tannins (Grosjean *et al.*, 1999). The beneficial effect of pelleting is explained by a better starch and protein digestibility (Carré *et al.*, 1987). The same effect has been observed in faba bean utilization (Lacassagne *et al.*, 1988).

DIGESTIBILITY AND ENERGY CONTENT IN MASH DIETS

Feed peas have a high coefficient of starch digestibility of 0.892 for adult cockerels in mash diets (Table 4). The mean AMEn value of feed peas is 11.81 MJ/kg DM in mash diets for adult cockerels. Protein is less digestible, even in feed peas (0.787) but values are similar to those found for the digestibility of soyabean meal protein (0.80–0.85, Carré *et al.*, 1997). Tannins have a strong negative impact on protein digestibility (coloured-flowered peas have a protein digestibility of 0.643 compared with 0.787 for feed peas), but they seem to have no impact on starch digestibility (Grosjean *et al.*, 1999). Consequently, the AMEn value of coloured-flowered peas is not very different from the AMEn value of feed peas (11.3MJ/kg DM vs. 11.81 MJ/kg DM). Broiler chickens use starch less efficiently and the AMEn values of broiler chickens are lower than for adult cockerels (12.29 vs. 13.12 MJ/kg DM for feed pea in a pelleted diet).

Table 4. Nutritive value of feed peas and coloured peas in poultry

Feed peas	Mash diet			Pelleted diet			
	Coefficient of Apparent digestibility		AMEn (MJ/kg)	Coefficient of Apparent digestibility		AMEn (MJ/kg)	
Cultivar	Starch	Protein		Starch	Protein		Reference
Adult cockerels							
Frisson	0.915	0.772	12.45	0.965	0.798	12.89	Carré *et al.*, 1987
			12.21				Askbrandt, 1988
Frisson	0.841	0.746	11.28	0.963	0.719	12.33	Carré *et al.*, 1991
Finale	0.846	0.753	11.77	0.969	0.817	12.84	
Commercial	0.808	0.787	11.7	0.945	0.851	13.36	Conan *et al.*, 1992
	(3)*	(3)*	(3)*	(3)*	(3)*	(3)*	
Commercial	0.885	0.792	12.87	0.939	0.810	13.3	
	(3)**	(3)**	(3)**	(3)**	(3)**	(3)**	
	0.903	0.789	11.99	0.985	0.855	13.18	Grosjean *et al.*, 1999
	(31)	(36)	(36)	(6)	(11)	(11)	
Baccara						12.6 (1)	Barrier-Guillot *et al.*, 2001
Mean	0.892	0.787	11.81	0.964	0.836	13.12	
Broiler chickens							
Frisson	0.809	0.759	10.86	0.957	0.808	12.52	Carré *et al.*, 1991
Finale	0.847	0.803	11.56	0.950	0.839	12.62	
Baccara						12.27 (26)	Barrier-Guillot *et al.*, 1999
Messire						12.41 (6)	
Victor						12.04 (5)	
Solara						12.77 (1)	
Baccara						12.2	Barrier-Guillot *et al.*, 2001
Mean	0.828	0.781	11.21	0.954	0.824	12.29	

* coarse ground
**fine ground

Table 4. Nutritive value of feed peas and coloured peas in poultry

Coloured peas	Mash diet		AMEn	Pelleted diet		AMEn	
	Coefficient of		AMEn	Coefficient of		AMEn	
Cultivar	Apparent digestibility		(MJ/kg)	Apparent digestibility		(kcal/kg)	Reference
	Starch	Protein		Starch	Protein		
Adult cockerels							
	0.885	0.643	11.3	0.984	0.743	12.72	Grosjean *et al.*, 1999
	(14)	(16)	(17)	(2)	(4)	(5)	

For faba beans (Table 5), it is necessary to distinguish four types since both vicine–convicine (VC) and tannins may have an impact on the nutritive value of faba beans for poultry. Vilariño *et al.* (unpublished) showed that tannins have a negative and significant impact on protein digestibility, as previously shown by Grosjean *et al.* (2000) and Lacassagne *et al.* (1991), and that vicine–convicine (VC) and tannins have a significant and additive impact on AMEn values in broiler chickens. Similar results have never been found in adult cockerels where the impact of vicine–convicine (VC) on nutritive value is less well documented. However, for high VC coloured-faba beans fed in mash diets to adult cockerels, the AMEn values average 11.22 MJ/kg DM, compared with 11.67 MJ/kg DM for low VC faba beans. For high VC white faba beans fed to adult cockerels in mash diets, the AMEn values average 11.68 MJ/kg DM compared with 12.49 MJ/kg DM for low VC white faba beans. AMEn values in broiler chicken are less well documented but, as for peas, AMEn values in broiler chicken are lower than in adult cockerels.

Table 5. Nutritive value of coloured and white faba beans in poultry

Coloured faba beans	Mash diet		AMEn	Pelleted diet		AMEn	
	Coefficient of		(MJ/kg	Coefficient of		(MJ/kg	
Cultivar	Apparent digestibility		DM)	Apparent digestibility		DM)	Reference
	Starch	Protein		Starch	Protein		
Adult cockerels							
High VC content							
Alfred						12.05	Grosjean *et al.*, 1995
Victor						12.48	
Castel						11.99	
NR	0.952	0.740	11.68	0.972	0.747	12.07	Grosjean *et al.*, 2000
cv Fabiola	0.917	0.713	10.63		0.785	11.57	
NR	0.923	0.843	11.65		0.816	12.01	
cv Robin	0.918	0.710	11.44				
cv Bourdon	0.905	0.684	10.71				
Maya						11.92	Brévault *et al.*, 2003
Marcel						12.81 (2)	Métayer *et al.*, 2006
Mean	0.923	0.738	11.222	0.972	0.783	12.19	

Table 5. Contd.

Coloured faba beans Cultivar	Mash diet Coefficient of Apparent digestibility		AMEn (MJ/kg DM)	Pelleted diet Coefficient of Apparent digestibility		AMEn (MJ/kg DM)	Reference
	Starch	Protein		Starch	Protein		
Adult cockerels							
Low VC content							
NR	0.926	0.844	11.67				Grosjean *et al.*, 2000
Divine						12.76	Brévault *et al.*, 2001
Divine						11.77	Métayer *et al.*, 2003
Mean	0.926	0.844	11.67			12.27	
Broiler chicken							
High VC content							
Alfred	0.856	0.669	11.16	0.915 (2)	0.706 (2)	11.53 (2)	Lacassagne *et al.*, 1988
Soravi	0.834	0.694	10.82	0.909 (2)	0.722 (2)	11.55 (2)	
Alfred*	0.902	0.698	9.55				Lacassagne *et al.*, 1991
Alfred**	0.703	0.694	12.38				
Marcel						12.83 (2)	Métayer *et al.*, 2006
Mean	0.824	0.689	10.98	0.912	0.714	11.97	
Low VC content							
Divine						12.31	Métayer *et al.*, 2003
Mean						12.31	

* fine grinding
**coarse grinding
(nb. of measures)

White faba beans Cultivar	Mash diet Coefficient of Apparent digestibility		AMEn (MJ/kg DM)	Pelleted diet Coefficient of Apparent digestibility		AMEn (MJ/kg DM)	Reference
	Starch	Protein		Starch	Protein		
Adult cockerels							
High VC content							
Albatross						12.01	Grosjean *et al.*, 1995
Caspar						12.32	
NR	0.958	0.839	11.83				Grosjean *et al.*, 2000
Fabiola	0.926	0.844	11.44		0.877	12.45	
NR	0.923	0.843	12.21		0.872	12.46	
cv Glacier	0.918	0.83	11.25				
Gloria						13.22	Brévault *et al.*, 2001
Gloria						13.38	Brévault *et al.*, 2003
Gloria						12.1	Métayer *et al.*, 2003
Gloria						13 (2)	Métayer *et al.*, 2006
Victoria						13.24 (2)	
Mean	0.9313	0.8390	11.68		0.8745	12.77	

Table 5. Contd.

White faba beans Cultivar	Mash diet Coefficient of Apparent digestibility		AMEn (MJ/kg DM)	Pelleted diet Coefficient of Apparent digestibility		AMEn (MJ/kg DM)	Reference
	Starch	Protein		Starch	Protein		
Adult cockerels							
Low VC content							
NR	0.933	0.817	12.21				Grosjean *et al.*, 2000
NR	0.957	0.844	12.77	0.988	0.879	13.45	
NR						12.56	Métayer *et al.*, 2003
Disco						13.08 (2)	Métayer et al., 2006
Mean	0.945	0.8305	12.49	0.988	0.879	13.04	
Broiler chicken							
High VC content							
Blandine	0.751	0.826	10.17	0.86 (2)	0.868 (2)	11.9	Lacassagne *et al.*, 1988
Blandine*	0.804	0.825	11.29				Lacassagne *et al.*, 1991
Blandine**	0.638	0.842	9.2				
Gloria						11.93	Métayer *et al.*, 2003
Gloria						12.99	Métayer *et al.*, 2006
Victoria						12.84	
Mean	0.731	0.831	10.22	0.86	0.868	12.42	
Low VC content							
NR						12.7	Métayer *et al.*, 2003
Disco						12.89	Métayer *et al.*, 2006
Mean						12.80	

(nb. of measures)

DIGESTIBILITY AND ENERGY CONTENT IN PELLETED DIETS

AMEn is on average 13.12 MJ/kg DM for feed peas, and 12.72 kg/DM for coloured-flowered peas (Table 4). Pelleting improves both starch digestibility (+0.085 absolute on average) and protein digestibility (+0.07 on average). The effect of pelleting is more important in coloured-flowered peas, especially for protein digestibility (+0.1 for coloured-flowered peas, compared with +0.05 for feed peas).

For high VC coloured-faba beans (Table 5), mean AMEn values are 12.19 MJ/kg DM compared with 12.27 MJ/kg DM for low VC faba beans. For high VC white-faba beans, mean AMEn values are 12.77 MJ/kg DM compared with 13.04 MJ/kg DM for low VC white faba beans.

Pea and faba bean in pig diets

PIGLETS (TABLES 6 AND 7)

Table 6. Feeding trials with feed pea in piglet (% of control diet)

Reference	Diet	Peas (g/kg)	Amino acid supplementation	Initial Weight (kg)	Average daily gain	Feed conversion ratio	Comments
Bertrand *et al.*, 1980	Wheat/Barley/ Maize	0		8.2	100 (513)	100 (1.91)	
		150			110.1	97.4	
		300			98.1	103.7	
	Wheat/Barley/ Maize	0		9	100 (533)	100 (1.72)	
		150	DL methionine		99.6	102.3	
		300	DL methionine		89.5	108.7	
		450	DL methionine		77.1	114.5	
	Wheat/Barley/ Maize	0	DL methionine	9.6	100 (562)	100 (1.83)	
		150	DL methionine		101.4	97.8	
Bouard *et al.*, 1980	Maize	0		6.4	100 (437)	100 (1.68)	
		200	DL methionine		90	103	
Bengala-Freire *et al.*, 1989	Wheat	0		6.7	100 (491)a	100 (1.54) a	
		150			90.2 b	109.7 ab	
		300	Lysine HCL DL methionine		83.9 b	111.7 b	
		450	Lysine HCL DL methionine		84.5 b	113.6 b	
		300 (extruded)	Lysine HCL DL methionine		99 a	103.9 a	
		450 (extruded)	DL methionine		101.8 a	102.6 a	
Gâtel *et al.*, 1989	Wheat	0		10.8	100 (561) a	100 (1.8) a	
		300			104 a	103.9 b	
		300	DL methionine		107.7 a	98.3 a	
Joindreville *et al.*, 1992	Wheat	0	Lysine HCL	7.5	100 (507) a		
		400	DL Methionine		93.9 b		TIA = 2.9
		400	L Threonine		87.6 c		TIA = 9.7
		400	Tryptophan		90.7 bc		TIA = 12.8
Van Cauwen- berghe *et al.*, 1997	Wheat	0	Lysine HCL DL Methionine	8	100 (402)	100 (1.85)	
	Wheat	305	DL methionine L Threonine		108.45 a	97.8 c	
	Wheat/Cassava	0	Lysine HCL DL Methionine L Threonine		98.2 b	104.3 b	

Table 6. Contd.

Reference	Diet	Peas (g/kg)	Amino acid supplementation	Initial weight (kg)	Average daily gain	Feed conversion ratio	Comments
	Wheat/Cassava	0	Lysine HCL DL Methionine L Threonine		96.8 b	109.7 a	
	Wheat/Cassava	300	DL Methionine Lysine HCL		100.2 b	100 bc	
	Wheat/Cassava	265	Lysine HCL DL Methionine L Threonine		102 ab	103.2 b	
Grosjean *et al.*, 1997	Wheat	0	Lysine HCL	8.2 (480)	100 (1.71) a		
	Wheat	400	DL Methionine		103.5	99.4 a	Raw
	Wheat	400	L Threonine		104.4	97 ab	Pelleted
	Wheat	400	Tryptophan		103.7	95.9 b	Extruded
	Wheat/Barley/ Maize	150		12.9	100 (609) a	100 (1.73) a	Cultivar Maxi
		400	Lysine HCL		100.4 a	95.9 a	Cultivar Maxi
		400	DL Methionine		97.2 a	97.7 a	Cultivar Santa
		400	L Threonine		76.7 b	110.9 b	Cultivar Progreta

Table 7. Feeding trials with faba beans in piglets (% of control diet)

Reference	Diet	Faba beans (g/kg)	Amino acid supple-mentation	Initial weight (kg)	Average daily gain	Feed conversion ratio	Comments
Fekete *et al.*, 1985	Wheat/Barley/Maize	0		10.8	100	100	
		100			101	102	No tannin
		200			92**	108**	No tannin
		300			85**	114**	No tannin
	Wheat/Barley/Maize	0		8.4	100	100	
		100			110**	98	No tannin
		200			104	99	No tannin
		300			96	112**	No tannin
	Wheat/Barley/Maize	0		9.15	100	100	
		100			100	107	No tannin
		200			99	102	No tannin
		300			85	104	No tannin
	Wheat/Barley/Maize	0		10.9	100	100	
		100			98	102	Tannins
		150			96	103**	Tannins
		200			93**	105**	Tannins
	Wheat/Barley/Maize	0		10.1	100	100	
		100			100	102	Tannins
		150			95	103**	Tannins
		200			93**	105**	Tannins

Table 7. Contd.

Reference	Diet	Faba beans (g/kg)	Amino acid supple-mentation	Initial weight (kg)	Average daily gain	Feed conversion ratio	Comments
	Wheat/Barley/Maize	0		10.9	100	100	
		150			98	104	No tannin
		150			100	104	Tannins
		150			97	105	Tannins
Skiba	Triticale/Barley/Maize	0		8	100 (511)	100 (1.82)	
et al.,		80			90	102.2	Tannins
2000		150			96	100	Tannins
		200			91.4	101.6	Tannins
Euronutrition, 2003		0		12.3	100 (578)	100 (1.71)	
		100			99.6	101.2	No tannin
		200			100.3	97.1	No tannin
Royer	Wheat/Barley	0		8	100 (544)	100 (1.52)	
et al., 2006		100	Lysine HCl		100.2	98	No tannin
		100	Methionine		97.6	100.6	Tannins
		200	Threonine		100.7	100.6	No tannin
		200	Tryptophan		99.6	101.3	Tannins

** significant

Trials have shown a decrease in daily growth and an deterioration in feed conversion ratio when feed peas were included at rates up to 150 g/kg (Bertrand *et al.*, 1980, Bouard *et al.*, 1980, Bengala-Freire *et al.*, 1989), except when peas were previously extruded. In that case, the same performance was obtained with the control diet as with diets containing extruded peas at rates of 300 g/kg or 450 g/kg (Table 6). This could be explained by a higher digestibility of energy and protein (Bengala-Freire *et al.*, 1989). Moreover, several trials showed that when diets have the correct amino acid balance, and the pea cultivar does not have high TIA (which could lead to a decrease in protein and amino acids digestibility), feed peas can be included in diets at rates up to 400g/kg, without decreasing performance (Grosjean *et al.*, 1997).

Contrasting results were obtained in ealier trials (Table 7) with piglets fed white and coloured faba beans. The trials described by Fekete *et al.* (1985) led to the recommendation that rates of faba beans should be limited to 100 g/kg in piglet diets whatever the type of faba beans. However recent trials showed that feeding piglets with faba beans at rates of 200 g/kg, with or without tannins, would lead to performances similar to those with control diets (Euronutrition, 2003; Royer *et al.*, 2006, unpublished). This may be due to a better amino acids balance in the diet.

GROWING AND FINISHING PIGS (TABLES 8 AND 9)

Table 8. Feeding trials with feed pea in pigs (% of control diet)

Reference/Diet	Peas (g/kg)	Amino acid supplementation	Average daily gain	Feed conversion ratio	Dressing percentage	Lean percentage	Backfat	Comments
Bourdon et al., 1976, Maize/Soyabean	0		100 (692)	100 (3.08)				Cultivar Frimas TIA 12.9
	150		98.9	100.9				
	300		97.9	102.9				
Castaing et al., 1981, Maize/Soyabean	0		100 (628) a	100 (3.2) a	100 (77.6)		100 (19.5)	
	120		100.4 a	100.6 a	100.8		103.6	
	240		98.9 a	100.6 a	100.2		105.1	
	360		94.3 b	105.9 b	99.6		103.8	
Maize/Soyabean	0		100 (746) a	100 (2.97)	100 (77.8)		100 (22.2)	
	260		95.8 b	105 b	99.3		101.3	Cultivar Frimas TIA 12.9
	260		99.3 a	100.7 a	99.5		103.6	Cultivar Amino TIA 3.7
	260		99.1 a	101 a	98.8		101.3	Cultivar Finale TIA 3.3
Palisse-Roussel et al., 1984, Wheat/Maize/Soyabean	0		100 (759) a	100 (2.75) a	100 (78.1)		100 (27.4)	
	370		89.4 b	106.9 b	101.7		97.8	
	370	Tryptophan (0.3g/kg)	100.3 a	99.3 a	101.2		101.4	
	370	Tryptophan (0.6g/kg)	101.4 a	98.5 a	100.9		98.2	
Edwards et al., 1987, Wheat/Barley/Soyabean	0		100 (633)	100 (2.64)	100 (76.5)		100 (24.9)	
	150		100.5	98.9	100		106	Cultivar Progreta
	300		97.3	103	99.4		106.4	Cultivar Progreta
	450		93.6	109.5	99.9		104.8	Cultivar Progreta
	0		100 (629)	100 (3.07)	100 (78.3)		100 (25.2)	
	150		99.2	100.6	100.5		102.3	Cultivar Birte
	300		96.5	102.9	101.1		105.1	Cultivar Birte
	450		95	105.2	100.5		103.9	Cultivar Birte
	0		100 (795)	100 (2.79)	100 (79.1)		100 (33.1)	
	300		103.6	103.6	99.9		99.4	Cultivar Birte
	300		99.1	99.3	99.7		94.2	Cultivar Progreta

Table 8. Contd.

Reference/Diet	Peas (g/kg)	Amino acid supplementation	Average daily gain	Feed conversion ratio	Dressing percentage	Lean percentage	Backfat	Comments
Gâtel et al., 1989								
Wheat	0		100 (725)	100 (3.15)	100 (78.9) a	100 (51.4)	100 (18.7)	
	250		99.4	99.4	100.9 ab	98.8	102.6	
	415	Methionine	101.4	96.8	101.1 b	99.4	102.1	
	415	Threonine Tryptophan	99.2	99	100.6 ab	98.6	102.6	
Maize	0		100 (745) ab	100 (2.92) ab	100 (77.3)	100 (50.5)	100 (20.5)	
	300	Methionine	99.6 ab	99.6 ab	100.1	99.2	102.9	
	300	Tryptophan Lysine	102.5 b	96.9 a	100.1	99.6	100.9	
	450	Methionine Tryptophan	98.6 a	101 b	100.2	98.8	106.3	
Wheat/Cassava	0		100 (764)	100 (2.95)	100 (77.9)	100 (51.8)	100 (17.5)	
	200	Methionine	100.4	98.9	99.2	99.4	100.6	
	300	Methionine	100	99.3	100.1	100	100.6	
	410	Methionine Tryptophan	98.2	101.3	100.8	101.1	96.6	

Table 9. Feeding trials with faba beans in pigs (% of control diet)

Reference/Diet	Faba bean (g/kg)	Amino acid supplementation	Average daily gain	Feed conversion ratio	Dressing percentage	Lean percentage	Backfat	Comments
Bourdon et al., 1976								
Maize	0		100 (692)	100 (3.08)	100 (74.3)			
	150		98.8	99	99.9			Tannins
	300		99.3	102.9	99.3			Tannins
Henry et al., 1978								
Barley	0		100 (525)	100 (3.76)				
	150		106.3	94.4				
	330		95	103.2				
	330	Methionine	95.6	103.7				
Maize	0		100 (567)	100 (3.39)				
	330		82.5	107.9				Tannins
	330	Methionine	75.8	113.6				Tannins
Maize	0		100 (616)	100 (3.12)				
	150		97.4	104.5				Tannins
	150	Tryptophan	100.3	100.6				Tannins
	300		91.9	110.6				Tannins
	300	Tryptophan	98.2	103.2				Tannins
ITCF, 1983	0		100 (761)	100 (2.92)	100 (77.4)	100 (50.6)	100 (22.5)	
Maize	175		94.9	105.8	99.7	100.6	97.3	No Tannin
	175		97.1	103.1	99.1	101.6	96	Tannins
	175		94.7	105.5	99.5	99.8	96	Tannins
ITCF-AGPM, 1985	0		100 (768) a	100 (2.88) a	100 (77.5)	100 (49.7)	100 (23.1)	
Maize	100		100.4 a	100.3 a	100.1	98.4	104.3	Tannins
	150		94.5 b	106.2 b	99.7	98.9	100	Tannins
	200		93.3 b	107.9 b	99.7	101.2	96.1	Tannins
ITCF-AGPM, 1986	0		100 (761)	100 (2.89)	100 (76.8)	100 (49.6)	100 (24.2)	
Maize	220	Methionine (0.4g/kg)	98.9	102.4	99.9	104	91.7	Tannins
	220	Methionine (0.8g/kg)	98.2	103.5	99.9	102.4	91.7	Tannins
	220		96.6	104.8	99.7	101	96.3	Tannins

Table 9. Contd

Reference/Diet	Faba bean (g/kg)	Amino acid supplementation	Average daily gain	Feed conversion ratio	Dressing percentage	Lean percentage	Backfat	Comments
Thacker *et al.*, 1985	0		100 (680)	100 (2.75)				
	100		97	106.2				
	150		95.5	105				
	200		95.5	106.9				
	250		89.7	118.5				
	300		85.3	123.6				
Euronutrition, 2003	0		100 (988)	100 (2.71)	100 (74.8)	100 (59.2)		
	150		97.8	101.5	100.5	100.3		No tannin
	300		100.2	98.1	100	101.5		No tannin
Royer *et al.*, 2006 Wheat/Barley/Maize	0		100 (962)	100 (2.76)		100 (60.3)		
	200	Methionine	100.1	100		98.8		No tannin
	350	Threonine	97.2	102.9		99.2		No tannin
	200	Tryptophan	96.2	103.9		99.8		Tannins
	350		98.7	101.4		99.3		Tannins

Numerous trials have been carried out with feed peas in pig diets (Table 8). Castaing and Leuillet (1981) reported that peas included at up to 250 g/kg in the diet can decrease feed intake and growth, especially in the growing period. The difference in growth performance between a control diet and a diet with peas can be explained first by a deficiency in tryptophan in the diet with peas, leading to a decrease in feed intake and growth, and by a poor digestibility of pea protein when the cultivar used has high TIA. Adding tryptophan to a diet containing 400 g peas/kg improved growth performance to the same level as that which was obtained with the control diet (Palisse-Roussel *et al.*, 1987; Gâtel *et al.*, 1989). Moreover, the use of peas with a high TIA (12.9) can decrease growth performance if peas are included at up to 250 g/kg, but the inclusion of peas with a low TIA (3.7) up to 300 g/kg results in performance similar to that obtained with the control diet (Castaing *et al.*, 1981). Varietal differences must be considered when formulating diets with peas, and if feeding values are not overestimated (due to a lack of knowledge about TIA for example) it is possible to include peas at up to 300 g/kg, even with a high TIA (Edwards *et al.*, 1987). Therefore, in most cases, the poor performance observed with diets containing feed peas is due either to unbalanced and/or a deficiency of amino acids, especially in maize-based diets, since maize is itself deficient in tryptophan. In diets supplemented with amino acids feed peas can be used at up to 400 g/kg without leading to any negative effects on pig performance and can substitute totally for soyabean meal.

Only a few trials have been carried out on coloured-flowered peas for pigs since feed peas are by far the major type of peas used in animal feed. It seems that the inclusion of up to 250 g coloured-flowered peas /kg in diets for growing–finishing pigs does not lead to a decrease in performance (Bourdon *et al.*, 1973). This result is in accordance with Swedish trials quoted by Gâtel and Grosjean (1990).

Former trials carried out with white or coloured faba beans in pig diets (Table 9) show that the use of faba beans at up to 100 g/kg does not alter growth performance. At rates in excess of 100 g/kg, the inclusion of faba beans tends to reduce growth and increase the feed conversion ratio, whatever the type of faba beans. Supplementation with tryptophan tends to reduce the difference in performance compared with the control diet (Henry *et al.*, 1978), whereas supplementation with methionine does not have any effect (ITCF-AGPM, 1986). However, two recent trials (unpublished) show that in diets supplemented with amino acids, the inclusion of white or coloured faba beans, at up to 350 g/kg, does not alter growth performance. This may be due to a better amino acid balance, formulation on the basis of digestible amino acids and a better knowledge of faba bean energy values.

GESTATING AND LACTATING SOWS

The use of pulses by gestating and lactating sows is not very well documented. The inclusion of feed pea in the diets of gestating sows up to 160 g/kg and in diets for lactating sows at up to 240 g/kg does not alter the reproductive performances (number of piglets born, number of litters weaned) or the longevity of sows (Gâtel *et al.*, 1987).

The introduction of coloured faba beans at a rate of 150 g/kg in the diets of gestating and lactating sows had no effect on reproductive performance (number of piglets born, number of litters weaned). The effect of faba bean on milk production has not been measured. (Buron *et al.*, 1992) but, according to Etienne *et al.* (1975), the inclusion of 150 g faba beans /kg, supplemented with methionine, does not affect the quantity and quality of milk produced.

Pea and faba bean in poultry diets

BROILER CHICKENS

Different feeding experiments carried out in France have shown that field peas could be introduced at rates of up to 300 g/kg in broiler diets (Lucbert *et al.*, 1988) if the diet is correctly balanced in amino acids, especially methionine and tryptophan. Broilers are not as sensitive as pigs to TIA. Diets containing 300 g peas with 'low' TIA (2.3 to 4.5 UTI/mg DM)/kg of allowed performance similar to those obtained with diets containing 300 g peas with 'high' TIA (from 8.2 to 15.9 UTI/mg DM) /kg (Barrier-Guillot *et al.*, 1992).

Coloured-flowered peas can be used in organic broiler diets at up to 250g/ kg, as shown by Bouvarel *et al.* (2001) without decreasing growth performance.

Lucbert (1986) reviewed several trials showing that the use of faba beans in broiler diets leads to a slight deterioration in feed conversion ratio, due to an increase in feed intake and a decrease in daily growth. Nevertheless, supplementing the diet with methionine dramatically improves performance (Marquardt *et al.*, 1981). In a more recent trial with coloured and white faba beans, it was shown that the inclusion of both these faba bean types at 250 g/ kg resulted in performance similar to that obtained with the control diet (Métayer *et al.*, 2003). These results are not in accordance with those obtained by Brévault *et al.* (2003), who noticed a significant decrease in performance with 200 g coloured faba bean (cultivar Maya)/kg compared with the control diet, or with the diet including white faba bean (cultivar Gloria).

Table 10. Recent feeding trials with faba beans in broiler diets

Reference	Control diet with soya	Diet with faba beans		P
Métayer et al., 2003		Gloria (white FB)	Divine (Coloured FB)	
Live weight gain (g/d)	52.1	51.1	51.8	NS
Food intake 1 to 56 d (g)	5844	5635	5716	NS
Feed conversion ratio 1 to 56 d	2	1.97	1.98	NS
Brévault et al., 2003		Gloria (white FB)	Maya (Coloured FB)	
Live weight gain (g/d)	31.4 ab	31.8 b	30.5 a	<0.01
Food intake 1 to 83 d (g)	7385 b	7341 b	7135 a	<0.001
Feed conversion ratio 1 to 83 d	2.87	2.82	2.85	NS

LAYING HENS

In several trials, reviewed by Maître (1987), a slight but significant reduction in egg weight was observed with diets including pea at rates up to 200 g/kg. However, more recently, Igbasan *et al.* (1997) comparing the influence of feeding yellow-, green- or brown-seeded peas on the performance of laying hens, concluded that the inclusion of any type of pea into the diets of laying hens at rates up to 400 g/kg did not affect production as long as diets were balanced carefully in order to meet the optimum nutrient requirements for laying hens, especially in methionine. The poor performance observed with peas in former trials may be attributed to an inadequate amino acids balance in the diets.

It has been demonstrated that vicine and convicine are factors depressing egg size (Olaboro, 1981). It has also been suggested that vicine may produce pro-oxidants that cause lipid peroxidation, erythrocyte haemolysis and interfere with normal lipid metabolism in the hen (Muduuli *et al.*, 1981). When faba bean is incorporated into the diets of laying hens at rates up to 70g/kg, a significant decrease in egg weight is noticed, and this can not be improved using tryptophan, methionine or linoleic acid supplements (Lacassagne, 1988). In a recent trial, Lessire *et al.* (2005) introduced of two cultivars of faba bean, one with a high content of vicine and convicine (cv Marcel) and the other with a low vicine–convicine content (cv Divine) at rates of 200g/kg. The laying rate was not modified by the two experimental diets, but egg weight was negatively correlated with dietary vicine–convcine content. Egg quality was not impaired by faba beans. The use of faba bean with a high vicine and convicine content must be limited to 70g/kg diet, but it is possible to include faba bean at up to 200g/kg if the cultivar used has a low vicine and convicine content.

Economic value of pulses

USE OF PEAS IN THE DIFFERENT FRENCH FORMULAS

The total quantity of peas used in the feed industry in France in 2005 was about 800,000 tonnes, whereas it reached 1.6 million tonnes in 1998. This decrease reflects the decrease in pea production in France from 1998 to 2005. During this period, the quantity of peas harvested has been reduced by 60%. The decrease in peas used in the industry does not indicate lower interest just reduced availability.

In France peas are used mainly in pig diets, where their nutritional value fits perfectly with the nutritional requirements of pigs. Of the 800,000 tonnes of peas used in the French feed industry in 2005, about 0.9 were used for pigs, and half of these were for finishing pig formulas. In these types of diet, 0.5 to 0.8 of the cost of the feed is attributed to the energy constraint, and in the case of peas the value is enhanced by its energy content. In other words, its shadow price is due mainly to its energy value (see Insert 1). Thus, although peas are a raw material rich in protein their price is determined mainly by energy content. In poultry diets, the shadow price of peas is decreased by a strong 'concentration' constraint (expressed by the last figure in bold). This constraint expresses the necessary concentration in components of raw materials used for poultry nutrition. The shadow price of peas is consequently lower in poultry than in pig formulations.

Indeed, while the mixed profile of peas (supply of protein and energy) is a strength for pig nutrition, its low nutrient concentration is a weakness for poultry nutrition where the main sources of protein used (soyabean meals) are very concentrated. However, when there is sufficient quantity of peas available, and when their price is low enough, peas can also be incorporated in broiler or laying hen formulations, and less frequently in dairy cows formulations (see Figure 1).

RELATIVE VALUE OF THE DIFFERENT PULSES

At present only white-flowered peas and coloured faba beans are available

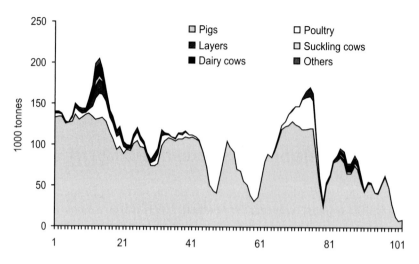

Figure 1. Uses of feed pea in different feed formulas in France (1998–2005)

on the market in significant quantities. Since their chemical composition and nutritional value are similar, they can compete with each other in feed formulations. The economic value of each one can be expressed by the shadow price in different feed formulations. As shown in Figure 2, the shadow price of white-flowered peas in finishing pig formulations is higher than that of coloured faba beans. This indicates a greater economic value for peas than for faba beans in this kind of formulation. In contrast, for finishing broiler formulations, the shadow price of coloured faba beans is higher than that of peas, which indicates a greater value of faba beans compared with peas for broilers, because of the higher level of crude protein in faba bean. Nevertheless, the shadow price of faba bean in a broiler formula is lower than its shadow price in a pig formula. For this reason faba beans, like peas, should first be allocated to pig formulations. If the available quantity is limited on the market, the market price will be determined mainly by the shadow prices of peas and faba beans in pig formulatrions, and so the market price of peas should be higher than that of faba beans for the feed market.

Environmental value of pulses for feed

The agronomic value of pulses in crop rotations is well known, because of their break-crop effect, but also because of their nitrogen-fixing capacity. Their environmental value in the rotation has been demonstrated by Nemecek *et al.* (2006) using the life cycle assessment method. Introducing grain

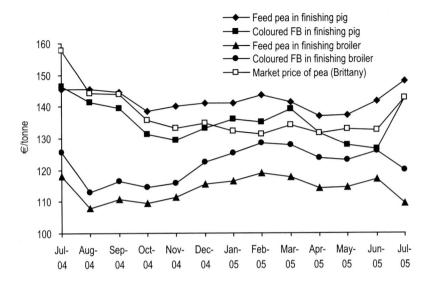

Figure 2. Shadow prices of feed pea and coloured faba bean in finishing pig and finishing broiler formulas in France (2004–2005)

legumes in rotations leads to a substantially lower energy demand, due to a reduction in N fertiliser use. The global warming potential is reduced for the same reason. The reduction in environmental burden is all the more important when grain legumes are introduced in intensive rotations. The environmental burdens of animal production are due mainly to the production of crop-based ingredients (Van der Werf *et al.*, 2004; Sonesson and Baumgartner, 2006). The use of grain legumes associated with rapeseed meal in a pig diet instead of soyabean meal alone reduced the energy demand and the global warming potential per kg of pig liveweight produced. These effects are explained by a reduction in the transport associated with the use of soyabean meal, by a lower energy demand (and global warming potential) to produce a mix of grain legumes and rapeseed meal than to produce soyabean meal, and by a lower content of cereals in the diet, due to the presence of pulses (Sonesson and Baumgartner, 2006).

Conclusion

For the most part, peas produced in the EU are feed peas, and faba beans are coloured faba beans. Both can be useful sources of protein and energy for animal feed.

Feed peas have a high nutritive value, which fits perfectly with pig nutritional requirements. Thanks to genetic improvement, white-flowered peas are not disadvantaged by antinutritional factors, such as trypsin-inhibiting factors. Their economic value in pig formulations is high, and it can replace soyabean meal completely in these formulations, when included at 400 g/kg diet. In poultry nutrition, due to an inadequate nutrient concentration, feed peas have a lower economic value and consequently are rarely used.

The use of coloured faba beans is more limited, due to the presence of tannins in the pericarp that decrease the energy content slightly. Despite this antinutritional factor, coloured faba beans are useful in pig diets, where they can be introduced up to 350 g/kg, but also in broiler diets, where they can be introduced up to 250 g/kg. When faba beans are included at levels as high as 250 g/kg in broiler diets, it can replace soyabean meal completely. Recent genetic improvements have enabled tannins and/or vicine and convicine to be removed from faba bean seeds. Removing the tannins from the seeds increases the energy value and the protein digestibility of faba beans for pigs and poultry. Removing vicine and convicine may increase the energy value of faba beans for broiler chickens, and increase the possible use of faba beans in laying hen diets. For faba beans, the more promising progress is to remove both tannins and vicine–convicine, since the effect of the two antinutritional factors on the nutritional value for broiler chickens is additive.

In addition to their obvious nutritional and economic value, the use of pulses instead of soyabean meal in the feed industry could decrease the burden of animal production on the environment. This is because pulses have environmental value at the crop production level, due to their nitrogen-fixation capacity and since they are produced locally. This considerable advantage is not recognised at present, but could be of great interest in the future in the context of increasing energy costs.

Acknowledgement

Many thanks are due to Corinne Peyronnet (UNIP) for her careful re-reading and to Gillian Craig for improving the English.

References

Askbrandt S.U.S. (1988). Metabolisable energy content of rapeseed meal, soyabean mea land white-flowered peas determined with laying hens and adult cockerels. *Bristish Poultry Science* **29**, 445-455

Barrier-Guillot B., Castaing J., Peyronnet C., Lucbert J. (1992). Comparison of pea varieties (Pisum sativum) varying in their trypsin inhibitor activity on broiler performance. In *1ère conférence européenne sur les protéagineux*, pp 447-448. Edited by AEP, Paris

Barrier-Guillot B., Grosjean F., Métayer J.P., Beaux M.F., Carrouée B. (1999). Valeur énergétique de 39 lots de pois protéagineux présentés en granulés chez le poulet de chair. In *3ième Journées de la Recherche Avicole*, pp 101-104, Edited by ITAVI, Paris

Barrier-Guillot B., Métayer J.P. (2001). Valeur alimentaire de cinq matières premières chez le coq adulte, le poulet de chair, le dindonneau et le canard. In *4ième Journées de la Recherche Avicole*, pp 131-134, Edited by ITAVI, Paris

Barrier-Guillot B., Métayer J.P., Grosjean F., Peyronnet C. (1995). Feeding value of pea presented in mash or pellets in adult cockerels, laying hens, broilers and turkeys poults. In *10th European symposium on poultry nutrition, Antalya, Turkey*, pp 286-287

Bastianelli D., Grosjean F., Peyronnet C., Duparque M., Régnier J.MM (1998) Feeding value of pea (*Pisum sativum* L.) 1. Chemical composition of different categories of pea. *Animal Science* **67,** 609-619

Bengala freire J., Aumaître A., Peiniau J. (1991). Effects of feeding raw and extruded peas on ileal digestibility, pancreatic enzymes and plasma glucose and insulin in early weaned pigs. Fahne Parey Tierphysiologie 53-64

Biarnès V. (2005).Intéractions génotype x milieu pour le rendement et la teneur en protéines. In *Agrophysiologie du pois protéagineux*, pp245-251. Edited by INRA éditions, Paris

Biarnès V., Dubois G. (2005). Protein content of registered European cultivars : variations among cultivars and trends over time and location. *Grain legumes* **44**, 10-11

Bond D.A., Duc G. (1993). Plant breeding as e means of reducing antinutritonal factors in grain legumes. In *Recent advances of research in antinutritional factors in legume seeds*, pp 379-396, Edited by Wageningen Pers, Wageningen

Bourdon D. and Perez J.M., 1976. Utilisation comparée du pois et de la féverole par le porc en croissance. In *Journées de la Recherche Porcine en France* pp 61-68. Edited by ITP, Paris

Bourdon D., Henry Y. (1973). Valeur énergétique du pois fourrager et utilisation par le porc en finition. In *Journées de la Recherche Porcine en France* pp 115-121. Edited by ITP, Paris

Bourdon D., Jung J., Perez J.M. (1977). Valeur énergétique et azotée de différentes variétés de pois (Pisum sativum L.) pour le porc. In *Journées* de la Recherche Porcine en France pp 265-269. Edited by ITP, Paris

Bourdon D., Perez J.M. (1976). Utilisation comparée du pois et de la féverol par le porc en croissance. In *Journées de la Recherche Porcine en France* 61-69

Bourdon D., perez J.M. (1982). Premiers résultats sur la valeur énergétique et azotée des pois protéagineux de printemps. In *Journées de la Recherche Porcine en France* **14**, pp 261-266. Edited by ITP, Paris

Bourdon D., Perez J.M. (1984). Valeur énergétique et azotée pour le porc de différents type de féverole pauvre ou riche en tanins. In *Journées de la Recherche Porcine en France* **16**, pp 401-408. Edited by ITP, Paris

Bouvarel I., Panhéleux M., Hatté C., Cherrière K., Jonis M. (2001). Le pois comme source principale de protéines dans l'aliment du poulet de chair biologique. In 4*ièmes Journées Techniques Avicoles*, pp 213-216, edited by ITAVI, Paris

Brévault N., Mansuy E., Crépon K., Bouvarel I., Lessire M., Rouillère H. (2003). Utilisation de différentes variétés de féveroles dans l'alimentation du poulet biologique. In 5*ièmes Journées Techniques Avicoles*, pp 221-224, edited by ITAVI, Paris

Buron G., Gâtel F. (1992). Utilisation de la féverole (*Vicia faba* L.) par la truie en reproduction. In *Journées de la Recherche Porcine en France* **24** pp 187-194. Edited by ITP, Paris

Canibe N., Bach Knudsen K.E. (1997). Digestibility of dried and toasted peas in pigs. 1. Ileal and total tract digestibilities of carbohydrates. *Animal Feed Science Technology* **64**, 293-310

Carré B. (1997). La qualité des graines de légumineuses en nutrition aviaire. In 2*ièmes journées de la recherche avicole*, pp 27-32. Edited by ITAVI, France

Carré B., Escartin R., Melcion J.P., Champ M., Roux G., Leclercq B. (1987). Effect of pelleting and associations with maize or wheat on the nutritive value of smooth pea (*Pisum sativum*) seeds in adult cockerels. *British Poultry Science* **28**, 219-229

Castaing J., Grosjean F. (1985). Effets de forts pourcentage de pois de printemps dans des regimes pour porcs charcutiers à base de maïs ou d'orge et en complément de tourteau de colza. In *Journées de la Recherche Porcine en France* **17** pp 407-418. Edited by ITP, Paris

Castaing J., Leuillet M; (1981). Etude de l'association maïs/pois protéagineux chez le porc charcutier. In *Journées de la Recherche Porcine en France* pp 151-162. Edited by ITP, Paris

Conan L., Barrier-Guillot B., Widiez J.L., Lucbert J. (1992). Effect of grinding and pelleting on the nutritional value of smooth pea seed (Pisum sativum) in adult cockerel. In *1ère conférence européenne sur les protéagineux*, pp 479-480. Edited by AEP, Paris

Crépon K. (2004) Protein supply in Europe and the challenge to increase grain legumes production: a contribution to sustainable agriculture. In *Grain legumes and the environment: how to assess benefits and impacts*, pp13-16. Edited by AEP, Paris

Crépon K., Pressenda F. (2005) Economic value of pea protein for feed *Grain legumes* **44**, 20-21

Duc G., Marget P., Esnault R., Le Guen J., Bastianelli D. (1999) Genetic variability for feeding value of faba bean seeds (Vicia faba) : comparative chemical composition of isogenics involving zero-tannin and zero-vicine genes. *Journal of Agricultural Science* **133**, 185-196

Duc G., Sixdenier G., Lila M., Furstoss V. (1989). Search of genetic variability for vicine and convicine content in VIcia faba L. A first report of a gene wich codes for nearly zero-vicine and zero-convicine contents. In *Recent advances of research in antinutritional factors in legume seeds*, pp 305-313, Edited by Wageningen Pers, Wageningen

Edwards S., Rogers-Lewis D.S., Fairbairn C.B. (1987). The effects of pea variety and inclusion rate in the diet on the performance of finishing pigs. *Journal of. agriultural. Sciences Cambridge* **108**, 383-388.

Etienne M., Duee P.H., Pastuszewska B. (1975). Nitrogen balance in lactating sows fed on diets containing soybean oil meal or horsebean (*Vicia faba*) as a protein concentrate. *Livestock production science*, **2**, 147-156

Fekete J., Willequet F., Gâtel F., Quemere P., Grosjean F. (1985). Utilisation de féverole par le porcelet sevré. In *Journées de la Recherche Porcine en France* **17** pp 397-406. Edited by ITP, Paris

Gâtel F., Buron G., Leuillet M. (1987). Utilisation du pois protéagineux de printemps par la truie en gestation – lactation. In *Journées de la Recherche Porcine en France* **19** pp 223-230. Edited by ITP, Paris

Gâtel F., Grosjean F.(1990) Composition and nutritive value of peas for pigs : a review of European results. *Livestock Production Science* **26**, 155-175

Gâtel F., Grosjean F., Castaing J. (1989). Utilisation par le porc charcutier de regimes à teneur élevée en pois de printemps (plus de 40 p. cent). In *Journées de la Recherche Porcine en France* **21** pp 69-74. Edited by ITP, Paris

Gdala J., Buraczewska L., Grala W. (1991). Factors influencing ileal and total digestibility of pea protein and amino acids in pigs. In *6ᵗʰ symp. Protein metabolism and nutrition*. Herning Denmark 1991, pp 240-242

Griffiths D.W., Ramsay G. (1993). The vicine and convicine content of faba bean (*Vicia faba* L.) plants from flowering to seed maturity. In *Recent advances of research in antinutritional factors in legume seeds*, pp 407-410, Edited by Wageningen Pers, Wageningen

Grosjean F., Barrier-Guillot B., Bastianelli D., Rudeaux F., Bourdillon A., Peyronnet C. (1999). Feeding value of three categories of pea (*Pisum sativum*, L.) for poultry. *Animal Science* **69**, 591-599

Grosjean F., Barrier-Guillot B., Joindreville C. Peyronnet C. (1995). Feeding value of different cultivars of faba beans (Vicia faba minor). In 2nd *European conference on Grain Legumes*, pp 308-309. Edited by AEP, Paris

Grosjean F., Bastianelli D., Bourdillon A., Cerneau P., Joindreville C. Peyronnet C. (1998a). Feeding value of pea (Pisum sativum L.) 2. Nutritional value in the pig. Animal Science **67**, 621-625

Grosjean F., Bourdillon A., Rudeaux F., Bastianelli D., Peyronnet C., Duc G., Lacassagne L. (2000). Valeur alimentaire pour la volaille de féveroles isogéniques (*Vicia faba* L.) avec ou sans tannins et avec ou sans vicine. *Sciences et techniques avicoles* **32**, 17-24

Grosjean F., Bourdon D., Isambert Ph., Peyronnet C., Joindreville C. (1992). Valeur alimentaire pour le porc charcutier de produits de décorticage de pois. In *Journées de la Recherche Porcine en France* **24**, pp 173-178. Edited by ITP, Paris

Grosjean F., Bourdon D., Kiener T., Castaing J., Gatel F. (1991). Valeur alimentaire pour les porcs des pois français et importés. In *Journées de la Recherche Porcine en France* **23**, pp 53-60. Edited by ITP, Paris

Grosjean F., Bourdon D., Theillaud-Rica V., Castaing J., Beague E. (1989). Comparaison des pois d'hiver et de printemps dans les aliments pour porc charcutier présentés en farine ou en granules. In *Journées de la Recherche Porcine en France* **21**, pp 59-68. Edited by ITP, Paris

Grosjean F., Castaing J., Gâtel F. (1986). Utilisation de différentes variétés de pois et d'une association pois de printemps-féverole par le porc charcutier. In *Journées de la Recherche Porcine en France* **18** pp 47-56. Edited by ITP, Paris

Grosjean F., Cerneau P., Bourdillon A., Bastianelli D., Peyronnet C., Duc G. (2001). Valeur alimentaire, pour le porc, de féveroles presque isogéniques, contenant ou non des tanins et à forte ou faible teneur en vicine et convicine. In *Journées de la Recherche Porcine en France* **33** pp 205-210. Edited by ITP, Paris

Grosjean F., Gâtel F. (1989). Utilisation des protéagineux par les porcins. SIMAVIP

Grosjean F., Joindreville C., Bogaert C., Bourdillon A., Peyronnet C., Le Guen M.P., Williate I. (1997). Utilisation d'aliments pour porcelets sevrés contenant 40% de pois. In *Journées de la Recherche Porcine en France* **29** pp 197-204. Edited by ITP, Paris

Grosjean F., Joindreville C., Williatte-Hazouard I., Skiba F., Carrouée B., Gâtel F. (2000). Ileal digestibility of protein and amino acids of feed peas with different trypsin inhibitor activity in pigs. Canadian Journal of animal science 643-652

Grosjean F., Métayer J.P., Peyronnet C., Carrouée B. (1993). Variability in trypsin inhibitor activity of peas (Pisum sativum) grown in France. In *Recent advances of research in antinutritional factors in legume seeds*, pp 411-415, Edited by Wageningen Pers, Wageningen

Grosjean F., Williatte-Houzouard I., Joindreville C., Skiba F., Peyronnet C. (1998b). Variabilité de la valeur alimentaire du pois pour les porcs, en liaison avec le milieu de production et les techniques culturales. In *Journées de la Recherche Porcine en France* **30**, pp 231-237. Edited by ITP, Paris

Henry Y. and Bourdon D. (1978). Utilization of legume seeds by the pig. *World review of animal production*, **14**, 1, 81-87.

Hess V., Thibault J.N., Duc G., Melcion J.P., Van Eys J., Sève B. (1998). Influence de la variété et du microbroyage sur la digestibilité iléale de l'azote et des acides amines du pois. In *Journées de la Recherche Porcine en France* **30**, pp 223-229. Edited by ITP, Paris

Huet J.C., Baudet J., Mossé J., (1987). Constancy of composition of storage proteins deposited in *Pisum sativum* seeds. *Phytochemistry* **26**, 47-50

Igbasan F.A., Guenter W (1997). The influence of feeding yellow, green and brown seeded peas on production performance of laying hens. *Journal of Science and Food Agriculture.*, **73**, 120-128.

ITCF, 1983. Féverole pour porcs charcutiers : comparaison de trois variétés, rapport d'activité

ITCF-AGPM, 1985. Féverole pour porcs charcutiers : incorporation de 10,15 ou 20% de féverole dans un régime à base de maïs, rapport d'activité

ITCF-AGPM, 1986. Féverole pour porcs charcutiers: effet de la supplémentation en méthionine, rapport d'activité

Jansman A.J.M., Longstaff M. (1993). Nutritional effects of tannins and vicine/convicine in legume seeds. In Recent advances of researcj in antinutritional factors in legume seeds, pp 301-316, Edited by Wageningen Pers, Wageningen.

Joindreville C., Grosjean F., Buron G., Peyronnet C., Beneytout J.L. (1992). Comparison of four pea varieties in pig feeding through digestibility and growth performance results. *J. Animal Physiology and Animal Nutrition.* **68**, 113-122

Lacassagne L. (1988). Alimentation des volailles : substituts au tourteau de soja 1. Les protéagineux. *INRA Production Animale* **1** (1), 47-57.

Lacassagne L., Francesch M., Carré B., Melcion J.P. (1988). Utilization of tannin-containing and tannin-free faba beans (Vicia faba) by young chicks :effects of pelletings feeds on energy, protein and starch digestibility. *Animal feed Science and Technology* **20**, 59-68

Lacassagne L., Melcion J.P., de Monredon F., Carrée B. (1991). The nutritional values of faba bean flours varying in their mean particle size in young chickens. *Animal Feed Science and Technology* **34**, 11-19

Lessire M., Hallouis J.M., Chagbeau A.M., Besnard J., travel A., Bouvarel I., Crépon K., Duc G., Dulieu P. (2005). Influence de la teneur en vicine et convicine de la féverole sur les performances de production de la poule pondeuse et la qualité de l'œuf. In *6ièmes Journées Techniques Avicoles*, pp 174-178, edited by ITAVI, Paris

Leterme P., Monmart T., Théwis A. (1992). Varietal distribution of the trypsin inhibitor activity in peas (*Pisum sativum* L.). *Animal Feed Science and Technology* **37**, 309-315

Leuillet M., Perez J.M. (1980). Le pois dans l'alimentation des porcelets : bilan des résultats et recommandations pratiques. *Les industries de l'alimentation animale* 332, 11-22.

Lucbert J. (1986). Utilisation des protéagineux par les volailles. SIMAVIP

Lucbert J., Castaing J. (1988). Du pois pour les volailles de chair. In *Le courrier avicole* n°858 novembre.

Maillard R., Kiener T., Bertrand S. (1990). Digestibilité "réelle" mesurée au niveau iléal, des acides amines de la féverole et du lupin. In *Journées de la Recherche Porcine en France* **23** pp 211-216. Edited by ITP, Paris

Maître I. (1987). Les protéagineux pour l'alimentation des pondeuses. *Dossiers techniques : études et expérimentations ITAVI*. Edited by ITAVI, Paris

Mariscal-Landin G., Lebreton Y., Sève B. (2002). Apparent ans tandardised true ileal digestibility of protein and amino acids from faba bean, lupin and pea, provided as whole seeds, dehulled or extruded in pig diets. *Animal feed Science and Technology*, **97** 183-198

Métayer J.P., Barrier-Guillot B., Skiba F., Crépon K., Bouvarel I., Marget P., Duc G, Lessire M. (2003), Valeur alimentaire et utilisation de différents types de féveroles chez le poulet et le coq adulte. In *5ième Journées de la Recherche Avicole*, pp 133-136, Edited by ITAVI, Paris

Métayer J.P., Grosjean F., Peyronnet C., Carrouée B. (1992). Composition of peas grown in France for animal feeding : results a survey. In *1ère conférence européenne sur les protéagineux*, pp 447-448. Edited by AEP, Paris

Métayer J.P., Vilariño M (2006). Effet de la variété et du lieu de culture sur la valeur énergétique des féveroles chez le poulet de chair et le coq adulte. Compte rendu d'essai ARVALIS-UNIP.

Mossé J., (1990) Acides amines de 16 céréales et protéagineux : variations et clés du calcul de la composition en function du taux d'azote des graines. Conséquences nutritionnelles. *INRA Production Animale* **3**, 103-119

Muduuli D., Marquardt R., Guenter W. (1981). Effect of dietary vicine on the productive performance of laying chickens. *Canadian Journal of Animal Sciences.* **61**, 757-764

Muel F., Carrouée B., Grosjean F. (1998). Trypsin inhibitors activity of pea cultivars :new data and a proposal strategy for breeding programme. In *3rd European conference on grain legumes*, pp 164-165 Edited by AEP, Paris

Nemecek T. (2006). Environmental impact of grain legumes in regional crop rotations. *Grain legumes* **45**, 20-22

Noblet J., Bourdon D. (1997). Valeur énergétique compare de onze matières premières chez le porc en croissance et la truie adulte. In *Journées de la Recherche Porcine en France* **29** pp 221-226. Edited by ITP, Paris

Olaboro G., Marquardt R., Campbell L., Fröhlich A. (1981). Putification, identification and quantification of an egg-weight-depressing factor (vicine) in fababeans (Vicia faba L.). *Journal of Science and Food Agriculture* **32**, 1163-1171

Palisse-Roussel M., Jacquot L., Maury Y. (1984). Intérêt de l'association pois de printemps et tryptophane de synthèse pour remplacer la totalité du tourteau de soja dans une formule porc engraissement. In *Journées de la Recherche Porcine en France* **16** pp 383-392. Edited by ITP, Paris

Perez J.M., Bourdon D. (1982). Essai de remplacement total du tourteau de soja dans le régime du porc en croissance : utilisation du pois supplémenté en tryptophane ou associé à un concentré de protéines de luzerne. In *Journées de la Recherche Porcine en France* **14** pp 283-296. Edited by ITP, Paris

Picard J. (1976). Aperçu sur l'hérédité du caractère absence de tannins dans les graines de féveroles (Vicia faba L.). *Annales de l'amélioration des plantes* **26**, 101-106

PROLEA (2006) *De la production à la consommation : Statistiques des oléagineux et protéagineux, huiles et protéines végétales.* PROLEA, Paris

Sauvant D., Perez J.M., Tran G., (2004). Table *de composition et de valeur nutritive des matières premières destinées aux animaux d'élevage.* INRA Editions, Paris

Sève B., Aumaître A., Bouchez P. (1985). Effet d'un traitement technologique sur la valeur nutritionnelle du pois pour le jeune porcelet. *Sciences des Aliments* **5**, 119-126.

Skiba F. (2000). Optimisation de l'utilisation de la féverole dans l'alimentation des porcelets biologiques. Compte rendu ARVALIS.

Skiba F. (2003). Digestibilité iléale des protéaines et des acides amines de lots de féveroles, d'un lot de pois et d'unh lot de lupin. Compte-rendu d'essai UNIP-ARVALIS.

Sonesson U., Baumgartner D. (2006). Environmental benefits of grain legumes for food and feed. In *Benefits of grain legumes for European agriculture and environment, new results and prospects*, Brussels 2006.

Thacker P.A. and Bowland J.P. (1985). Faba beans : an alternative protein supplement for use in pig diets. *Pig new and information*, **6**, n°1, 25-30

UNIP (1995). *Peas in animal feeding.* Editions UNIP-ITCF, Paris

Valdebouze P., Bergeron E., Gaborit T., Delort-Laval J. (1980). Content and distribution of trypsin inhibitors and hemagglutinins in some legume seeds. *Canadian Journal of Plant Sciences.* **60**, 695-701

Van Cauwenberghe S., Joindreville C., Beaux M.F., Grosjean F., Peyronnet C., Williate I., Gâtel F. (1997a). Performances de croissance du porcelet en post-sevrage obtenues avec des régimes à base de pois et de manioc. In *Journées de la Recherche Porcine en France* **29** pp 189-196. Edited by ITP, Paris

Van Cauwenberghe S., Joindreville C., Beaux M.F., Grosjean F., Williate I., Gâtel F. (1997b). Estimation de la valeur énergétique des aliments et des matières premières chez le porcelet en post-sevrage et chez le porc charcutier. In *Journées de la Recherche Porcine en France* **29** pp 205-212. Edited by ITP, Paris

Vilariño M., Skiba F., Callu P., Crépon K. (2004). Valeur énergétique et digestibilité iléale des acides aminés de différents types de féveroles chez le porc charcutier. In *Journées de la Recherche Porcine en France* **36** pp 211-216. Edited by ITP, Paris

LIST OF PARTICIPANTS

The fortieth University of Nottingham Feed Conference was organised by the following committee:

MR N.J. CHANDLER *(National Renderers Association)*
DR Z. DAVIS *(Defra)*
MR M. HAZZLEDINE *(Premier Nutrition)*
MR M. ROGERS *(Volac International)*
DR D. PARKER *(Novus International)*
MR J.R. PICKFORD
DR I.H. PIKE *(IFOMA)*
MR J. TWIGGE *(Trouw Nutrition Ltd)*
DR R. TEN DOESCHATE *(ABNA Ltd)*
DR M.A. VARLEY *(Provimi Ltd)*

DR J.M. BRAMELD
PROF P.J. BUTTERY
DR P.C. GARNSWORTHY *(Secretary)*
DR T. PARR ⎫ *University of Nottingham*
DR A.M. SALTER
DR K.D. SINCLAIR
PROF R. WEBB
DR J. WISEMAN *(Chairman)*

The conference was held at the University of Nottingham Sutton Bonington Campus, 12-14 September 2006. The following persons registered for the meeting.

Agnew, Dr K	United Feeds Ltd, 8 Norther Road, Belfast BT3 9AL, UK
Aguilar Perez, Mr C	Universitad Autonoma de Yucatan, Merida, Yucatan, Mexico
Archer, Mrs V	University of Nottingham, Sutton Bonington Campus, Loughborough, Leics LE12 6UZ, UK
Bartram, Dr C	Southern Valley Feeds, Huntworth Mill, Bridgwater TA6 6LQ, UK
Beaumont, Mr D	Lohmann Animal Health, Maple Lodge, Ryknield Hill, Denby, DE5 8NW, UK
Bewley, Mr J	Ice Robotics, Logan Building, Roslin Biocentre, Roslin, Midlothian EH25 9TT, UK
Brameld, Dr J M	University of Nottingham, Sutton Bonington Campus, Loughborough LE12 5RD, UK
Brown, Mr G	DSM Nutritional Products (UK) Ltd, Heanor Gate, Heanor, Derbys DE75 7SG, UK
Buttery, Prof P	University of Nottingham, Sutton Bonington Campus, Loughborough LE12 5RD, UK
Caldier, Mr P	Independent Journalist, 26 bld Carmat, Saint-Denis 93200, France
Castillejos, Dr L	Diamond V Europe, P O Box 14, Marum 9363 ZG, The Netherlands
Chandler, Mr N J	National Renderers Association, 52 Packhorse Road, Gerrards Cross SL9 8EF, UK

Chaosap, Miss C	University of Nottingham, Sutton Bonington Campus, Loughborough, Leics LE12 5RD, UK
Charrie, Mrs C	Newport Scientific Europe Ltd, Unit 454, Silk House, Macclesfield SH11 7QJ, UK
Choun, Mr M	James and Son GM Ltd, Olmar Court, 3 Regent Park, Booth Dr, Park Farm, Wellingborough, Northants NN8 6GR, UK
Clarke, Mr A N	Britphos Ltd, Rawdon House, Green Lane, Yeadon, Leeds LS19 7BY, UK
Close, Dr W	Close Consultancy, 129 Barkham Road, Wokingham, Berks RG41 2RS, UK
Cole, Mr J	BFI Innovations, 1 Telford Court, Chester Gates, Dunkirk Lea, Chester CH1 6LT, UK
Connerton, Prof I	University of Nottingham, Sutton Bonington Campus, Loughborough, Leics LE12 5RD, UK
Cook, Mr B	Calibre, 5/6 Asher Court, Lyncastle Way, Appleton, Warrington WA4 4ST, UK
Cooke, Dr B C	1 Jenkins Orchard, Wick St Lawrence, Weston-S-Mare BS22 7YP, UK
Crepon, Mrs K	UNIP, 12 avenue George V, 75008 Paris , France
Dale, Mr T N	Scotmin Nutrition, 26 Whitehouse Dale, York YO24 1EB, UK
Davies, Dr Z	DEFRA, Area 4B, Nobel House, 17 Smith Square, London SW1P 3JR, UK
De Smet, Dr K	Nutrition Sciences/Vitamex, Booiebos 5, Drongen 9031, Belgium
Doppenberg, Dr J	Schothorst Feed Research, P O Box 533, Lelystad 8200AM, The Netherlands
Doucet, Dr F	University of Nottingham, Sutton Bonington Campus, Loughborough, Leics LE12 5RD, UK
Eldridge, Mr J	Three Counties Feeds, Old School House, 79 Chapel St, Tiverton, Devon, UK
Fjermedal, Dr A	Fiska Molle A/S, Grooseveien 94, Grimstad 4879, Norway
Flint, Prof A P F	University of Nottingham, Sutton Bonington Campus, Loughborough LE12 5RD, UK
Fowers, Miss R	Frank Wright Ltd, Blenheim House, Blenheim Road, Ashbourne DE6 1HA, UK
Fullarton, Mr P	Forum Bioscience, 41-51 Brighton Road, Redhill, Surrey RH1 6YS, UK
Gardner, Dr D	University of Nottingham, Sutton Bonington Campus, Loughborough Leics, LE12 5RD, UK
Garnsworthy, Dr P C	University of Nottingham, Sutton Bonington Campus, Loughborough, Leics LE12 5RD, UK
Gibson, Dr M	Dakota Gold Marketing, 4506 N. Lewis Ave, Sioux Falls South Dakota 57104, USA

Golds, Mrs S P	University of Nottingham, Sutton Bonington Campus, Loughborough LE12 5RD, UK
Goodman, Mrs T	Farmsense Ltd, Docklands, Dock Road, Lytham FY8 5AQ, UK
Gould, Mrs M	Volac International Ltd, Volac House, Orwell, Royston SG8 5QX, UK
Green, Mrs K	Fishmeal Information Network, 4 The Forum, Minerva Business Park, Peterborough PE2 6FT, UK
Green, Prof M	University of Nottingham, Sutton Bonington Campus, Loughborough, Leics LE12 5RD, UK
Green, Dr S	Adisseo, Berkhamsted House, 121 High Street, Berkhamsted HP4 2DJ, UK
Gregson, Miss E	University of Nottingham, Sutton Bonington Campus, Loughborough, Leics LE12 5RD, UK
Hall, Miss C	BOCM Pauls, First Ave, Royal Portbury Dock, Portbury, Bristol BS20 9XS, UK
Halls, Mr R	Roquette UK Ltd, Sallow Road, Corby NN17 5JX, UK
Hayler, Mrs R	BASF Aktiengesellschaft, E-MEE/LT - J550, Ludwigshafen 67056, Germany
Hazzledine, Dr M	Premier Nutrition, Ivanhoe, Lodge Lane, Nailsea, Bristol BS48 2BB, UK
Henckel, Dr P	Danish Inst of Agricultural Sciences, Food Sc, Research Centre Foulum, Blinchers Alle, P O Box 50, DK-8830 Tjele, Denmark
Hernandez Medrano, Mr J	University of Nottingham, Sutton Bonington Campus, Loughborough, Leics LE12 5RD, UK
Hill, Dr S	University of Nottingham, Sutton Bonington Campus, Loughborough, Leics LE12 5RD, UK
Holder, Dr P	SVG Intermol, Alexandra House, Regent Road, Liverpool L20 1ES, UK
Holma, Mrs M	Raisio Feed, P O Box 101, Raisio 21201, Finland
Hooley, Mrs E	University of Nottingham, Sutton Bonington Campus, Loughborough LE12 5RD, UK
Hoste, Dr S	ACMC Ltd, Upton House, Beeford, Driffield, East Yorks YO25 8AF, UK
Huxley, Dr J	University of Nottingham, Sutton Bonington Campus, Loughborough, Leics LE12 5RD, UK
Ingham, Mr R	Kemira Growth UK Ltd, Ince, Chester CH2 4LB, UK
Issac, Mr P	Mole Valley Farmers, Huntworth Mill, Bridgewater TA6 6LQ, UK
Jagger, Dr S	ABNA, ABN House, Oundle Road, Peterborough PE2 9PW, UK
Jones, Dr G	Zintec Feed Supplements, Downwood, Shobdon, Hertfordshire HR6 9NH, UK
King, Mr C	Three Counties Feeds, Old School House, 79 Chaple St, Tiverton, Devon , UK

Kirkland, Dr R	Volac, Volac House, Fishers Lane, Orwell, Royston, Herts SG8 5QX, UK
Knowles, Mr A	Meat & Livestock Commission, P O Box 44, Winterhill House, Snowdon Drive, Milton Keynes MK6 1AX, UK
Koeleman, Mrs E	Feed Mix Magazine, Reed Business Information, P O Box 4, Doetinchem 7000BA, The Netherlands
Lapierre, Dr H	Agriculture and Agri-Food Canada, P O Box 90, Lennoxville J1M 1Z3, Canada
Lee, Miss E	University of Nottingham, Sutton Bonington Campus, Loughborough, Leics LE12 5RD, UK
Lowe, Dr J	Dodson and Horrell Ltd, Kettering Road, Islip, Kettering NN14 3JW, UK
Lucey, Mr P	Dairy Gold Quality Feeds, Lombardstown, Co Cork , Ireland
Macmillan, Mrs E	University of Melbourne, 250 Princes Highway, Werribee 3030, Australia
Macmillan, Prof J	University of Melbourne, Victoria, 3010, Australia
Mafo, Mr A	Hi Peak Feeds Ltd, Hi Peak Feeds Mill, Sheffield Road, Killamarsh SZ1 1ED, UK
Malo, Mr J J	Nutreco, Boxmeerseweg 30, Sint Anthonis 5845ET, The Netherlands
Masey O'Neill, Miss H	University of Nottingham, Sutton Bonington Campus, Loughborough, Leics LE12 5RD, UK
Mavromichalis, Dr I	Nutral (Provimi), c/ Cobalto, p 261-263, Pol Industrial Sur Colmenar Viejo (Madrid) 28770, Spain
Max, Dr R	Sokoine Univ of Agriculture, Dept of Veterinary Physiology, P O Box 3017, Morogoro POB 3017, Tanzania
Mayne, Dr S	Agri Food & Biosciences Institute, Hillsborough, Co Down BT26 6DR, UK
McIlmoyle, Dr D	Rumenco, Stretton House, Derby Road, Burton upon Trent DE13 0DW, UK
Mellor, Miss S	Nottingham University Press, Manor Farm, Church Lane, Thrumpton, Notts NG11 0AX, UK
Morris, Mr W	BOCM Pauls Ltd, First Ave, Royal Portbury Dock, Portbury, Bristol BS20 9XS, UK
Mul, Mr A J	CCL Research, P O Box 107, Veghel 5460 AC, The Netherlands
Mullholland, Mr M	College of Agric, Food & Rural Enterprise, Grenmount Campus, 22 Grenmount Rd, Antrim BT41 4PU, UK
Newbold, Dr J	Provimi Research and Tech Centre, Lenneka Marelaan 2, Sint-Stevens-Woluwe 1932, Belgium
Nohr, Dr D	University of Hohenheim, Fruwirthstr 12, D-70593 Stuttgart, Germany
Oliver, Dr T	ABNA, P O Box 250, Oundle Road, Peterborough PE2 9PW, UK

Overend, Dr M	Forum Animal Nutrition and Health, 41-51 Brighton Rd, Redhill, Surrey RH1 6YS, UK
Paganga, Dr G	AASC Ltd, Unit 5, Stanton Road, Southampton S015 4HU, UK
Parker, Dr D	Novus Europe, 200 Avenue Marcel Thiry, Building D, Brussels B-1200, Belgium
Parr, Dr T	University of Nottingham, Sutton Bonington Campus, Loughborough LE12 5RD, UK
Pedersen, Dr C	Danisco Animal Nutrition, Market House, Court High St, Marlborough SN8 1AA, UK
Pierse, Miss E	Kerry Ingredients, R & D, Tralee Road, Listowel Co Kerry, Ireland
Pike, Dr I H	FGC/IFFO, Chard, Bovington Green, Marlow SL7 2JL, UK
Pike, Mr S	Calibre, 5/6 Asher Court, Lyncastle Way, Appleton, Warrington WA4 4ST, UK
Pine, Mr A	Premier Nutrition, The Levels, Rugeley WS15 1GB, Uk
Piva, Dr G	Faculty of Agriculture, Via E Parmense 84, Piacenza, Italy 29100, UK
Reeve, Dr A	C & H Nutrition, Alexander House, Crown Gate, Runcorn WA7 2UP, UK
Relandeau, Mrs C	Ajinomoto Eurolysine S A S, 153 Rue de Courcelles, Paris Cedex 17 75817, France
Richards, Dr S	SCA Nutec, Dalton Airfield Industrial Estate, Dalton, Thirsk YO7 3HE, UK
Roele, Mr R	Persorp Franklin BV, Industrieweg 8, Waspik 516S NH, The Netherlands
Rogers, Mr M	Volac International Ltd, Volac House, Orwell, Royston SG8 5QX, UK
Rudd, Mr G	AIC, Confederation House, East of, England Showground, Peterborough PE2 6XE, UK
Salter, Prof A	University of Nottingham, Sutton Bonington Campus, Loughborough LE12 5RD, UK
Seppala, Miss S	Raisio Plc, P O Box 101, Raisio 21201, FINLAND
Shilton, Mrs L	Wheyfeed Ltd, Hill Farm, Melton Road, Stanton on the Wolds NG12 5PJ, UK
Short, Dr F	ADAS Gleadthorpe, Meden Vale, Mansfield, Notts NG2 9PF, UK
Sinclair, Dr K D	University of Nottingham, Sutton Bonington Campus, Loughborough LE12 5RD, UK
Sterzen, Mr H	Felleskjopet Fortutvikling, N-7005 Trondheim, Norway
Studley, Mr D	Three Counties Feeds, Old School House, 79 Chaple St, Tiverton, UK
Tansini, Dr G	Vetagrow SRL, Via Colletta 12, Reggio Emilia 42100, Italy

Taylor-Pickard, Dr J A	Alltech, Tudor Oaks, 26 Milner Drive, Whitton, Twickenham, Middlesex TW2 7PJ, UK
Ten Doeschate, Dr R	ABNA Ltd, ABN House, Oundle Road, Peterborough PE2 9PW, UK
Thatcher, Prof B	University of Florida, Gainesville, FL 32611 Florida, USA
Thatcher, Mrs M-J	University of Florida, College of Veterinary Medicine, Dept LACS P O Box 100136 Gainesville FL, 32610-0136, USA
Thornber, Miss V	Premier Nutrition, Brereton Business Park, The Levels, Rugeley WS15 1RO, UK
Trebble, Mr J	Mole Valley Farmers, Huntworth Mill, Bridgewater TA6 6LQ,
Tsunoda, Mr A	6-18-2-401 Minami Oi Shinagawa, TOKYO 140-0013, Japan
Upton, Ms E	Kemira Growhow, Industrigatan 70, Helsingborg 25109, Sweden
Van der Drift, Miss S	Schothorst Feed Research, P O Box 533, Lelystad 8200AM, The Netherlands
Varley, Dr M	Provimi Ltd, Eastern Ave, Lichfield, Staffs WS13 7SE, UK
Webb, Prof R	University of Nottingham, Sutton Bonington Campus, Loughborough LE12 5RD, UK
White, Mr G	University of Nottingham, Sutton Bonington Campus, Loughborough, Leics LE12 5RD, UK
Whitney, Miss H	BQP, 36 Station Rd, Framlingham, Suffolk IP13 9EE, UK
Wilde, Mr D	Alltech, Alltech House, Ryhall Road, Stamford PE9 1TZ, UK
Williams, Mr J	Norfeed UK Ltd, Station Terrace, Langthorpe, Boroughbridge, North Yorkshire, YO51 9BU, UK
Wilson, Dr T	ABNA, P O Box 250, Oundle Road, Peterborough PE2 9PW, UK
Wiseman, Prof J	University of Nottingham, Sutton Bonington Campus, Loughborough LE12 5RD, UK
Wonnacott, Miss K	University of Nottingham, Sutton Bonington Campus, Loughborough, Leics LE12 5RD, UK
Woodworth, Dr J	Lonza Inc, 1376 1500 Ave, Enterprise, Kansas 67441, USA

INDEX

Additives regulation	159-160
Amino acids	
biofuels by-products	216-218
peas and beans	333, 344-351
responses	
boars	306
milk protein	19-32
sows	294-301
Animal breeding	275-286, 290-292
Anti-nutritional factors	
peas and beans	334-335
Antioxidants	
animal products	103-113
Avian influenza virus	256-260
Bacteriophage	
poultry	266-268
Beans	
nutritional value	331-354
Biofuels	
by-products	199-207, 209-226
legislation	168
Biohydrogenation	
rumen	9-11
Boar	
amino acids	306
DHA	307
energy requirements	305-306
EPA	307
PUFA	307
vitamins	306-307
Body condition score	
dairy cows	37-38, 61-78
Broilers	
peas and beans	353-354
BST	
fertility dairy cows	47-55
By-products	
biofuels	199-207, 209-226
Calving interval	
body condition score	68-70
extended lactation	87-100
fertility	37-56
Campylobacter	
poultry	263-266
Cancer	
protective effects of meat	122-129
Cardiovascular disease	2-5
Carnitine	
meat quality	
pigs	243-249
Cereal starch	
digestibility	
pigs	313-327
Conjugated linoleic acid	
milk	1-14
Dairy cows	
body condition score	61-78
extended lactations	87-100
fertility	37-56, 95-96
milk	
fatty acids	1-14
protein	19-32
Desaturase	
mammary gland	5-9
DHA	
Fertility	
boar	307
dairy cows	44
in milk	7
Digestibility	
peas and beans	
pigs	335-340
poultry	340-344
starch, pigs	313-327
Distillers grains	
biofuels	199-207, 209-226
Dry period	
body condition score	
dairy cows	73-75
Economic value	
peas and beans	355-356

Energy
  balance
    body condition score
      dairy cows   61-78
  requirements
    boar   305-306
    sow   294-300
Environmental impact of animals   284-285
Environmental legislation   166-167
EPA
  fertility
    boar   307
    dairy cows   44
  in milk   7
Ethanol
  biofuels   199-207, 209-226
European Union enlargement   189-197
Extended lactation
  dairy cows   87-100

Faba beans
  nutritional value   331-354
Fat
  fertility dairy cows   44-47
  human health   1-14, 119-120
Feed
  hygiene legislation   156-157
  intake
    dairy cows   61-78
    sow   245-246
  labelling legislation   153-156, 173
  processing, starch, pigs   313-327
Feed/food products legislation   167, 180-187
Fertility
  dairy cows   37-56, 95-96
Fish oil
  effect on milk fatty acids   7
Folic acid
  in meat   122-123, 136-137

Genetic merit
  dairy cows
    body condition score   70-73
    extended lactation   91-93
Genetics
  nutrition
    challenges   275-286
    pigs   289-308
Glycogen
  meat quality, pigs   229-239
GM feeds
  legislation   161-162

Health
  dairy cows
    body condition score   68-70
    reproduction   37-56

Hormones
  meat quality, pigs   244-245
  reproduction, dairy cows   37-56
Human health
  fat   119-120
  meat   117-139
  milk fatty acids   1-14
  protein   118-119
  zoonoses   255-269

Immune system
  antioxidants   109-113
  fertility, dairy cows   41-44
Iodine
  legislation   160
Iron
  in meat   135-136

Layers
  peas and beans   354-355
Legislation   153-187
Legumes
  nutritional value   331-354
Lysine
  boar   306
  biofuels by-products   216-218
  dairy cows   19-32
  sow   294-300

Meat
  folic acid   122-123, 136-137
  iron   135-136
  protective effects against cancer 122-129
  PUFA   119-120
  selenium   125-127, 137-138
  vitamins   123-125, 129-135, 137
  world trade   189-197
  zinc   127-129, 138
Methionine
  biofuels by-products   216-218
  dairy cows   19-32
  pigs   216-218
Metritis   38-40
Milk, dairy cows
  amino acids   19-32
  body condition score   61-78
  extended lactation   87-100
  fatty acids   1-14
  protein   19-32
  world trade   189-197
Mineral requirements
  boar   306-307
  sow   302-304
Muscle
  development, pigs   243-249
  glycogen, pigs   229-239

Mycotoxins
  legislation   158-159, 174

Nutrition
  amino acids
    boars   306
    biofuels by-products   216-218
    milk protein   19-32
    peas and beans   333, 344-351
    sows   294-301
  by-products   199-207, 209-226
  dairy cows
    milk fatty acids   1-14
    body condition score   61-78
    extended lactation   93-95
    fertility   37-56
    milk protein   19-32
  genetics, challenges   275-286
  human
    fat   119-120
    meat   117-139
    milk fatty acids   1-14
    protein   118-119
  peas and beans   331-354
  pigs
    by-products   215-224
    starch   313-327
  sow and boar   289-308

Organic production legislation   165-166

Peas
  nutritional value   331-354
Pigs
  meat quality
    muscle glycogen   229-239
    carnitine   243-249
  nutritional value of
    by-products 216-222, 209-225
  sow and boar nutrition   289-308
  starch digestibility   313-327
Poultry
  bacteriophage   266-268
  campylobacter   263-266
  salmonella   260-263
  zoonoses   255-269
Pregnancy rate
  dairy cows   37-56
Processing
  effect on starch digestibility
    pigs   313-327
Protein
  boars   306
  biofuels by-products 216-218
  human health   118-119

milk   19-32
peas and beans   333, 344-351
sows   294-301
PUFA
  fertility
    boar   307
    dairy cows   44-47
  in meat   119-120
  in milk   5-14

Rapid Alert System legislation 162-163
Repeat breeders
  dairy cows   40
Reproduction
  health
    dairy cows   37-56
Rumen biohydrogenation   9-11

Salmonella
  poultry   260-263
SCD
  mammary gland   5-9
Selenium
  in meat 125-127, 137-138
Sow
  amino acids   294-301
  energy requirements 294-300
  feed intake   245-246
  peas and beans   353-330
  vitamins   304-305
Starch
  digestibility pigs 313-327

Trans fatty acids in milk   9-10
TSE legislation   164-165

Undesirable substances legislation 157-159

Veterinary Medicines Regulations
  legislation 163-164, 175-179
Vitamins
  boar   306-307
  in meat 123-125, 129-135, 137
  sow   304-305

Waste
  legislation   180-187
Weaning
  pigs   313-327

Zinc
  in meat 127-129, 138
Zoonoses
  poultry   255-269